T0263117

Hepatocellular Carcinoma

Editors

ADAM C. YOPP
MARIA B. MAJELLA DOYLE

SURGICAL ONCOLOGY CLINICS OF NORTH AMERICA

www.surgonc.theclinics.com

Consulting Editor
TIMOTHY M. PAWLIK

January 2024 • Volume 33 • Number 1

ELSEVIER

1600 John F. Kennedy Boulevard • Suite 1800 • Philadelphia, Pennsylvania, 19103-2899

http://www.theclinics.com

SURGICAL ONCOLOGY CLINICS OF NORTH AMERICA Volume 33, Number 1
January 2024 ISSN 1055-3207, ISBN-13: 978-0-443-18396-6

Editor: John Vassallo (j.vassallo@elsevier.com)
Developmental Editor: Malvika Shah

Surgical Oncology Clinics of North America (ISSN 1055-3207) is published quarterly by Elsevier Inc., 360 Park Avenue South, New York, NY 10010-1710. Months of publication are January, April, July, and October. Business and Editorial Offices: 1600 John F. Kennedy Blvd., Ste. 1800, Philadelphia, PA 19103-2899. Customer Service Office: 3251 Riverport Lane, Maryland Heights, MO 63043. Periodicals postage paid at New York, NY and additional mailing offices. Subscription prices are $345.00 per year (US individuals), $100.00 (US student/resident), $385.00 (Canadian individuals), $100.00 (Canadian student/resident), $499.00 (foreign individuals), and $205.00 (foreign student/resident). For institutional access pricing please contact Customer Service via the contact information below. Foreign air speed delivery is included in all *Clinics* subscription prices. All prices are subject to change without notice. **POSTMASTER**: Send address changes to *Surgical Oncology Clinics of North America,* Elsevier Health Science Division, Subscription Customer Service, 3251 Riverport Lane, Maryland Heights, MO 63043. **Customer Service: 1-800-654-2452 (US and Canada). 314-447-8871 (outside US and Canada). Fax: 314-447-8029. E-mail: journalscustomerservice-usa@elsevier.com (for print support); journalsonlinesupport-usa@elsevier.com (for online support)**.

Reprints. For copies of 100 or more, of articles in this publication, please contact the Commercial Reprints Department, Elsevier Inc., 360 Park Avenue South, New York, New York 10010-1710. Tel. 212-633-3874; Fax: 212-633-3820; E-mail: reprints@elsevier.com.

Surgical Oncology Clinics of North America is covered in *MEDLINE/PubMed (Index Medicus)* and *EMBASE/ Excerpta Medica, Current Contents/Clinical Medicine,* and *ISI/BIOMED.*

Contributors

CONSULTING EDITOR

TIMOTHY M. PAWLIK, MD, MPH, PhD, FACS, FRACS (Hon.)
Professor and Chair, Department of Surgery; The Urban Meyer III and Shelley Meyer Chair for Cancer Research; Professor of Surgery, Oncology, and Health Services Management and Policy; Surgeon in Chief; The Ohio State University, Wexner Medical Center, Columbus, Ohio, USA

EDITORS

ADAM C. YOPP, MD
Professor of Surgery, Occidental Chemical Chair in Cancer Research, Chief, Division of Surgical Oncology, The University of Texas Southwestern Medical Center, Dallas, Texas, USA

MARIA B. MAJELLA DOYLE, MD, MBA
Professor, Division of General Surgery, Division of Abdominal Organ Transplantation, Department of Surgery, Washington University School of Medicine, St Louis, Missouri, USA

AUTHORS

ASEEL Y. ABUALNIL, MD
Department of Radiation Oncology, Rutgers Cancer Institute of New Jersey, Rutgers Robert Wood Johnson Medical School, Rutgers University, New Brunswick, New Jersey, USA

ANTHONY BEJJANI, MD
Division of Hematology/Oncology, VA Greater Los Angeles Health System, Los Angeles, California, USA

GLORIA Y. CHANG, MD
General Surgery Resident, Division of Surgical Oncology, Department of Surgery, The University of Texas Southwestern Medical Center, Dallas, Texas, USA

MARIANA CHAVEZ-VILLA, MD
Research Fellow, Division of Transplantation, Department of Surgery, University of Rochester Medical Center, Rochester, New York, USA

VICTORIA CHERNYAK, MD, MS
Professor, Department of Radiology, Memorial Sloan Kettering Cancer Center, New York, New York, USA

MATTHEW P. DEEK, MD
Department of Radiation Oncology, Rutgers Cancer Institute of New Jersey, Rutgers Robert Wood Johnson Medical School, Rutgers University, New Brunswick, New Jersey, USA

ISMAEL DOMÍNGUEZ-ROSADO, MD, MSc
Assistant Professor, Department of Surgery, Instituto Nacional de Ciencias Médicas y Nutrición Salvador Zubirán, Mexico City, Mexico

MARIA B. MAJELLA DOYLE, MD, MBA
Professor, Division of General Surgery, Division of Abdominal Organ Transplantation, Department of Surgery, Washington University School of Medicine, St Louis, Missouri, USA

IFRAH FATIMA, MD
Resident, Department of Internal Medicine, University of Missouri-Kansas City, Kansas City, Missouri, USA

RICHARD S. FINN, MD
Professor, Division of Hematology/Oncology, Department of Medicine, Geffen School of Medicine at UCLA, Santa Monica, California, USA

MRIDULA A. GEORGE, MD
Department of Medical Oncology, Rutgers Cancer Institute of New Jersey, Rutgers Robert Wood Johnson Medical School, Rutgers University, New Brunswick, New Jersey, USA

JASON S. HAWKSWORTH, MD
Surgical Director, Adult Liver Transplantation and Hepatobiliary Surgery, Associate Professor, Division of Abdominal Organ Transplantation, Columbia University Irving Medical Center, New York, New York, USA

DAVID HSIEHCHEN, MD
Assistant Professor, Division of Hematology/Oncology, Department of Medicine, The University of Texas Southwestern Medical Center, Dallas, Texas, USA

SALMA K. JABBOUR, MD
Professor, Vice Chair of Clinical Research Department of Radiation Oncology, Rutgers Cancer Institute of New Jersey, Rutgers Robert Wood Johnson Medical School, Rutgers University, New Brunswick, New Jersey, USA

EDEN KOO, MD
Department of Internal Medicine, The University of Texas Southwestern Medical Center, Dallas, Texas, USA

RITESH KUMAR, MD
Resident, Department of Radiation Oncology, Rutgers Cancer Institute of New Jersey, Rutgers Robert Wood Johnson Medical School, Rutgers University, New Brunswick, New Jersey, USA

ALEXANDER LALOS, MD
Assistant professor, Division of Gasteroenterology and Hepatology, Rutgers Robert Wood Johnson Medical School, Rutgers University, New Brunswick, New Jersey, USA

ALISA LIKHITSUP, MD, MPH
Clinical Assistant Professor, Department of Gastroenterology and Hepatology, University of Michigan, Ann Arbor, Michigan, USA

JESSICA LINDEMANN, MD, PhD
Post-Graduate Year 9, Department of Surgery, Division of Abdominal Organ Transplantation, Washington University School of Medicine, St Louis, Missouri, USA

NEIL MEHTA, MD
Associate Professor, Department of Medicine, University of California, San Francisco, Connie Frank Transplant Center, San Francisco, California, USA

ARADHYA NIGAM, MD
Resident, Department of Surgery, MedStar Georgetown University Hospital, Washington, DC, USA

NEEHAR D. PARIKH, MD, MSc
Assistant Professor, MM Internal Medicine - Gastroenterology University of Michigan, Ann Arbor, Michigan, USA

MIKIN PATEL MD
Assistant Professor, Department of Radiology, University of Chicago Medicine, Chicago, Illinois, USA

ANJANA PILLAI, MD
Associate Professor, Department of Medicine, University of Chicago Medicine, Chicago, Illinois, USA

NICOLE E. RICH, MD, MS
Assistant Professor of Medicine, Division of Digestive and Liver Diseases, Department of Internal Medicine, Associate Director of Liver Tumor Program, Harold C. Simmons Comprehensive Cancer Center, The University of Texas Southwestern Medical Center, Dallas, Texas, USA

MIHIR M. SHAH, MD
Associate Professor, Division of Surgical Oncology, Department of Surgery, Emory University School of Medicine, Atlanta, Georgia, USA

AMIT G. SINGAL, MD, MS
Division of Digestive and Liver Diseases, Professor, Department of Internal Medicine, The University of Texas Southwestern Medical Center, Dallas, Texas, USA

ZACHARY WHITHAM, MD
Division of Surgical Oncology, Resident, Department of Surgery, University of Texas Southwestern Medical Center, Dallas, Texas, USA

EMILY R. WINSLOW, MD
Department of Transplant Surgery, MedStar Georgetown University Hospital, Washington, DC, USA

MIGNOTE YILMA, MD, MAS
Resident Physician, Department of Surgery, National Clinician Scholars Program, University of California, San Francisco, San Francisco, California, USA

ADAM C. YOPP, MD
Professor of Surgery, Occidental Chemical Chair in Cancer Research, Chief, Division of Surgical Oncology, The University of Texas Southwestern Medical Center, Dallas, Texas, USA

JENNIFER YU, MD, MPHS
Assistant Professor, Division of Abdominal Organ Transplantation, Department of Surgery, Washington University School of Medicine, St Louis, Missouri, USA

Contents

Globally, hepatocellular carcinoma (HCC) is a major cause of cancer-related death and a leading cause of morbidity and mortality in patients with chronic liver disease and cirrhosis. The predominant cause of HCC is shifting from viral to nonviral causes, in parallel with the high global prevalence of nonalcoholic fatty liver disease and increasing alcohol consumption in many countries. There have been promising recent advances in the treatment of all stages of HCC; however, improvements in early detection, increased utilization of HCC surveillance, and equitable access to HCC therapies are needed to curb increases in HCC mortality.

Hepatocellular carcinoma (HCC) surveillance is recommended by professional society guidelines given a consistent association with reduced HCC-related mortality. HCC surveillance should be performed using semi-annual abdominal ultrasound and alpha-fetoprotein, although this combination has suboptimal sensitivity and can miss more than one-third of HCC at an early stage. There are promising emerging blood-based and imaging-based strategies, including abbreviated MRI and biomarker panels; however, these require further validation before routine use in clinical practice. HCC surveillance is underused in clinical practice due to patient-related and provider-related barriers, highlighting a need for interventions to improve surveillance utilization in clinical practice.

Multiple hepatocellular carcinoma (HCC) staging systems have been proposed and used clinically over time. These may consider clinical, pathological, radiological, or treatment response factors, depending on the model. Given the heterogeneity of HCC treatment in its different stages and the validation of the systems in different populations, they are not universal. Likewise, the improvement in diagnostic tools, as well as novel therapeutic alternatives, have made these models more complex. Despite this, some have been modified over time in line with advances in the field, and although there is no universally accepted one, each has its usefulness, strengths, and weaknesses.

Therapy for chronic hepatitis C virus infection with direct-acting antiviral agents (DAAs) has been highly successful in achieving sustained virological response (SVR) with associated improvements in liver dysfunction, liver-related mortality, and transplant-free survival. There is a high risk of hepatocellular carcinoma (HCC) with an annual incidence of 2% to 4% in patients with cirrhosis. Following DAAs treatment and achievement of SVR, the risk of incident and recurrent HCC drops significantly over time, with risk associated with demographic and liver disease-related factors. Several risk factors have been described including age, male, diabetes comorbidities, alcohol abuse, hepatitis B virus or human immunodeficiency virus-coinfection, and advanced liver disease or increased liver fibrosis. Recurrence risk after DAA therapy has been associated with baseline tumor burden, with increased risk with larger lesion(s), multifocal disease, elevated alpha-fetoprotein level, treatment type (curative vs palliative), and shorter interval between HCC complete response and DAA initiation. Overall, due to the heterogeneity among individual patient data and lack of adequately controlled data, there are no conclusive statements that can be drawn that DAAs exposure is directly associated with HCC occurrence or recurrence. However, the best available data suggest a decreased risk of incident HCC with DAA therapy and no increased risk of recurrence with DAAs after complete tumor response.

This article overviews Liver Imaging Reporting and Data System (LI-RADS), a system that standardizes techniques, interpretation and reporting of imaging studies done for hepatocellular carcinoma surveillance, diagnosis, and locoregional treatment response assessment. LI-RADS includes 4 algorithms, each of which defines ordinal categories reflecting probability of the assessed outcome. The categories, in turn, guide patient management. The LI-RADS diagnostic algorithms provide diagnostic criteria for the entire spectrum of lesions found in at-risk patients. In addition, the use of LI-RADS in clinical care improves clarity of communication between radiologists and clinicians and may improve the performance of inexperienced users to the levels of expert liver imagers.

The recognition that hepatocellular carcinoma (HCC) is a rising problem globally dates back decades; however, the development of effective medical treatment for the disease has only led to robust improvements in patient outcomes in the recent past. As knowledge evolves and regimens are proven to be more active, the importance of multidisciplinary management in patients with all stages of HCC will become more important to optimize patient outcomes. Key to optimizing patient outcomes is an understanding of the evolution and current role of these therapies in the HCC landscape.

Hepatocellular carcinoma (HCC) continues to be a leading cause of cancer-related death in the United States. With advances in locoregional therapy for unresectable HCC during the last 2 decades and the recent expansion of transplant criteria for HCC, as well as ongoing organ shortages, patients are spending more time on the waitlist, which has resulted in an increased usage of locoregional therapies. The plethora of molecularly targeted therapies and immune checkpoint inhibitors under investigation represent the new horizon of treatment of HCC not only in advanced stages but also potentially at every stage of diagnosis and management.

Intermediate-stage hepatocellular carcinoma (HCC) comprises a heterogeneous group of patients with varying levels of tumor burden. Transarterial chemoembolization was traditionally the mainstay of treatment for intermediate-stage HCC for almost 2 decades. New and emerging treatment options have revolutionized HCC therapy, allowing for broader application to patients with intermediate- and advanced-stage disease. Accordingly, new guidelines acknowledge these options, and intermediate stage HCC can now be treated with surgical, locoregional or systemic therapies, or a combination thereof. Patients will continue to benefit from the development of complex treatment strategies in a multidisciplinary setting to optimize individual outcomes.

Hepatocellular carcinoma (HCC)is a common type of liver cancer with a poor prognosis, especially in patients with advanced stages or underlying liver disease. While surgical resection, liver transplantation, and ablation therapies have traditionally been the mainstay of treatment for HCC, radiation therapy has become increasingly recognized as an effective alternative, particularly for those who are not surgical candidates. Stereotactic Body Radiation Therapy (SBRT) is a highly precise form of radiation therapy that delivers very high doses of radiation to the tumor while sparing surrounding healthy tissue. Several studies have reported favorable outcomes with SBRT in HCC treatment. Moreover, SBRT can be used to treat recurrent HCC after prior treatment, offering a potentially curative approach in select cases. While SBRT has demonstrated its efficacy and safety in treating HCC, future studies are needed to further investigate the potential role of SBRT in combination with other treatments for HCC.

SURGICAL ONCOLOGY CLINICS OF NORTH AMERICA

SERIES OF RELATED INTEREST

Advances in Surgery
https://www.advancessurgery.com
Surgical Clinics of North America
https://www.surgical.theclinics.com
Thoracic Surgery Clinics
https://www.thoracic.theclinics.com

THE CLINICS ARE AVAILABLE ONLINE!
Access your subscription at:
www.theclinics.com

Foreword

Hepatocellular Carcinoma

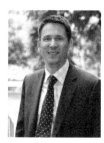

Timothy M. Pawlik, MD, MPH, PhD, FACS, FRACS (Hon.)
Consulting Editor

This issue of the *Surgical Oncology Clinics of North America* focuses on Hepatocellular Carcinoma (HCC). HCC is the most common type of primary liver cancer, and the fourth leading cause of cancer-related deaths worldwide. Approximately 60% to 70% of HCCs develop in the setting of chronic liver disease and cirrhosis. The pathogenesis of HCC is variable, yet it is primarily based on an inflammatory process related to hepatotropic virus infections (ie, hepatitis B or C virus), ethanol consumption (ie, alcoholic cirrhosis), or fatty infiltration of the liver (ie, nonalcoholic steatohepatitis). Surgery in the form of resection or liver transplantation offers the best chance of long-term survival among patients with HCC. Unfortunately, many patients present with either advanced stage disease or poorly compensated liver function and are not candidates for surgery. Other modalities to treat HCC include locoregional therapy with intra-arterial therapy, ablation, or stereotactic radiation. Response to systemic chemotherapy traditionally has been poor. More recently, the IMbrave150 trial demonstrated that atezolizumab and bevacizumab had activity and a survival benefit for patients with advanced HCC. In turn, a new era of research on identifying ways to leverage the unique immune microenvironment of the liver to treat HCC not only in the advanced stage but also in the neoadjuvant/adjuvant settings to downstage patients or prevent recurrence has emerged. Given the rapidly changing landscape of HCC treatment, as well as the multiple treatment options available to these patients, a true multidisciplinary approach is needed. In turn, providers who care for patients with HCC should be knowledgeable about the most recent treatment approaches to HCC. To that end, this current issue of *Surgical Oncology Clinics of North America* is an important practical resource that offers a timely update on the topic. We are fortunate to have Maria B. Majella Doyle, MD, MBA and Adam C. Yopp, MD as our Guest Editors. Dr Doyle is the Mid-America Transplant/Department of Surgery Distinguished Endowed Chair in Abdominal Transplantation at Washington University School of Medicine in St. Louis. Dr Doyle completed her MD at the Royal College of Surgeons in Dublin, Ireland

Surg Oncol Clin N Am 33 (2024) xiii–xiv
https://doi.org/10.1016/j.soc.2023.08.001
1055-3207/24/© 2023 Published by Elsevier Inc.

followed by clinical fellowships in Cork, as well as in Washington University, St. Louis. Dr Doyle's research interests include clinical outcomes, HCC, liver transplantation, and donor management. Dr Yopp is the Chief of the Division of Surgical Oncology at UT Southwestern Medical Center, where he is also the Surgical Director of the Liver Tumor Program. Dr Yopp earned his medical degree at St. George's University. Following completion of a general surgery residency at Maimonides Medical Center in New York, he received advanced training in hepatopancreatobiliary malignancies as a surgical oncology fellow at Memorial Sloan Kettering Cancer Center.

The issue covers multiple important topics, including the changing epidemiology of HCC, overview of the different staging systems, as well as imaging and various treatment approaches to HCC. In particular, this issue addresses the controversies related to direct-acting antivirals, as well as the evolution of systemic therapies with emphasis on immunotherapy and locoregional therapies. The role of surgical resection for early- and intermediate-stage disease and a discussion about optimal liver transplantation criteria are included.

I want to thank Drs Doyle and Yopp for amassing a fantastic group of coauthors to contribute to this issue of *Surgical Oncology Clinics of North America*. The authors aptly highlighted the important clinical topics related to HCC. This issue of *Surgical Oncology Clinics of North America* provides surgeons and all members of the multidisciplinary team with critical information to advance the care of patients with HCC. Again, thank you to Drs Doyle and Yopp, as well as to the contributing authors.

Timothy M. Pawlik, MD, MPH, PhD, FACS, FRACS (Hon.)
Professor and Chair
Department of Surgery
The Urban Meyer III and Shelley Meyer
Chair for Cancer Research
The Ohio State University
Wexner Medical Center
395 West 12th Avenue, Suite 670
Columbus, OH 43210, USA

E-mail address:
tim.pawlik@osumc.edu

Preface

Hepatocellular Carcinoma

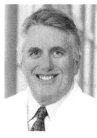 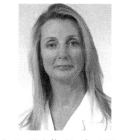

Adam C. Yopp, MD   Maria B. Majella Doyle, MD, MBA
Editors

Hepatocellular carcinoma is the fourth leading cause of cancer deaths worldwide and the fastest growing cause of cancer mortality in the United States. Patients diagnosed with hepatocellular carcinoma are a heterogenous group due to underlying chronic liver dysfunction and the presence of a concomitant malignancy. This heterogeneity requires a multifaceted cancer care approach, including surgical, locoregional, systemic, and supportive treatment options encompassing the specialties of surgery, radiology, oncology, hepatology, and palliative care. Over the last decade, large strides have been made in the diagnosis and treatment of hepatocellular carcinoma.

In this issue of *Surgical Oncology Clinics of North America*, we have asked some of the leading experts in the field of hepatocellular carcinoma representing medical specialties across the cancer care continuum to reflect on the need for multidisciplinary care in this patient population. The contributing authors address the changing epidemiology of hepatocellular carcinoma in the United States and worldwide with the advent of new treatments for hepatitis C virus and the growing epidemic of morbid obesity leading to NASH-related disease. Additional contributions discuss tailoring surveillance programs for patients at risk for hepatocellular carcinoma in an effort to raise the rather dismal screening rates to identify patients at an earlier stage where curative treatments can be utilized. Further contributions highlight the novel role of the LI-RADS radiologic system in the diagnosis of hepatocellular carcinoma, a cancer where biopsy is oftentimes not needed to guide treatment decisions. As hepatocellular carcinoma oftentimes occurs in the background of chronic liver dysfunction, staging systems used in other malignancies may not be useful, and alternative staging systems that may be more appropriate are discussed in detail. A recent development in the treatment of hepatitis C virus with direct-acting antivirals and the potential role in the pathogenesis of hepatocellular carcinoma are discussed, and the controversy is addressed. Finally, multiple articles discuss hepatocellular carcinoma treatments illustrating the multifaceted and nuanced approach encompassing surgery (resection and transplantation), locoregional, and systemic treatments, especially in light of exciting novel treatment approaches.

Although hepatocellular carcinoma is clearly a worldwide cancer problem, with the recent progress that has been made across the cancer care continuum by the article contributors and others, there is optimism that continued strides can be made, improving the prognosis for patients at risk for and with hepatocellular carcinoma.

Adam C. Yopp, MD
Division of Surgical Oncology
UT Southwestern Medical Center
5323 Harry Hines Boulevard
Dallas, TX 75390-8548, USA

Maria B. Majella Doyle, MD, MBA
Division of General Surgery
Abdominal Transplantation Section
Washington University
4921 Parkview Place
St Louis, MO 63110, USA

E-mail addresses:
adam.yopp@utsouthwestern.edu (A.C. Yopp)
doylem@wustl.edu (M.B. Majella Doyle)

Changing Epidemiology of Hepatocellular Carcinoma Within the United States and Worldwide

Nicole E. Rich, MD, MS

KEYWORDS

- Liver cancer • Epidemiology • Risk factors • Incidence • Mortality • Disparities

KEY POINTS

- Globally, hepatocellular carcinoma (HCC) is a major cause of cancer-related death and a leading cause of morbidity and mortality in patients with chronic liver disease and cirrhosis.
- HCC incidence and mortality rates are increasing in many countries despite advances in antiviral treatment and HCC therapies.
- The predominant cause of HCC is shifting both in the United States and worldwide from viral to nonviral causes in parallel with the high global prevalence of nonalcoholic fatty liver disease and increasing alcohol consumption in many countries.
- Primary prevention (through treatment of viral hepatitis, lifestyle modifications) and early detection are key to reducing the burden of HCC.

INTRODUCTION

Hepatocellular carcinoma (HCC), the most common type of primary liver cancer, is the third most common cause of cancer-related death worldwide and a leading cause of death in patients with chronic liver disease and cirrhosis, accounting for an estimated 830,200 deaths globally in 2020.[1] Alarmingly, it is projected to surpass colorectal cancer and breast cancer to become the third leading cause of cancer-related death in the United States by 2040.[2] HCC risk factors, prevalence, and survival vary across regions. There has been an etiologic shift in the major risk factors for HCC over the past few decades, both in the United States and throughout the world. Herein, the authors discuss the current trends in HCC incidence and mortality.

Division of Digestive and Liver Diseases, Department of Internal Medicine, Harold C. Simmons Comprehensive Cancer Center, UT Southwestern Medical Center, 5959 Harry Hines Boulevard, Professional Office Building 1, Suite 4.420G, Dallas, TX 75390-8887, USA
E-mail address: Nicole.rich@utsouthwestern.edu

Surg Oncol Clin N Am 33 (2024) 1–12
https://doi.org/10.1016/j.soc.2023.06.004
1055-3207/24/© 2023 Elsevier Inc. All rights reserved.

HEPATOCELLULAR CARCINOMA INCIDENCE AND MORTALITY TRENDS IN THE UNITED STATES

Dramatic increases in HCC incidence have been observed in the United States over the past 3 decades, although recent data suggest incidence rates have plateaued or begun to decrease, particularly among younger and middle-aged adults, with a Surveillance, Epidemiology and End Results (SEER) analysis through 2015 demonstrating a 6.2% per year decrease in individuals aged 40 to 49 years and 10.3% per year decrease in individuals aged 50 to 59 years.[3] Conversely, incidence has continued to increase steadily since the mid-2000s among older adults aged 60 years or older, in both men and women and across all racial and ethnic groups, except among Asian/Pacific Islanders older than 70 years.[3]

Overall, HCC mortality rates increased in the United States during the 2000s until around 2013, when rates began to plateau and subsequently started to decline around 2016. Recent improvements in overall survival are attributed to increasing efforts toward early detection and significant advances in surgical, locoregional, and systemic therapies.[4]

RACIAL, ETHNIC, SOCIOECONOMIC, AND GEOGRAPHIC DIFFERENCES WITHIN THE UNITED STATES

The disease burden of HCC is distributed unequally in the United States, with generally higher incidence and mortality rates among racial and ethnic minority groups compared with non-Hispanic White individuals.[5,6] Historically, Asian/Pacific Islanders have had the highest age-adjusted HCC incidence rates in the United States but have recently been surpassed with the highest age-adjusted incidence rates now observed among Hispanic individuals and American Indian/Alaskan Native (AI/AN) populations.[7,8] Nativity, or country of birth origin, has been demonstrated to affect HCC risk, with US-born Hispanic individuals (particularly men) having higher HCC risk compared with those born outside the United States, whereas the converse is true for Asian/Pacific Islanders, with individuals born outside the United States having higher HCC risk than those born in the United States.[9] There is also significant geographic variation in HCC incidence in the United States, with Texas, Hawaii, New Mexico, and California having the highest rates.[10,11] HCC incidence and mortality rates are also increasing at an increased rate among rural areas compared with urban areas, particularly in Southern states.[12]

Overall, HCC mortality is declining in the United States, across sexes and most racial and ethnic groups, particularly among Asian/Pacific Islanders and individuals younger than 50 years.[4] However, mortality rates have continued to increase in older adults (aged >65 years) and American Indian/Alaskan Natives.[4] There is also significant state-level variation in HCC outcomes, with 33 of the 50 US states reporting increases in mortality rates, with these states predominately clustered in the Southern United States.[4]

HEPATOCELLULAR INCIDENCE AND MORTALITY TRENDS WORLDWIDE

Historically, HCC incidence and mortality rates have been highest in East Asia, South Asia, and parts of Africa, with more than half of the world's HCC cases and deaths occurring in East Asia and 45% of the world's cases and 47% of deaths occurring in China alone in the year 2020 (**Fig. 1**).[1] In the same year, the highest HCC age-standardized rates in the world were observed in Mongolia (85.6 new cases per 100,000 persons) followed by Egypt (34.1 new cases per 100,000 persons), with the

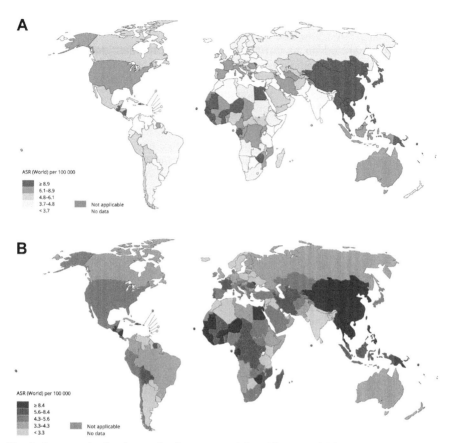

Fig. 1. Age-standardized rates for liver cancer. (*A*) Incidence and (*B*) mortality per 100,000 persons, by country. All rights reserved. The designations used and the presentation of the material in this publication do not imply the expression of any opinion whatsoever on the part of the World Health Organization/International Agency for Research on Cancer concerning the legal status of any country, territory, city or area, or of its authorities or the delimitation of its frontiers or boundaries. Dotted and dashed lines on maps represent approximate borderlines for which there may not yet be full agreement. (Based on 2020 GLOBOCAN data from the World Health Organization and International Agency for Research on Cancer (IARC). Figure created at gco.iarc.fr/today/online-analysis-map.)

lowest rates in Sri Lanka, St. Lucia, and Algeria (1.2, 1.3, and 1.5 new cases per 100,000 persons, respectively).[1] Greater than 60% of HCC cases and deaths occurred in high Human Development Index countries—a group that includes China, Mongolia, and Egypt.[1] These rates reflect the high burden of established HCC risk factors in these regions, including hepatitis B virus (HBV), hepatitis C virus (HCV), nonalcoholic fatty liver disease (NAFLD), and aflatoxin exposure. HCC incidence rates have begun to decline in recent years in some East Asian and South Asian countries, including Japan, China, Republic of Korea, and the Philippines. Efforts toward universal vaccination of newborns, as well as improvements in HCV antiviral therapy have dramatically reduced the burden of HBV-related HCC in some Asian countries. Conversely, several Middle Eastern countries have observed sharp increases in HCC incidence in recent years, including Iran, Iraq, Afghanistan, and Qatar. Significant etiologic changes in HCC have also been observed in South American countries, owing to dramatic increases in NAFLD-related HCC.[13]

Despite significant advances in HCC treatment over the past decade, its overall prognosis remains poor, with 5-year survival rates less than 20%.[14] Thus, trends in incidence and mortality rates of HCC (both overall and by region/territory) are relatively similar (see **Fig. 1**), with global incidence and mortality rates of 9.5 per 100,000 persons and 8.7 per 100,000 persons in the year 2020, respectively.[15]

SEX DIFFERENCES

HCC is more common in men than in women (with a 2:1 to 4:1 male-female [M:F] ratio) across nearly all regions of the world and among all races, ethnic groups, and time periods. Given this consistent trend, it is hypothesized that sex hormones may play an important role in HCC pathogenesis; this has been demonstrated in animal models, with estrogens being protective against HCC via suppression of proinflammatory cytokines such as IL-1 and IL-6[16,17] and testosterone promoting tumorigenesis via androgen signaling pathways, leading to upregulation of vascular endothelial growth factor, one of the key molecular targets of HCC-directed therapy.[18] However, there is insufficient data to confirm this hypothesis in humans, with one population-based study finding no association between endogenous estrogens and HCC risk in postmenopausal women.[19] In addition, several established HCC risk factors (eg, alcohol consumption, smoking, injection drug use, diabetes) are historically more prevalent in men compared with women.[20] In the United States, HCC rates were highest in men in HCV epidemic birth cohorts (eg, baby boomers, individuals born between 1945–1965). However, recent data suggest that HCC is trending toward less male predominance, especially in younger birth cohorts, in parallel with declining rates of HCV in subsequent generations of men and rates of NAFLD-related HCC increasing more rapidly in women.[5,21] In parallel with incidence trends, there is a significant and consistent sex disparity in HCC mortality, with higher age-adjusted mortality rates in men compared with women in all regions of the world (M:F ratio ranging from 1:2 in Central America to 3:2 in Southern Europe) in the year 2020.[15]

TRENDS IN HEPATOCELLULAR RISK FACTORS

The major risk factors for HCC, aside from male sex and older age, include HBV, HCV, NAFLD, diabetes, alcohol consumption, and smoking. The risk of HCC varies across etiologies, and the prevalence (and age at acquisition) of these risk factors varies geographically and between men, women, and different racial and ethnic groups.

Hepatitis B virus

Chronic HBV is the most common cause of HCC worldwide, responsible for greater than 50% of cases globally. HBV is highly carcinogenic due to integration of its viral proteins into the host genome. Although most cases occur in patients with underlying cirrhosis, HBV can result in HCC in the absence of cirrhosis.[22,23] It is estimated between 10% to 25% of HBV carriers will develop HCC during their lifetime.[24] The prevalence of HBV in the World Health Organization (WHO) Western Pacific and African regions are 6.2% and 6.1%, respectively, with significantly higher prevalence in some African countries including Somalia, Sudan, Liberia, and Nigeria.[25] In the United States, prevalence of chronic HBV is much lower, estimated at approximately 0.3%.[26] Ongoing viral replication and liver injury are key risk factors for HBV-related HCC, with HBV viral load (ie, serum HBV DNA levels) correlating directly with HCC risk. Other viral factors associated with HCC risk include elevated quantitative hepatitis B surface antigen levels, HBV genotype C, and some basal core promoter mutations.[27,28] In addition, demographics (eg, male sex, older age) and exposure to other known HCC risk factors (ie, alcohol consumption, aflatoxin exposure, diabetes, and obesity) are predictors of individual HCC risk.[29] Several HCC risk prediction models have been developed and validated in patients with HBV and may be useful in tailoring HCC surveillance protocols and identifying low-risk patients who may not require ongoing surveillance.[30]

Treatment of HBV with nucleos(t)ide analogues, including entecavir and tenofovir, results in significant reduction in HCC incidence rates.[31,32] Universal HBV vaccination of newborns and catch-up programs have been implemented in several countries and have served as key prevention strategies to reduce the burden of HBV (and HBV-related HCC). For example, a national program implemented in Taiwan in the mid-1980s led to significant declines in HCC incidence and mortality in subsequent birth cohorts, exceeding 80% and 90%, respectively.[33]

Hepatitis C virus

HCV is a strong risk factor for HCC, with annual incidence ranging from 3% to 8%.[34] Globally, an estimated 20% of total HCC cases are related to HCV, and it is the most common cause of HCC in North America, Europe, and Japan.[35] Achieving HCV cure (ie, sustained virologic response, SVR) with highly effective and well-tolerated oral direct-acting antivirals (DAAs) has been a major step to decrease the burden of HCV-related HCC. Most importantly, DAAs provide a chance at HCV cure for more than 95% of patients, including who were either ineligible or did not achieve SVR with previous interferon-based regimens, such as older patients and those with decompensated cirrhosis, human immunodeficiency virus, polysubstance abuse, and other medical or psychiatric comorbidities.[36] Once SVR has been achieved with DAAs, HCC risk declines significantly, and this lower risk remains stable over time, including among patients with advanced fibrosis or cirrhosis.[37,38] In a large Veterans Affairs (VA) study, compared with patients who did not achieve SVR, those who achieve SVR with DAAs had a 76% reduction in risk of incident HCC.[37] Despite this impressive risk reduction, the absolute risk of HCC following DAA-induced SVR is not zero and persists up to 10 years post-SVR in patients with advanced fibrosis or cirrhosis.[39] In the aforementioned VA study, 183 patients developed with an annual incidence of 0.9%, and post-SVR HCC risk was highest among patients with cirrhosis, with annual incidence ranging from 1.0% to 2.2% per year,[37] exceeding the current threshold at which HCC surveillance is considered cost-effective.[40] Despite the efficacy of DAAs, a significant proportion of patients in the United States with HCV remain untreated, which has led to the proposal of a national HCV elimination program, which if implemented, would positively affect HCC burden in the future.[41] The WHO has set an ambitious goal of HCV elimination worldwide by the year 2030,[42] and similar programs have been implemented or are currently underway in other nations, including Egypt, Georgia, Cameroon, Iceland, India, Malta, Mongolia, Rwanda, and the Netherlands.

Nonalcoholic fatty liver disease

NAFLD is a common condition both in the United States and worldwide, with an estimated prevalence exceeding 34% in the United States and 30% globally.[43,44] Exact estimates vary,[45,46] but a subset of patients with NAFLD (up to 40%) will progress from simple hepatic steatosis to nonalcoholic steatohepatitis (NASH), the more severe form of the disease characterized by hepatocyte injury and inflammation, with 10% to 20% of patients with NASH progressing to fibrosis and eventually cirrhosis.[47] The presence of cirrhosis remains the strongest risk factor of HCC in patients with NAFLD.[48] Diabetes is a major risk factor for NAFLD[49] and is also as an independent risk factor for HCC (associated with 2- to 3-fold increase in risk).[50] Although NAFLD is a weaker risk factor for HCC compared with HBV or HCV (annual incidence estimated 0.5%–2.6% among individuals with cirrhosis[51]), its high prevalence drives the large disease burden, and it is the fastest increasing cause of HCC in the United States. Further, it is increasingly recognized that a not insignificant proportion of HCC occur in patients with NAFLD without cirrhosis,[52] although the absolute individual risk is low at less than 0.1% per year, raising significant challenges when considering which individuals to enroll in an HCC surveillance program.[53] Previously recognized as the fastest increasing cause of HCC among individuals listed for liver transplant,[54] a recent analysis of 2022 United Network for Organ Sharing data demonstrated that NAFLD has now surpassed HCV as the leading cause of HCC among waitlisted liver transplant candidates in the United States.[55] This dramatic shift is related to the increasing prevalence of obesity and NAFLD occurring in parallel to the rapid decline in liver transplant candidates waitlisted with HCV-related HCC by nearly 50% from 2017 to 2021, owing in large part to the success of direct-acting antivirals.

Similar to Western countries, the epidemiology of HCC in Asia is also shifting from predominately viral hepatitis to nonviral causes, including NAFLD.[56] In parallel to the increasing prevalence of obesity and diabetes in Asia, the prevalence of NAFLD in South Asia (33.8%), South East Asia (33.1%), East Asia (29.7%), and Asia Pacific (28.0%) regions is now estimated to be similar or higher to the prevalence of NAFLD in North America (31.2%).[44] Concomitant NAFLD is also common among Asian patients with current (or prior) HBV infection, further increasing the risk of progression to cirrhosis and risk of incident HCC.[57] Within the United States, there are significant racial and ethnic disparities in NAFLD prevalence, with the highest burden in Hispanic individuals and lowest burden in Black individuals.[58] Hispanic individuals are also at highest risk of progression to NASH compared with other racial and ethnic groups[58]; this has translated into increases in NAFLD-related HCC in these populations and is likely driving the relative fastest increases in overall HCC incidence observed in Hispanic men compared with other populations.[8]

Alcohol-Related Liver Disease

Along with NAFLD-related HCC, the burden of alcohol-related HCC has increased significantly over the past decade. The annual incidence of HCC in individuals with alcohol-related cirrhosis varies significantly across studies, with estimates ranging from 0.8% to 5.6%,[59,60] and a meta-analysis of 18 studies (n = 148,333 patients) demonstrated the 5-year and 10-year cumulative risk of HCC in patients with alcohol-related cirrhosis to be 3% and 9%, respectively.[61] It is estimated that approximately 30% of HCC cases worldwide are related to alcohol use,[35] and alcohol-related cause has been associated with worse prognosis compared with viral-related HCC, largely related to later stage detection and lower rates of curative treatment receipt.[62–64]

Alcohol use is commonplace across the globe. According to the WHO, an estimated 2.3 billion individuals currently drink alcohol, and per-capita alcohol consumption has steadily increased since 1990, projected to reach 7.6 liters (6.5–10.2 liters) by 2030.[65] Alcohol consumption varies across gender, race, ethnicity, and by geographic region, with highest consumption in Central and Eastern Europe and lowest rates in North African Middle Eastern countries.[65] However, global patterns of alcohol use began to change significantly since 1990, with decreasing alcohol consumption in European countries and certain Asian countries reporting recent increases in alcohol consumption, notably India.[65] Alcohol consumption and its impact on health is complex and is influenced by individual-level (eg, genetics), neighborhood-level (eg, home and work environment, peer networks), and societal-level factors (eg, social norms, culture, policy related to alcohol)[66]; alcohol use patterns are also linked to social determinants of health.[67] Policy changes to reduce access to alcohol including decreased exposure to alcohol advertising, taxes, and limits on alcohol sales have been associated with lower alcohol-related liver disease mortality[68] and may help mitigate continued increases in the burden of alcohol-related HCC in the future.

Aflatoxin Exposure

Aflatoxins comprise a group of carcinogens produced by fungal species, particularly in warm, humid conditions, including *Aspergillus*. These toxins are found in many locations throughout the world, most commonly in Asian and African countries, and may contaminate the food supply (eg, rice, corn, soybeans).[69] Notably, aflatoxins increase HCC risk substantially when co-occurring with HBV infection due to an observed synergistic effect.[70] Aflatoxin reduction programs (ie, improvements in grain storage and crop substitution), such as those implemented in China and Philippines, have contributed to remarkable decreases in incident HCC cases.[71–73]

LIMITATIONS OF CANCER REGISTRY DATA

Precisely estimating HCC incidence and mortality by cause can be challenging, as most data on HCC incidence and mortality in the United States are collected from cancer registry data (eg, SEER, US Cancer Statistics Database), which lacks granular information on underlying liver disease cause, as well as information on health behaviors and liver function, an important determinant of HCC prognosis.[74] Further, individuals often have multiple risk factors for HCC, and there is the additional possibility of misclassification and/or several risk factors being attributed to the same incident cases or deaths, affecting population estimates. As HCC can be diagnosed radiographically in many cases rather than depending on a histologic diagnosis,[75] there is also the possibility of ascertainment bias in some published studies and estimates of disease burden. Globally, the exact frequencies of liver cancer incidence and deaths are likely underestimated and/or underreported in low-income countries with poor access to health care, limited resources, and lack of surveillance and diagnostic capacity.

FUTURE TRENDS

The epidemiologic landscape of HCC is rapidly evolving. Given the shift in prevalence of known HCC risk factors in the United States and worldwide, a multifaceted approach is needed to improve identification, risk stratification, and management of patients with chronic liver disease and cirrhosis who are at risk for HCC.

Given the complexity of HCC pathogenesis and evolving epidemiology, it remains difficult to precisely predict future HCC trends. The effects of HCV and HBV treatment and prevention are only recently being reflected in current estimates of HCC burden. In addition, it remains unclear if HCC incidence rates will continue to decline among younger adults, owing to increased efforts to screen for and treat HBV and HCV, or if rates will increase given significant increases in metabolic syndrome, obesity, and NAFLD among children and younger adults. Although highly effective direct active antivirals have revolutionized the treatment of HCV, widespread opioid use has led to significant increases in acute HCV treatment among younger adults who use injection drugs. Recent data from a large prospective cohort of US patients with cirrhosis indicate that, in parallel with the shift in HCC risk factors and cirrhosis cause observed in clinical practice, HCC incidence seems to be lower than previously observed.[76] There have been promising recent advances in the treatment of all stages of HCC, including advanced stage HCC with the advent of effective immunotherapy regimens; however, improvements in early detection, increased utilization of HCC surveillance, and equitable access to HCC therapies are needed to curb increases in HCC mortality. To curb the tide of HCC, future efforts should focus not just on viral hepatitis elimination but also on primary prevention of obesity, treatment of diabetes and NAFLD, and modifying behavioral risk factors such as alcohol consumption and smoking.

CLINICS CARE POINTS

- The etiology of HCC is shifting from viral hepatitis (hepatitis B virus, hepatitis C virus) to non-viral causes (nonalcoholic fatty liver disease and alcohol-related liver disease).
- Patients with hepatitis C who have been treated and cured (i.e., achieved sustained virologic response) have a significantly lower risk of HCC compared to those who remain untreated; however, the absolute risk of HCC in patients with cured HCV who have already developed advanced fibrosis or cirrhosis is >1%, exceeding currently accepted thresholds at which HCC surveillance is considered cost-effective.
- Pharmacologic and behavioral interventions are needed to reduce the increasing burden of nonalcoholic fatty liver disease and alcohol-related liver disease, which are emerging as the dominant causes of HCC.

DISCLOSURES

N.E. Rich has served as a consultant for AstraZeneca. N.E. Rich's research is supported by National Cancer Institute, United States K08CA259536, the American College of Gastroenterology, United States Junior Faculty Development Award, and the Texas Health Resources Clinical Scholar Award.

REFERENCES

1. Sung H, Ferlay J, Siegel RL, et al. Global cancer statistics 2020: GLOBOCAN estimates of incidence and mortality worldwide for 36 cancers in 185 countries. CA: a cancer journal for clinicians 2021;71:209–49.
2. Rahib L, Wehner MR, Matrisian LM, et al. Estimated projection of US cancer incidence and death to 2040. JAMA Netw Open 2021;4:e214708.
3. Rich NE, Yopp AC, Singal AG, et al. Hepatocellular carcinoma incidence is decreasing among younger adults in the United States. Clin Gastroenterol Hepatol 2020;18:242–8.e5.
4. Lee YT, Wang JJ, Luu M, et al. The mortality and overall survival trends of primary liver cancer in the United States. J Natl Cancer Inst 2021;113:1531–41.
5. Myers S, Neyroud-Caspar I, Spahr L, et al. NAFLD and MAFLD as emerging causes of HCC: a populational study. JHEP Rep 2021;3:100231.
6. Rich NE, Carr C, Yopp AC, et al. Racial and ethnic disparities in survival among patients with hepatocellular carcinoma in the United States: a systematic review and meta-analysis. Clin Gastroenterol Hepatol 2022;20:e267–88.
7. Melkonian SC, Jim MA, Reilley B, et al. Incidence of primary liver cancer in American Indians and Alaska Natives, US, 1999-2009. Cancer Causes Control 2018; 29:833–44.

8. Petrick JL, Kelly SP, Altekruse SF, et al. Future of hepatocellular carcinoma incidence in the United States forecast through 2030. J Clin Oncol 2016;34:1787–94.

9. Setiawan VW, Wei PC, Hernandez BY, et al. Disparity in liver cancer incidence and chronic liver disease mortality by nativity in hispanics: the multiethnic cohort. Cancer 2016;122:1444–52.

10. El-Serag HB, Sardell R, Thrift AP, et al. Texas has the highest hepatocellular carcinoma incidence rates in the USA. Dig Dis Sci 2021;66:912–6.

11. White DL, Thrift AP, Kanwal F, et al. Incidence of hepatocellular carcinoma in all 50 United States, from 2000 through 2012. Gastroenterology 2017;152: 812–20.e5.

12. Zhou K, Gainey CS, Dodge JL, et al. Diverging incidence trends for hepatocellular carcinoma in rural and urban settings in the United States. Clin Gastroenterol Hepatol 2022;20:1180–5.e2.

13. Farah M, Anugwom C, Ferrer JD, et al. Changing epidemiology of hepatocellular carcinoma in South America: a report from the South American liver research network. Ann Hepatol 2023;28:100876.

14. Siegel RL, Miller KD, Jemal A. Cancer statistics, 2018. CA Cancer J Clin 2018; 68:7–30.

15. Rumgay H, Arnold M, Ferlay J, et al. Global burden of primary liver cancer in 2020 and predictions to 2040. J Hepatol 2022;77:1598–606.

16. Iavarone M, Lampertico P, Seletti C, et al. The clinical and pathogenetic significance of estrogen receptor-β expression in chronic liver diseases and liver carcinoma. Cancer 2003;98:529–34.

17. Naugler WE, Sakurai T, Kim S, et al. Gender disparity in liver cancer due to sex differences in MyD88-dependent IL-6 production. Science 2007;317:121–4.

18. Kanda T, Jiang X, Yokosuka O. Androgen receptor signaling in hepatocellular carcinoma and pancreatic cancers. World J Gastroenterol 2014;20:9229–36.

19. Petrick JL, Florio AA, Zhang X, et al. Associations between prediagnostic concentrations of circulating sex steroid hormones and liver cancer among postmenopausal women. Hepatology 2020;72:535–47.

20. Makarova-Rusher OV, Altekruse SF, McNeel TS, et al. Population attributable fractions of risk factors for hepatocellular carcinoma in the United States. Cancer 2016;122:1757–65.

21. Zhang X, El-Serag HB, Thrift AP. Sex and race disparities in the incidence of hepatocellular carcinoma in the united states examined through age–period–cohort analysis. Cancer Epidemiol Biomarkers Prev 2020;29:88–94.

22. Chayanupatkul M, Omino R, Mittal S, et al. Hepatocellular carcinoma in the absence of cirrhosis in patients with chronic hepatitis B virus infection. Journal of hepatology 2017;66:355–62.

23. Kim JM, Kwon CHD, Joh J-W, et al. Differences between hepatocellular carcinoma and hepatitis B virus infection in patients with and without cirrhosis. Ann Surg Oncol 2014;21:458–65.

24. McGlynn KA, Petrick JL, London WT. Global epidemiology of hepatocellular carcinoma: an emphasis on demographic and regional variability. Clin Liver Dis 2015;19:223–38.

25. Available at: https://www.who.int/westernpacific/health-topics/hepatitis/regional-hepatitis-data. Accessed June 17, 2023.

26. Hyun Kim B, Ray Kim W. Epidemiology of hepatitis B virus infection in the United States. Clin Liver Dis 2018;12:1–4.

27. Liu S, Zhang H, Gu C, et al. Associations between hepatitis B Virus mutations and the risk of hepatocellular carcinoma: a meta-analysis. JNCI: J Natl Cancer Inst 2009;101:1066–82.
28. Tseng TC, Liu CJ, Yang HC, et al. High levels of hepatitis B surface antigen increase risk of hepatocellular carcinoma in patients with low HBV load. Gastroenterology 2012;142:1140–9.e3.
29. Campbell C, Wang T, McNaughton AL, et al. Risk factors for the development of hepatocellular carcinoma (HCC) in chronic hepatitis B virus (HBV) infection: a systematic review and meta-analysis. J Viral Hepat 2021;28:493–507.
30. Kim H-s, Yu X, Kramer J, et al. Comparative performance of risk prediction models for hepatitis B-related hepatocellular carcinoma in the United States. J Hepatol 2022;76:294–301.
31. Hosaka T, Suzuki F, Kobayashi M, et al. Long-term entecavir treatment reduces hepatocellular carcinoma incidence in patients with hepatitis B virus infection. Hepatology 2013;58:98–107.
32. Singal AK, Salameh H, Kuo YF, et al. Meta-analysis: the impact of oral anti-viral agents on the incidence of hepatocellular carcinoma in chronic hepatitis B. Aliment Pharmacol Ther 2013;38:98–106.
33. Chiang C-J, Yang Y-W, You S-L, et al. Thirty-year outcomes of the national hepatitis B immunization program in Taiwan. JAMA 2013;310:974–6.
34. El-Serag HB, Kanwal F. Epidemiology of hepatocellular carcinoma in the United States: where are we? Where do we go? Hepatology 2014;60:1767–75.
35. Akinyemiju T, Abera S, Ahmed M, et al. The burden of primary liver cancer and underlying etiologies from 1990 to 2015 at the global, regional, and national level: results from the global burden of disease study 2015. JAMA Oncol 2017;3: 1683–91.
36. Falade-Nwulia O, Suarez-Cuervo C, Nelson DR, et al. Oral direct-acting agent therapy for hepatitis C virus infection: a systematic review. Ann Intern Med 2017;166:637–48.
37. Kanwal F, Kramer J, Asch SM, et al. Risk of hepatocellular cancer in HCV patients treated with direct-acting antiviral agents. Gastroenterology 2017;153: 996–1005.e1.
38. Lockart I, Yeo MGH, Hajarizadeh B, et al. HCC incidence after hepatitis C cure among patients with advanced fibrosis or cirrhosis: A meta-analysis. Hepatology 2022;76:139–54.
39. Ioannou GN, Beste LA, Green PK, et al. Increased risk for hepatocellular carcinoma persists up to 10 years after HCv eradication in patients with baseline cirrhosis or high FIB-4 scores. Gastroenterology 2019;157:1264–78.e4.
40. Parikh ND, Singal AG, Hutton DW, et al. Cost-effectiveness of hepatocellular carcinoma surveillance: an assessment of benefits and harms. Am J Gastroenterol 2020;115:1642–9.
41. Fleurence RL, Collins FS. A national hepatitis c elimination program in the United States: a historic opportunity. JAMA 2023;329:1251–2.
42. Available at: https://www.who.int/health-topics/hepatitis/elimination-of-hepatitis-by-2030. 2023. Accessed June 19, 2023.
43. Younossi ZM, Koenig AB, Abdelatif D, et al. Global epidemiology of nonalcoholic fatty liver disease—meta-analytic assessment of prevalence, incidence, and outcomes. Hepatology 2016;64:73–84.
44. Younossi ZM, Golabi P, Paik JM, et al. The global epidemiology of nonalcoholic fatty liver disease (NAFLD) and nonalcoholic steatohepatitis (NASH): a systematic review. Hepatology 2023;77(4):1335–47.

45. Allen AM, Therneau TM, Ahmed OT, et al. Clinical course of non-alcoholic fatty liver disease and the implications for clinical trial design. J Hepatol 2022;77: 1237–45.
46. Loomba R, Wong R, Fraysse J, et al. Nonalcoholic fatty liver disease progression rates to cirrhosis and progression of cirrhosis to decompensation and mortality: a real world analysis of Medicare data. Aliment Pharmacol Ther 2020;51:1149–59.
47. Loomba R, Adams LA. The 20% rule of NASH progression: the natural history of advanced fibrosis and cirrhosis caused by NASH. Hepatology 2019;70:1885–8.
48. Kanwal F, Kramer JR, Mapakshi S, et al. Risk of hepatocellular cancer in patients with non-alcoholic fatty liver disease. Gastroenterology 2018;155:1828–37.e2.
49. Younossi ZM, Stepanova M, Younossi Y, et al. Epidemiology of chronic liver diseases in the USA in the past three decades. Gut 2020;69:564–8.
50. Davila JA, Morgan RO, Shaib Y, et al. Diabetes increases the risk of hepatocellular carcinoma in the United States: a population based case control study. Gut 2005;54:533–9.
51. Huang DQ, El-Serag HB, Loomba R. Global epidemiology of NAFLD-related HCC: trends, predictions, risk factors and prevention. Nat Rev Gastroenterol Hepatol 2021;18:223–38.
52. Mittal S, El-Serag HB, Sada YH, et al. Hepatocellular carcinoma in the absence of cirrhosis in united states veterans is associated with nonalcoholic fatty liver disease. Clin Gastroenterol Hepatol 2016;14:124–31.e1.
53. Loomba R, Lim JK, Patton H, et al. AGA clinical practice update on screening and surveillance for hepatocellular carcinoma in patients with nonalcoholic fatty liver disease: expert review. Gastroenterology 2020;158:1822–30.
54. Goff C, Shaikh A, Goli K, et al. Contemporary Changes in Etiology for Hepatocellular Carcinoma in Liver Transplantation. Clin Gastroenterol Hepatol 2023;21(9): 2410–2.e1.
55. Koh JH, Ng CH, Nah B, et al. NASH is the Leading Cause of Hepatocellular Carcinoma in Liver Transplant Candidates. Clin Gastroenterol Hepatol 2023. https://doi.org/10.1016/j.cgh.2023.05.019.
56. Yip TC, Lee HW, Chan WK, et al. Asian perspective on NAFLD-associated HCC. J Hepatol 2022;76:726–34.
57. Chan TT, Chan WK, Wong GL, et al. Positive hepatitis B Core antibody is associated with cirrhosis and hepatocellular carcinoma in nonalcoholic fatty liver disease. Am J Gastroenterol 2020;115:867–75.
58. Rich NE, Oji S, Mufti AR, et al. Racial and ethnic disparities in nonalcoholic fatty liver disease prevalence, severity, and outcomes in the United States: a systematic review and meta-analysis. Clin Gastroenterol Hepatol 2018;16:198–210.e2.
59. Hagström H, Thiele M, Sharma R, et al. Risk of cancer in biopsy-proven alcohol-related liver disease: a population-based cohort study of 3410 persons. Clin Gastroenterol Hepatol 2022;20:918–29.e8.
60. Jepsen P, Ott P, Andersen PK, et al. Risk for hepatocellular carcinoma in patients with alcoholic cirrhosis: a Danish nationwide cohort study. Ann Intern Med 2012; 156:841–7.
61. Huang DQ, Tan DJH, Ng CH, et al. Hepatocellular carcinoma incidence in alcohol-associated cirrhosis: systematic review and meta-analysis. Clin Gastroenterol Hepatol 2023;21:1169–77.
62. Costentin CE, Mourad A, Lahmek P, et al. Hepatocellular carcinoma is diagnosed at a later stage in alcoholic patients: Results of a prospective, nationwide study. Cancer 2018;124:1964–72.

63. Bucci L, Garuti F, Camelli V, et al. Comparison between alcohol- and hepatitis C virus-related hepatocellular carcinoma: clinical presentation, treatment and outcome. Aliment Pharmacol Ther 2016;43:385–99.
64. Reggidori N, Bucci L, Santi V, et al. Landscape of alcohol-related hepatocellular carcinoma in the last 15 years highlights the need to expand surveillance programs. JHEP Rep 2023;5(8):100784.
65. Manthey J, Shield KD, Rylett M, et al. Global alcohol exposure between 1990 and 2017 and forecasts until 2030: a modelling study. Lancet 2019;393:2493–502.
66. Sudhinaraset M, Wigglesworth C, Takeuchi DT. Social and cultural contexts of alcohol use: Influences in a social–ecological framework. Alcohol Res Curr Rev 2016;38(1):35–45.
67. Schmidt LA, Mäkelä P, Rehm J, et al. Alcohol: equity and social determinants. Equity, social determinants and public health programmes 2010;11:30.
68. Parikh ND, Chung GS, Mellinger J, et al. Alcohol policies and alcohol-related liver disease mortality. Gastroenterology 2021;161:350–2.
69. McGlynn KA, Petrick JL, El-Serag HB. Epidemiology of hepatocellular carcinoma. Hepatology 2021;73(Suppl 1):4–13.
70. Liu Y, Chang C-CH, Marsh GM, et al. Population attributable risk of aflatoxin-related liver cancer: systematic review and meta-analysis. Eur J Cancer 2012; 48:2125–36.
71. Chen J-G, Egner PA, Ng D, et al. Reduced aflatoxin exposure presages decline in liver cancer mortality in an endemic region of China. Cancer Prev Res 2013;6: 1038–45.
72. Vaghela S, Afshari R. Comparative cancer risk assessment to estimate risk of hepatocellular carcinoma attributable to dietary exposure of aflatoxin through a surrogate (Maize) in eastern mediterranean region (Iran) as compared to east (Canada) and west pacific (China) regions. Asia Pac J Med Toxicol 2017;6: 67–73.
73. Sun Z, Chen T, Thorgeirsson SS, et al. Dramatic reduction of liver cancer incidence in young adults: 28 year follow-up of etiological interventions in an endemic area of China. Carcinogenesis 2013;34:1800–5.
74. Reig M, Forner A, Rimola J, et al. BCLC strategy for prognosis prediction and treatment recommendation: the 2022 update. J Hepatol 2022;76:681–93.
75. Marrero JA, Kulik LM, Sirlin CB, et al. Diagnosis, staging, and management of hepatocellular carcinoma: 2018 practice guidance by the american association for the study of liver diseases. Hepatology 2018;68:723–50.
76. Kanwal F, Khaderi S, Singal AG, et al. Risk factors for HCC in contemporary cohorts of patients with cirrhosis. Hepatology 2023;77:997–1005.

Hepatocellular Carcinoma Surveillance
Evidence-Based Tailored Approach

Eden Koo, MD[a], Amit G. Singal, MD, MS[a,b,*]

KEYWORDS

- Liver cancer • Screening • Early detection • Ultrasound • Biomarkers
- Alpha fetoprotein

KEY POINTS

- There is a consistent association between hepatocellular carcinoma (HCC) surveillance and improved early HCC detection and reduced HCC-related mortality.
- HCC surveillance should be performed using semiannual abdominal ultrasound with serum alpha-fetoprotein.
- Ongoing studies are examining novel imaging-based and blood-based strategies for HCC surveillance.
- Efforts are needed to overcome patient-level and provider-level barriers to surveillance and increase surveillance use.

INTRODUCTION

Hepatocellular carcinoma (HCC), the most common primary liver malignancy in adults, is now the third leading cause of cancer-related deaths worldwide and projected to be the third leading cause of death in the United States by 2035.[1,2] Overall prognosis of HCC remains dismal, with a 5-year survival-rate less than 20%,[3] primarily because most HCC cases are diagnosed at an advanced stage, thereby only allowing palliative therapies as feasible options.[4]

The primary at-risk cohort for HCC is patients with cirrhosis regardless of underlying cause, which is present in 90% of patients with HCC in the Western world.[5,6] Surveillance programs have been implemented with the hopes of increasing early tumor detection and decreasing mortality. Professional society guidelines including those from the American Association for the Study of Liver Diseases (AASLD), European Association for the Study of the Liver (EASL), and Asian Pacific Association for the

[a] Department of Internal Medicine, UT Southwestern Medical Center, Dallas, TX, USA;
[b] Division of Digestive and Liver Diseases, Department of Internal Medicine, UT Southwestern Medical Center, 5959 Harry Hines Boulevard, POB 1, Suite 420, Dallas, TX 75390-8887, USA
* Corresponding author.
E-mail address: amit.singal@utsouthwestern.edu

Surg Oncol Clin N Am 33 (2024) 13–28
https://doi.org/10.1016/j.soc.2023.06.005
surgonc.theclinics.com
1055-3207/24/© 2023 Elsevier Inc. All rights reserved.

Study of the Liver (APASL) recommend semi-annual HCC surveillance in high-risk individuals.[7–9]

Despite these established practice guidelines, there are several issues that impair the effectiveness of HCC surveillance in clinical practice.[10–12] Herein, we discuss the evidence supporting the rationale for HCC surveillance, review established and emerging surveillance methods, and comment on the implementation of surveillance programs in clinical practice. We also describe potential harms of HCC surveillance and identify measures that may improve the overall value of surveillance programs in the future.

AT-RISK POPULATION FOR HEPATOCELLULAR CARCINOMA

There is geographic variation in risk factors for HCC, with hepatitis B virus (HBV) infection being the most common cause worldwide–particularly in East Asia and Africa. Conversely, hepatitis C virus (HCV) and nonviral causes such as alcohol-related cirrhosis and nonalcoholic steatohepatitis are the most common liver disease causes in the Western World, including the United States and Europe. Whereas HBV is a DNA virus and can cause HCC in the absence of cirrhosis, more than 80% of known HCC cases in the Western world have cirrhosis at the time of diagnosis, and cirrhosis is the strongest risk factor for HCC. Based on cost-effectiveness analyses, both the AASLD and EASL define high-risk populations in which annual HCC risk exceeds 1.5% per year in the presence of cirrhosis and exceeds 0.2% per year in the absence of cirrhosis (**Table 1**).

Among patients *without* an established diagnosis of cirrhosis, HCC surveillance is recommended in specific HBV-carriers. The AASLD and EASL have moved away from race and age-based recommendations and now recommend surveillance based on risk stratification models. Both societies recommend surveillance in patients with HBV who are at intermediate or high risk of HCC according to the PAGE-B score (comprising platelet count, age, and gender). Specifically, the EASL defines individuals with a PAGE-B score of 10 to 17 to be at intermediate risk for HCC, and those above 18 to be at high risk for HCC.

HCC surveillance is recommended in most patients with cirrhosis, although those with Child-Pugh C cirrhosis who are not on the transplant waiting list are not recommended to undergo surveillance due to high competing risk of liver-related mortality. Although risk of HCC is higher in viral causes of cirrhosis than nonviral causes, all causes are thought to have sufficient risk to warrant HCC surveillance.[13] Two emerging populations bear in-depth discussion—patients with HCV infection postsustained virological response (SVR) to direct acting antiviral therapy and those with nonalcoholic fatty liver disease (NAFLD).

Several studies have demonstrated significant reductions in HCC risk of ~70% among patients with and without cirrhosis who achieve SVR.[14,15] However, patients with cirrhosis continue to have some persistent risk of HCC greater than 1% per year, extending years after SVR.[16] Therefore, it is recommended that these patients continue to undergo surveillance indefinitely.[17] There has been debate about the value of surveillance in patients with advanced fibrosis who achieve SVR because some of these patients can develop HCC over time; however, decision analyses have shown that this practice is not cost effective on a population level.[18] However, professional society guidelines differ in their recommendation for surveillance in this population, with AASLD recommending against this practice but EASL and APASL saying this can be considered.

NAFLD is now the fastest growing cause of chronic liver disease, cirrhosis, and HCC in Western populations.[19–22] Several cohort studies have shown that up to one-third of HCC cases in the setting of NAFLD can occur in the absence of cirrhosis.[23,24] This was

Table 1
High-risk populations indicated for hepatocellular carcinoma surveillance, by professional society

Professional Society	High-Risk Surveillance Population	Surveillance Modality
AASLD 2023	All patients with Child-Pugh A or B liver cirrhosis of any cause Child-Pugh C liver cirrhosis of any cause if awaiting liver transplant Noncirrhotic HBV-infected persons if: • Man from endemic country[a] >40 y age • Woman from endemic country >50 y age • Persons from Africa >30 y age • Family history of HCC • PAGE-B[b] score ≥10 Stage 4 PBC	US with AFP[c]
EASL 2018	All patients with Child-Pugh A or B liver cirrhosis of any cause Child-Pugh C liver cirrhosis of any cause if awaiting liver transplant Noncirrhotic HBV-infected persons at intermediate or high risk of HCC (PAGE-B score 10–17 and ≥ 18, respectively) Noncirrhotic HCV-infected persons with evidence of F3 fibrosis	US only
APASL 2017	All patients with cirrhosis of any cause Noncirrhotic HBV-infected persons if: • Asian men age >40 y • Asian women age >50 y • African men age >20 y • Family history of HCC	US with or without AFP[d]

Abbreviations: AASLD, American Association for the Study of Liver Diseases; AFP, Alpha-fetoprotein; APASL, Asian Pacific Association for the Study of the Liver; EASL, European Association for the Study of the Liver; HBV, Hepatitis B; HCV, Hepatitis C; US, ultrasound.
[a] Defined by AASLD hepatitis B virus guidance.
[b] Platelet, age, gender, HBV.
[c] Cutoff: 20 ng/mL.
[d] Cutoff: 200 ng/mL.

concerning given the large population of patients with noncirrhotic NAFLD and how this would influence surveillance programs. However, subsequent cohort studies have demonstrated that the annual incidence of HCC in noncirrhotic NAFLD is lower than 1% annually, across various subgroups, and therefore does not meet criteria for surveillance.[25,26] However, these data highlight the need for risk stratification in this population to identify which patients with noncirrhotic NAFLD may benefit in the future. There has been ongoing work examining risk models based on clinical risk factors, genomics, and emerging risk stratification biomarkers, although all have limited external validation currently so are not ready for routine use in clinical practice.[27–30]

EVIDENCE AND RATIONALE FOR HEPATOCELLULAR CARCINOMA SURVEILLANCE

The goal of any cancer-screening program is to detect either asymptomatic or early-stage disease with the hopes of improving available treatment options and overall survival.[31] Surveillance is the application of screening at regular intervals in at-risk populations. An ideal program is established with considerations of identifiable patient populations, screening test availability and accuracy, patient and provider acceptance of the screening test, differential treatments based on cancer stage including potential curative options if detected at an early stage, and cost effectiveness.[32]

The theoretical benefit of HCC surveillance is based on the strong association between tumor stage and HCC prognosis.[6] Curative options including surgical resection, ablation, and liver transplantation afford 5-year survival exceeding 70% if patients are detected at early stages.[11] Conversely, patients with intermediate and advanced-stage HCC tumors are treated with palliative options such as transcatheter arterial chemoembolization or systemic therapies,[33] with a median survival of only 1 to 3 years.[34]

Despite the understanding that earlier tumor detection affords curative treatment options, there have been limited randomized controlled trial (RCT) data supporting the effectiveness of HCC surveillance programs in reducing disease-related mortality. The commonly cited landmark RCT for HCC surveillance was conducted in China among more than 18,000 HBV-infected persons. The study concluded that those randomized to surveillance were more likely to have HCC detected at an early stage and thus receive curative therapy. Although study adherence was suboptimal (60%), there was a 37% reduction in HCC-related mortality among the surveillance cohort.[35] Another RCT from China among 17,820 patients with HBV similarly found significant improvements in 1 and 2-year survival rates (88.1% and 77.5%, respectively, vs 0% for the nonsurveillance arm).[36] Overall, these RCTs provide evidence that HCC surveillance improves early tumor detection and reduction in mortality among patients with HBV; however, it is unclear if one can extrapolate the conclusions to modern-day populations with cirrhosis from the Western world. Patients with cirrhosis are often older, have more comorbid conditions, have higher competing risk of liver-related mortality, and may be of larger habitus thus reducing the sensitivity of abdominal ultrasound (US), which is inherently an operator-dependent modality.[37]

There are currently no published RCTs investigating HCC surveillance in patients with cirrhosis. When one was attempted in the past, it had to be prematurely closed given poor acceptance and enrollment by both patients and providers.[38] However, observational data consistently suggest a survival benefit with HCC surveillance in patients with cirrhosis. A meta-analysis of 47 studies (including 15,158 patients with cirrhosis) found that surveillance was associated with improved early-stage detection (OR, 2.08; 95% CI: 1.80–2.37), curative treatment rates (OR, 2.24; 95% CI, 1.99–2.52), and prolonged survival (3-year pooled survival, 50.8% vs 27.9% [$P < .01$] in surveillance vs nonsurveillance arms).[11] Among the subset of data that could be adjusted for lead-time bias, the association between HCC surveillance and improved survival was sustained (3-year survival rate: 39.7% vs 29.1% [$P < .05$]). An updated meta-analysis in 2022 identified 59 studies including 154,396 patients with HCC, 41,052 (28.2%) of whom were diagnosed via surveillance programs.[39] Surveillance was associated with improved early-stage detection (RR 1.86; 95% CI: 1.73–1.98), receipt of curative treatment (RR 1.83; 95% CI: 1.69–1.97), and overall survival (HR 0.67; 95% CI: 0.61–0.72), even after adjusting for lead-time bias.

However, there are some discordant data that warrant discussion. A US Department of Veteran Affairs (VA) affiliated case-control study in 2018 performed a 1:1 match of 238 patients with cirrhosis who died of HCC to 238 patients with cirrhosis who did not die of HCC.[40] Patients were matched by age, sex, cirrhosis etiology, and Model for End-Stage Liver Disease score. The study did not find significant difference between cases or controls who underwent screening US, screening measurement of serum alpha-fetoprotein (AFP), or the screening combination of the 2 (US + AFP), suggesting screening exposure was not associated with decreased HCC-related mortality. The study that has been criticized for the low screening exposure (average of 1 US per patient every 2 years), far less than the recommended semiannual interval.[41] Additionally, less than 15% of cases underwent curative therapies, likely lowering the observed benefits of surveillance due to those downstream failures that are likely not as problematic in other health-care settings.[42]

Largely due to impracticality, it is unlikely we can expect future RCTs to compare effectiveness of HCC surveillance versus non-HCC surveillance. Ethical concerns would render any attempt to randomize patients into a nonsurveillance group impossible. It would also be difficult to enroll patients informed of the risks and benefits of HCC surveillance, thus unlikely to consent to a trial involving substandard of care measures. As a result, society guidelines have largely relied on observational data to shape current recommendations. These studies, however, are vulnerable to methodological biases such as lead-time bias, length time bias, and residual confounding.[43]

SURVEILLANCE-RELATED HARMS

The choice to establish any surveillance program should balance benefits with any potential psychological, financial, and physical harms.[44] With regards to HCC surveillance, patients may be subject to physical harms ranging from discomfort due to a venipuncture to radiation and contrast imaging due to diagnostic testing. Psychological harms can include fear while awaiting surveillance results to depression and anxiety if the surveillance result is positive. Financial burden of HCC surveillance can include direct medical costs such as copays or deductibles, indirect costs such as parking and transportation, and opportunity costs due to missed work.[45]

A few studies have attempted to quantify HCC surveillance harms. One study among 680 patients with cirrhosis followed for 3 years examined the balance of benefits and harms. Of 48 patients diagnosed with HCC, 34 were diagnosed at an early stage, that is, achieved benefit.[46] However, 187 (27.5%) patients experienced surveillance-related physical harms, defined as receipt of "unnecessary" diagnostic testing for false positive or indeterminate results. Of these, 59 patients underwent repeated diagnostic imaging (ie, repeated radiation and contrast exposure) or invasive testing via biopsy. An additional study single-center study found that 15% of patients in an HCC surveillance program underwent diagnostic testing for suspicious liver nodules later determined to be benign or remained indeterminate.[47] In contrast, in a secondary analysis of a clinical trial evaluating HCC surveillance among patients with cirrhosis, Singal and colleagues[48] quantified surveillance related harms during an 18-month period. Of 614 patients, "mild" physical harms were observed in only 54 (8.8%) patients—namely involving 1 "unnecessary" diagnostic computed tomography (CT) or MRI—and none experiencing invasive testing such as biopsy. Earlier studies highlight that some patients underwent diagnostic evaluation for indeterminate surveillance tests (such as subcentimeter lesions on US), suggesting that harm may be mitigated by closer observation of guideline recommendations.[49]

Surveillance Interval

Guidelines recommend semiannual, that is, 6-month interval surveillance in the previously aforementioned high-risk populations.[7–9] The basis of this interval was initially derived from the expected HCC tumor growth rate (~117 days).[50] This interval was then supported by a few studies comparing patients undergoing semiannual surveillance with those undergoing annual surveillance.[51,52] The semiannual surveillance group was associated with higher detection rates of early-stage HCC tumors, thus leading to higher curative therapy receipt rates. Wang and colleagues[53] similarly found that 4-month surveillance intervals were superior to annual surveillance among patients with viral-mediated liver disease. Additional studies have supported semiannual surveillance as superior to annual surveillance and noninferior to quarterly surveillance.[54–56]

Surveillance Modalities

Abdominal US is considered the standard modality for HCC surveillance by the AASLD, EASL, and APASL, mostly due to advantages such as its noninvasive approach, inexpensive operation, and that it poses no risk of radiation or contrast exposure for the patient. In a meta-analysis, sensitivity of US alone was estimated to be 84% for HCC at any stage and 47% for early-stage HCC.[57] The effectiveness of US heavily depends on operator experience as well as patient factors such as truncal obesity and liver disease severity.[58] A single-center retrospective analysis of 941 cirrhotic patients undergoing HCC surveillance concluded that nearly 1 in 5 US examinations had impaired visualization for the exclusion of liver masses.[59] Although visualization can improve for a portion of patients, many patients with impaired visualization at baseline continue to have impaired visualization on repeat examination.[60] Persistent limitations in US visualization were associated with nonviral causes of cirrhosis and obesity. Although impaired visualization has minimal impact on specificity, examinations with severe visualization limitations can miss nearly three-fourths of HCC at an early stage.[61] These findings are of particular concern given epidemiologic shifts with NAFLD-related cirrhosis poised to become an increasingly common cause of HCC.[62]

AFP is the best-studied serum biomarker to date for HCC screening. When used alone, AFP has suboptimal performance, with sensitivities for early HCC of only 32% to 49% and specificities of 80% to 94%.[63] However, there continues to be debate regarding its added value to US for early HCC detection. The AASLD recommends surveillance using US with AFP, whereas the EASL recommends US alone.[7,8] The prior meta-analysis by Tzartzeva and colleagues[57] found US plus AFP had superior sensitivity than US alone (RR 1.23; 95% CI: 1.08–1.41). For early-stage HCC, pooled sensitivity of US plus AFP was superior to US alone (63% vs 45%). Despite AFP having a lower reported specificity than US, harms of surveillance related to false positives and in-determinate tests also seem to be more associated with US than AFP.[46] This discordance is thought to be partly related to provider behavior and interpretation of low-level false-positive AFP levels that can mitigate surveillance harms and potential excessive workup for indeterminate lesions on US. These data suggest that US + AFP may be the optimal strategy for early HCC detection.

Conversely, EASL cites Biselli and colleagues[64] who reported that adding AFP only provides an additional detection of 6% to 8% of cases not identified by US, which does not counterbalance the financial costs associated with false-positive results that are inherently associated with AFP. A cost-effectiveness study found that US plus AFP was superior to US alone in more than 80% of simulations, at a traditional cost-effectiveness threshold of US$100,000 per quality adjusted life year.[65]

There have been proposals to use methods such as AFP-adjusted panels, differences in cutoffs by liver disease etiology, and longitudinal interpretation of AFP values. For example, Gopal and colleagues[66] suggested performance of AFP could be improved by using a lower threshold in patients with nonviral liver disease and higher thresholds in the setting of active viremia. Using AFP in a longitudinal manner with a parametric Bayesian screening algorithm, rather than as a single threshold assessment, has also been shown to enhance performance.[67]

Other imaging-based surveillance approaches

Other imaging modalities traditionally used in the diagnostic setting include CT and MRI scans. Given increasing recognition of US's limitations, there has been an increasing interest to see if these modalities may be applied to the surveillance setting (**Table 2**).

A cohort study from South Korea of 407 patients with cirrhosis compared US to multiphase MRI (with liver-specific contrast) for the surveillance of HCC. During a follow-up of 1.5 years, 43 patients were diagnosed with HCC, of whom 42 were found at an early stage. MRI-based surveillance had a lower false-positive rate compared with US (3.0% vs 5.6%) as well as superior sensitivity for early HCC detection (83.7% vs 25.65%).[68] A similar study from South Korea compared 2-phase low-dose CT imaging (arterial phase and 3-minute delayed phase) versus US in 139 patients at high risk of developing HCC.[69] During a follow-up of 1.5 years, 24 participants developed HCC, with 2-phase CT having significantly better sensitivity (83.3% vs 29.2%, $P < .001$) and specificity (95.6% vs 87.7%, $P = .03$). However, it should be noted that the primary studied populations in both studies are HBV-infected patients with an average BMI lower than typically observed in Western world patients. Further research is needed evaluating MRI performance in non-HBV individuals as well as its

Table 2 Summary of established and emerging surveillance methods			
Category	Surveillance Method	Pros	Cons
Imaging	Noncontrast US	Low cost, ease of access, noninvasive	Operator-dependent, limited detection in larger habitus
	CT	Superior efficacy	Radiation exposure, cost, barriers to access
	MRI	Superior efficacy	Cost, barriers to access
	AMRI	Reduced study time, acquisition time, reporting time compared with MRI	Barriers to access and unclear cost-effectiveness
Single biomarkers	AFP	Low cost, ease of access, improved detection when combined with US	Lack of consensus among professional societies on cost-effectiveness, marginal analysis
	1. AFP-L3 2. DCP 3. GP73 4. GPC3 5. Osteopontin 6. Fucosylated kininogen	Early studies reporting superior sensitivity and/or specificity compared with AFP	Limited phase II biomarker validation studies. Further phase III and phase IV cohort studies needed
Biomarker panels	Gender, age, biomarkers, AFP, AFP-L3, DCP (GALAD)	Good sensitivity of early-stage HCC	Further phase III and phase IV cohort studies needed
Liquid biopsy biomarkers	1. Methylated cell-free DNA 2. Extracellular vesicles 3. Circulating tumor cells	Good sensitivity of early-stage HCC	Further phase III and phase IV cohort studies needed

suitability in those with truncal obesity. Further, the use of these studies must be considered in light of possible physical harms with repeated testing (radiation and contrast exposure), cost-effectiveness although costs for these modalities is starting to decrease over time, and limited radiologic capacity if expanded to broad populations with cirrhosis. The latter point may be particularly relevant for rural areas or safety-net health systems, in which MRI capacity may be lower than other areas.

Abbreviated MRI (AMRI) protocols have been proposed as an option to mitigate the financial costs associated with traditional MRI. These protocols theoretically reduce acquisition time for the patient as well as impression reporting time from radiologists.[70,71] Certain proposed protocols include noncontrast, diffusion-weighted imaging, dynamic contrast-enhanced, and hepatobiliary phase. A meta-analysis evaluated the effectiveness of various AMRI protocols and reported pooled sensitivity and sensitivity of 86% and 94%, respectively.[72] Other retrospective studies based in Europe and Asia have reported high AMRI sensitivity and specificity rate for early-stage HCC but mostly in nonsurveillance cohorts.[73] A recent multisite radiologic-pathologic comparing AMRI to pathology gold standard from resection and transplant patient found that AMRI had a high sensitivity and specificity for early-stage HCC (88.2% and 89.1%, respectively).[74] Although sensitivity for early-stage HCC was preserved in patients with nonviral liver disease and obese individuals, it was markedly lower in those with Child Pugh B or C cirrhosis compared with Child A cirrhosis (64.1% vs 94.2%, $P < .001$), suggesting AMRI may not have optimal performance for all patients. The prospective, multicenter MAGNUS-HCC trial is an ongoing trial that aims to be the first study comparing the feasibility of noncontrast MRI with US in a surveillance population.[75] Patients enrolled in HCC surveillance will undergo US every 6 months in addition to noncontrast MRI every 12 months, with rates of HCC detection compared during a 3-year follow-up period. Similar trials are now being launched with other AMRI protocols.

Emerging blood-based biomarker panels

In addition to AFP, several alternative serum biomarkers have been proposed for HCC surveillance. The *lens culinaris* lectin-binding subfractions of AFP (AFP-L3) and des gamma carboxy prothrombin (DCP) are the 2 most-studied biomarkers outside of AFP. The specificity of AFP-L3 for HCC has been reported to be as high as 99.4%.[76,77] The sensitivity and specificity of AFL-L3 (at a cutoff of 1.7%) has been reported as 37% and 94%, respectively.[78] Liebman and colleagues[79] first reported the presence of DCP, a prothrombin variant, in more than 90% of studied patients with HCC. Although DCP is widely used in Japan for HCC diagnosis and surveillance, it has been poorly studied in Western populations.[80] In a case-control study by Lok and colleagues,[81] the combination of DCP and AFP measured at 2 time points (0 and 12 months) resulted in higher sensitivities but lower specificities. Other HCC serum biomarkers that have been proposed include Golgi protein 73 (GP73), Glypican 3 (GPC3), Osteopontin, and Fucosylated kininogen, although these have largely only undergone limited phase II biomarker validation.[82] Further validation in phase III and phase IV cohort studies are needed before consideration in clinical practice.[83]

Given the heterogeneity of HCC, it is increasingly recognized that a single biomarker will not be sufficient and biomarker panels are likely needed. A biomarker panel has been proposed that incorporates gender, age, biomarkers, AFP, AFP-L3%, and DCP (GALAD). In a multinational phase II case-control biomarker study, GALAD has a sensitivity of 60% to 80% for the detection of early-stage HCC.[84] A subsequent pilot phase III study among 397 patients with cirrhosis reported that GALAD had a c-statistic of 0.79 (95%CI 0.71–0.87) and sensitivity of 53.8% with specificity fixed at 90% for early-stage HCC detection.[85] GALAD is completing phase III evaluation in the Early Detection Research Network HCC Early Detection Strategy Study and has been proposed for a randomized phase IV trial compared with US-based surveillance.

Methylated cell-free DNA markers, an important "culprit" in carcinogenesis, may be detected via "liquid biopsy," or assessment of circulating tumor cells and DNA or exosome products.[86,87] National phase II studies have further explored the utility of these biomarkers, although they still require validation in phase III cohort studies. A prospective validation study evaluated the performance of HelioLiver, commercialized as a multianalyte blood test combining 77 cell-free DNA methylation pattern targets, clinical variables, and 3 protein tumor markers. In this blinded, multicenter study, HelioLiver demonstrated high sensitivity (85% for HCC of any stage and 76% for early-stage HCC) and specificity (91%).[88] Another panel including 3 methylated DNA markers, AFP, and sex was validated in a phase II study with an overall sensitivity of 88%, early-stage sensitivity of 82%, and specificity of 87%. Early stage sensitivity of this panel was superior to AFP with cutoff at 20 ng/mL (40%, $P < .01$) and GALAD (71%, $P = .03$).[89,90]

Utilization of Hepatocellular Carcinoma Surveillance

Despite the demonstrated benefits of HCC surveillance on early tumor detection, it is estimated that only 24.0% of patients with cirrhosis undergo surveillance.[91] Surveillance use is significantly higher among patients followed in subspecialty clinics, with surveillance utilization in ~74% of patients followed by subspecialists, compared with only ~30% of those followed by primary care providers alone. Surveillance use seems to be particularly underused in racial and ethnic minority populations and those of low socioeconomic status, contributing to observed disparities in overall survival.[92–95]

There are multiple avenues that may lead to "surveillance failure," such as patients not being engaged in clinical care, providers failing to identify at-risk patients, provider nonadherence to surveillance recommendations, and patient nonadherence to surveillance recommendations.[96,97] The most common points of failure are patients not being engaged in routine clinical care before HCC diagnosis and provider failure to order surveillance in patients with known cirrhosis.[98,99] There are several patient and provider-level barriers to HCC surveillance including patients reporting scheduling difficulties, costs of surveillance, and transportation as notable barriers.[100,101] Providers report issues including knowledge gaps, time constraints in clinic, and competing clinical demands.[102]

There have been multiple published studies reporting quality improvement measures to promote utilization of HCC surveillance. One reported model involving electronic medical record (EMR) clinical reminders has been shown to be successful. In a study involving 2884 VA patients with cirrhosis, Beste and colleagues[103] reported significantly improved surveillance rates (18.2%–27.6%) in patients with cirrhosis who were cared for at a VA facility in which an EMR reminder was implemented. In an RCT of 1800 patients with cirrhosis, mailed outreach for screening US, mailed outreach plus patient navigation (barrier assessment, motivational education), and usual care with visit-based screening were compared. HCC surveillance during an 18-month period was completed more frequently in both outreach and outreach/navigation arms compared with usual care (23.3% and 17.8% vs 7.3%, respectively).[104,105] A subsequent multicenter trial evaluating mailed outreach across 3 types of health systems similarly found increased use of HCC surveillance with mailed outreach compared with usual care (35.1% vs 21.9%) during a 12-month period, with further evaluation during a 36-month period ongoing.[106]

Although these strategies have proven efficacious, surveillance continues to be underused in the intervention arms, highlighting that improvements in HCC surveillance in clinical practice will likely require a multidisciplinary network targeting patient and provider education, as well as a more deliberate integration of HCC surveillance into health systems.

SUMMARY

Although the body of evidence supporting HCC surveillance is sufficient to be recommended by professional expert societies, there is a continued need for high-level data examining benefits and harms of surveillance in contemporary patient populations. Surveillance should currently be performed using semiannual abdominal US with serum AFP, although there is increasing recognition that this strategy misses more than one-third of HCC at an early stage. Ongoing studies are examining novel imaging-based and blood-based strategies such as AMRI and biomarker panels for HCC surveillance, although validation in prospective studies is still needed. While awaiting those data, efforts are needed to overcome patient-level and provider-level barriers to surveillance and optimize surveillance utilization in clinical practice.

CLINICS CARE POINTS

- HCC surveillance is associated with improved early tumor detection and reduced cancer-related mortality in patients with cirrhosis and those with chronic hepatitis B infection.
- HCC surveillance should be performed using abdominal ultrasound and AFP every 6 months in at-risk patients.
- Utilization rates of HCC surveillance in clinical practice are low due to several patient- and provider-level barriers.

FINANCIAL SOURCE

Dr A.G. Singal's research is in part supported by National Institute of Health, United States R01 CA212008, U01 CA230694, and R01 CA222900. The content is solely the responsibility of the authors and does not necessarily represent the official views of the NIH. The funding agencies had no role in design and conduct of the study; collection, management, analysis, and interpretation of the data; or preparation of the article.

CONFLICT OF INTEREST

Dr A.G. Singal has served as a consultant or on advisory boards for Genentech, AstraZeneca, Bayer, Eisai, Exelixis, FujiFilm Medical Sciences, Exact Sciences, Glycotest, Universal Diagnostics, Roche, Freenome, GRAIL, and TARGET RWE.

REFERENCES

1. Global Burden of Disease Cancer Collaboration, Fitzmaurice C, Abate D, et al. Global, regional, and national cancer incidence, mortality, years of life lost, years lived with disability, and disability-adjusted life-years for 29 cancer groups, 1990 to 2017: a systematic analysis for the global burden of disease study. JAMA Oncol 2019;5(12):1749–68.

2. Liu Y, Zheng J, Hao J, et al. Global burden of primary liver cancer by five etiologies and global prediction by 2035 based on global burden of disease study 2019. Cancer Med 2022;11(5):1310–23.

3. Villanueva A. Hepatocellular Carcinoma. N Engl J Med 2019;380(15):1450–62.

4. Moon A, Singal AG, Tapper E. Contemporary epidemiology of chronic liver disease and cirrhosis. Clin Gastroenterol Hepatol 2020;18(12):2650–66.

5. Yang JD, Hainaut P, Gores GJ, et al. A global view of hepatocellular carcinoma: trends, risk, prevention and management. Nat Rev Gastroenterol Hepatol 2019; 16(10):589–604.

6. Llovet JM, Kelley RK, Villanueva A, et al. Hepatocellular carcinoma. Nat Rev Dis Prim 2021;7(1):1–28.

7. Marrero JA, Kulik LM, Sirlin CB, et al. Diagnosis, staging, and management of hepatocellular carcinoma: 2018 practice guidance by the american association for the study of liver diseases. Hepatol Baltim Md 2018;68(2):723–50.

8. Galle PR, Forner A, Llovet JM, et al. EASL clinical practice guidelines: management of hepatocellular carcinoma. J Hepatol 2018;69(1):182–236.

9. Omata M, Cheng AL, Kokudo N, et al. Asia–Pacific clinical practice guidelines on the management of hepatocellular carcinoma: a 2017 update. Hepatol Int 2017;11(4):317–70.

10. Kansagara D, Papak J, Pasha AS, et al. Screening for hepatocellular carcinoma in chronic liver disease: a systematic review. Ann Intern Med 2014;161(4): 261–9.

11. Singal AG, Pillai A, Tiro J. Early detection, curative treatment, and survival rates for hepatocellular carcinoma surveillance in patients with cirrhosis: a meta-analysis. PLoS Med 2014;11(4):e1001624.

12. Jepsen P, West J. We need stronger evidence for (or against) hepatocellular carcinoma surveillance. J Hepatol 2021;74(5):1234–9.

13. Kanwal F, Khaderi S, Singal AG, et al. Risk factors for HCC in contemporary cohorts of patients with cirrhosis. Hepatol Baltim Md 2023;77(3):997–1005.

14. Ioannou GN, Green PK, Berry K. HCV eradication induced by direct-acting antiviral agents reduces the risk of hepatocellular carcinoma. J Hepatol 2017. https://doi.org/10.1016/j.jhep.2017.08.030. S0168-8278(17)32273-0.

15. Kanwal F, Kramer J, Asch SM, et al. Risk of hepatocellular Cancer in HCV patients treated with direct-acting antiviral agents. Gastroenterology 2017; 153(4):996–1005.e1.

16. Ioannou GN, Beste LA, Green PK, et al. Increased risk for hepatocellular carcinoma persists up to 10 years after HCV eradication in patients with baseline cirrhosis or high FIB-4 scores. Gastroenterology 2019;157(5):1264–78.e4.

17. Singal AG, Lim JK, Kanwal F. AGA clinical practice update on interaction between oral direct-acting antivirals for chronic hepatitis C infection and hepatocellular carcinoma: expert review. Clin Liver Dis 2020;15(6):211–2.

18. Farhang Zangneh H, Wong WWL, Sander B, et al. Cost effectiveness of hepatocellular carcinoma surveillance after a sustained virologic response to therapy in patients with hepatitis C virus infection and advanced fibrosis. Clin Gastroenterol Hepatol 2019;17(9):1840 9.e16.

19. El-Serag HB, Kanwal F, Feng Z, et al. Risk factors for cirrhosis in contemporary hepatology practices-findings from the texas hepatocellular carcinoma consortium cohort. Gastroenterology 2020;159(1):376–7.

20. Parikh ND, Marrero WJ, Wang J, et al. Projected increase in obesity and non-alcoholic-steatohepatitis-related liver transplantation waitlist additions in the United States. Hepatology 2019;70(2):487–95.

21. Younossi Z, Stepanova M, Ong JP, et al. Nonalcoholic steatohepatitis is the fastest growing cause of hepatocellular carcinoma in liver transplant candidates. Clin Gastroenterol Hepatol 2019;17(4):748–55.e3.
22. Huang DQ, Singal AG, Kono Y, et al. Changing global epidemiology of liver cancer from 2010 to 2019: NASH is the fastest growing cause of liver cancer. Cell Metab 2022;34(7):969–77.e2.
23. Stine JG, Wentworth BJ, Zimmet A, et al. Systematic review with meta-analysis: risk of hepatocellular carcinoma in non-alcoholic steatohepatitis without cirrhosis compared to other liver diseases. Aliment Pharmacol Ther 2018; 48(7):696–703.
24. Mittal S, El-Serag HB, Sada YH, et al. Hepatocellular carcinoma in the absence of cirrhosis in united states veterans is associated with nonalcoholic fatty liver disease. Clin Gastroenterol Hepatol 2016;14(1):124–31.e1.
25. Kanwal F, Kramer JR, Mapakshi S, et al. Risk of hepatocellular cancer in patients with non-alcoholic fatty liver disease. Gastroenterology 2018;155(6): 1828–37.e2.
26. Lee TY, Wu JC, Yu SH, et al. The occurrence of hepatocellular carcinoma in different risk stratifications of clinically noncirrhotic nonalcoholic fatty liver disease. Int J Cancer 2017;141(7):1307–14.
27. Ioannou GN, Green P, Kerr KF, et al. Models estimating risk of hepatocellular carcinoma in patients with alcohol or NAFLD-related cirrhosis for risk stratification. J Hepatol 2019;71(3):523–33.
28. Bianco C, Jamialahmadi O, Pelusi S, et al. Non-invasive stratification of hepatocellular carcinoma risk in non-alcoholic fatty liver using polygenic risk scores. J Hepatol 2021;74(4):775–82.
29. Fujiwara N, Kubota N, Crouchet E, et al. Molecular signatures of long-term hepatocellular carcinoma risk in nonalcoholic fatty liver disease. Sci Transl Med 2022;14(650):eabo4474.
30. Fujiwara N, Kobayashi M, Fobar AJ, et al. A blood-based prognostic liver secretome signature and long-term hepatocellular carcinoma risk in advanced liver fibrosis. Med 2021;2(7):836–50.e10.
31. Pinsky PF. Principles of Cancer Screening. Surg Clin North Am 2015;95(5): 953–66.
32. Ryerson AB, Massetti GM. CDC's Public Health Surveillance of Cancer. Prev Chronic Dis 2017;14:160480. doi: http://dx.doi.org/10.5888/pcd14.160480.
33. Llovet JM, Villanueva A, Marrero JA, et al. Trial design and endpoints in hepatocellular carcinoma: AASLD consensus conference. Hepatology 2021;73(S1): 158–91.
34. Reig M, Forner A, Rimola J, et al. BCLC strategy for prognosis prediction and treatment recommendation: The 2022 update. J Hepatol 2022;76(3):681–93.
35. Zhang BH, Yang BH, Tang ZY. Randomized controlled trial of screening for hepatocellular carcinoma. J Cancer Res Clin Oncol 2004;130(7):417–22.
36. Yang B, Zhang B, Xu Y, et al. Prospective study of early detection for primary liver cancer. J Cancer Res Clin Oncol 1997;123(6):357–60.
37. Jepsen P. Comorbidity in cirrhosis. World J Gastroenterol WJG 2014;20(23): 7223–30.
38. Poustchi H, Farrell GC, Strasser SI, et al. Feasibility of conducting a randomized control trial for liver cancer screening: is a randomized controlled trial for liver cancer screening feasible or still needed? Hepatology 2011;54(6):1998–2004.

39. Singal AG, Zhang E, Narasimman M, et al. HCC surveillance improves early detection, curative treatment receipt, and survival in patients with cirrhosis: A meta-analysis. J Hepatol 2022;77(1):128–39.
40. Moon AM, Weiss NS, Beste LA, et al. No association between screening for hepatocellular carcinoma and reduced cancer-related mortality in patients with cirrhosis. Gastroenterology 2018;155(4):1128–39.e6.
41. Singal AG, Murphy CC. Hepatocellular carcinoma surveillance: an effective but complex process. Gastroenterology 2019;156(4):1215.
42. Singal AG, Lok AS, Feng Z, et al. Conceptual model for the hepatocellular carcinoma screening continuum: current status and research agenda. Clin Gastroenterol Hepatol 2022;20(1):9–18.
43. Rich NE, Singal AG. Overdiagnosis of hepatocellular carcinoma: prevented by guidelines? Hepatology 2022;75(3):740–53.
44. Harris RP, Wilt TJ, Qaseem A. High value care task force of the american college of physicians. A value framework for cancer screening: advice for high-value care from the American college of physicians. Ann Intern Med 2015;162(10): 712–7.
45. Petrasek J, Singal AG, Rich NE. Harms of hepatocellular carcinoma surveillance. Curr Hepatol Rep 2019;18(4):383–9.
46. Atiq O, Tiro J, Yopp AC, et al. An assessment of benefits and harms of hepatocellular carcinoma surveillance in patients with cirrhosis. Hepatology 2017; 65(4):1196–205.
47. Konerman MA, Verma A, Zhao B, et al. Frequency and outcomes of abnormal imaging in patients with cirrhosis enrolled in a hepatocellular carcinoma surveillance program. Liver Transpl 2019;25(3):369–79.
48. Singal AG, Patibandla S, Obi J, et al. Benefits and harms of hepatocellular carcinoma surveillance in a prospective cohort of patients with cirrhosis. Clin Gastroenterol Hepatol 2021;19(9):1925–32.e1.
49. Singal AG, Ghaziani TT, Mehta N, et al. Recall patterns and risk of primary liver cancer for subcentimeter ultrasound liver observations: a multicenter study. Hepatol Commun 2023;7(3):e0073.
50. Sheu JC, Sung JL, Chen DS, et al. Growth rate of asymptomatic hepatocellular carcinoma and its clinical implications. Gastroenterology 1985;89(2):259–66.
51. Trevisani F, De Notariis S, Rapaccini G, et al. Semiannual and annual surveillance of cirrhotic patients for hepatocellular carcinoma: effects on cancer stage and patient survival (Italian experience). Am J Gastroenterol 2002;97(3):734–44.
52. Santi V, Trevisani F, Gramenzi A, et al. Semiannual surveillance is superior to annual surveillance for the detection of early hepatocellular carcinoma and patient survival. J Hepatol 2010;53(2):291–7.
53. Wang J-H, Chang K-C, Kee K-M, et al. Hepatocellular carcinoma surveillance at 4- vs. 12-month intervals for patients with chronic viral hepatitis: a randomized study in community. Am J Gastroenterol 2013;108(3):416–24.
54. Nathani P, Gopal P, Rich N, et al. Hepatocellular carcinoma tumour volume doubling time: a systematic review and meta-analysis. Gut 2021;70(2):401–7.
55. Rich NE, John BV, Parikh ND, et al. Hepatocellular carcinoma demonstrates heterogeneous growth patterns in a multicenter cohort of patients with cirrhosis. Hepatology 2020;72(5):1654–65.
56. Trinchet JC, Chaffaut C, Bourcier V, et al. Ultrasonographic surveillance of hepatocellular carcinoma in cirrhosis: a randomized trial comparing 3- and 6-month periodicities. Hepatology 2011;54(6):1987–97.

57. Tzartzeva K, Obi J, Rich NE, et al. Surveillance imaging and alpha fetoprotein for early detection of hepatocellular carcinoma in patients with cirrhosis: a meta-analysis. Gastroenterology 2018;154(6):1706–18.e1.

58. Fetzer DT, Browning T, Xi Y, et al. Associations of ultrasound LI-RADS Visualization score with examination, sonographer, and radiologist factors: retrospective assessment in over 10,000 examinations. AJR Am J Roentgenol 2022;218(6): 1010–20.

59. Simmons O, Fetzer DT, Yokoo T, et al. Predictors of adequate ultrasound quality for hepatocellular carcinoma surveillance in patients with cirrhosis. Aliment Pharmacol Ther 2017;45(1):169–77.

60. Schoenberger H, Chong N, Fetzer DT, et al. Dynamic changes in ultrasound quality for hepatocellular carcinoma screening in patients with cirrhosis. Clin Gastroenterol Hepatol 2022;20(7):1561–9.e4.

61. Chong N, Schoenberger H, Yekkaluri S, et al. Association between ultrasound quality and test performance for HCC surveillance in patients with cirrhosis: a retrospective cohort study. Aliment Pharmacol Ther 2022;55(6):683–90.

62. Estes C, Anstee QM, Arias-Loste MT, et al. Modeling NAFLD disease burden in China, France, Germany, Italy, Japan, Spain, United Kingdom, and United States for the period 2016-2030. J Hepatol 2018;69(4):896–904.

63. Gupta S, Bent S, Kohlwes J. Test characteristics of alpha-fetoprotein for detecting hepatocellular carcinoma in patients with hepatitis C. A systematic review and critical analysis. Ann Intern Med 2003;139(1):46–50.

64. Biselli M, Conti F, Gramenzi A, et al. A new approach to the use of α-fetoprotein as surveillance test for hepatocellular carcinoma in patients with cirrhosis. Br J Cancer 2015;112(1):69–76.

65. Parikh ND, Singal AG, Hutton DW, et al. Cost-effectiveness of hepatocellular carcinoma surveillance: an assessment of benefits and harms. Am J Gastroenterol 2020;115(10):1642–9.

66. Gopal P, Yopp AC, Waljee AK, et al. Factors that affect accuracy of α-fetoprotein test in detection of hepatocellular carcinoma in patients with cirrhosis. Clin Gastroenterol Hepatol 2014;12(5):870–7.

67. Tayob N, Lok ASF, Do KA, et al. Improved detection of hepatocellular carcinoma by using a longitudinal alpha-fetoprotein screening algorithm. Clin Gastroenterol Hepatol 2016;14(3):469–75.e2.

68. Kim SY, An J, Lim YS, et al. MRI with liver-specific contrast for surveillance of patients with cirrhosis at high risk of hepatocellular carcinoma. JAMA Oncol 2017;3(4):456–63.

69. Yoon JH, Lee JM, Lee DH, et al. A comparison of biannual two-phase low-dose liver CT and US for HCC surveillance in a group at high risk of HCC development. Liver Cancer 2020;9(5):503–17.

70. Khatri G, Pedrosa I, Ananthakrishnan L, et al. Abbreviated-protocol screening MRI vs. complete-protocol diagnostic MRI for detection of hepatocellular carcinoma in patients with cirrhosis: an equivalence study using LI-RADS v2018. J Magn Reson Imaging JMRI 2020;51(2):415–25.

71. Park HJ, Kim SY, Singal AG, et al. Abbreviated magnetic resonance imaging vs ultrasound for surveillance of hepatocellular carcinoma in high-risk patients. Liver Int 2022;42(9):2080–92.

72. Gupta P, Soundararajan R, Patel A, et al. Abbreviated MRI for hepatocellular carcinoma screening: a systematic review and meta-analysis. J Hepatol 2021; 75(1):108–19.

73. An JY, Peña MA, Cunha GM, et al. Abbreviated MRI for hepatocellular carcinoma screening and surveillance. Radiographics 2020;40(7):1916–31.

74. Yokoo T, Masaki N, Parikh ND, et al. Multicenter validation of abbreviated MRI for detecting early-stage hepatocellular carcinoma. Radiology 2023;307(2): e220917.

75. Kim HA, Kim KA, Choi JI, et al. Comparison of biannual ultrasonography and annual non-contrast liver magnetic resonance imaging as surveillance tools for hepatocellular carcinoma in patients with liver cirrhosis (MAGNUS-HCC): a study protocol. BMC Cancer 2017;17(1):877.

76. Kudo M. Alpha-fetoprotein-L3: useful or useless for hepatocellular carcinoma? Liver Cancer 2013;2(3–4):151–2.

77. Lee HA, Lee YR, Lee YS, et al. Lens culinaris agglutinin-reactive fraction of alpha-fetoprotein improves diagnostic accuracy for hepatocellular carcinoma. World J Gastroenterol 2021;27(28):4687–96.

78. Marrero JA, Feng Z, Wang Y, et al. Alpha-fetoprotein, des-gamma carboxyprothrombin, and lectin-bound alpha-fetoprotein in early hepatocellular carcinoma. Gastroenterology 2009;137(1):110–8.

79. Liebman HA, Furie BC, Tong MJ, et al. Des-gamma-carboxy (abnormal) prothrombin as a serum marker of primary hepatocellular carcinoma. N Engl J Med 1984;310(22):1427–31.

80. Kudo M, Kawamura Y, Hasegawa K, et al. Management of hepatocellular carcinoma in Japan: JSH consensus statements and recommendations 2021 update. Liver Cancer 2021;10(3):181–223.

81. Lok AS, Sterling RK, Everhart JE, et al. Des-gamma-carboxy prothrombin and alpha-fetoprotein as biomarkers for the early detection of hepatocellular carcinoma. Gastroenterology 2010;138(2):493–502.

82. Wang W, Wei C. Advances in the early diagnosis of hepatocellular carcinoma. Genes Dis 2020;7(3):308–19.

83. Singal AG, Hoshida Y, Pinato DJ, et al. International liver cancer association (ILCA) white paper on biomarker development for hepatocellular carcinoma. Gastroenterology 2021;160(7):2572–84.

84. Berhane S, Toyoda H, Tada T, et al. Role of the GALAD and BALAD-2 serologic models in diagnosis of hepatocellular carcinoma and prediction of survival in patients. Clin Gastroenterol Hepatol 2016;14(6):875–86.e6.

85. Singal AG, Tayob N, Mehta A, et al. GALAD demonstrates high sensitivity for HCC surveillance in a cohort of patients with cirrhosis. Hepatology 2022; 75(3):541–9.

86. Chen VL, Xu D, Wicha MS, et al. Utility of liquid biopsy analysis in detection of hepatocellular carcinoma, determination of prognosis, and disease monitoring: a systematic review. Clin Gastroenterol Hepatol 2020;18(13):2879–902.e9.

87. Kisiel JB, Dukek BA, R Kanipakam R VS, et al. Hepatocellular carcinoma detection by plasma methylated DNA: discovery, phase I pilot, and phase II clinical validation. Hepatology 2019;69(3):1180–92.

88. Lin N, Lin Y, Xu J, et al. A multi-analyte cell-free DNA–based blood test for early detection of hepatocellular carcinoma. Hepatol Commun 2022;6(7):1753–63.

89. Chalasani NP, Ramasubramanian TS, Bhattacharya A, et al. A novel blood-based panel of methylated DNA and protein markers for detection of early-stage hepatocellular carcinoma. Clin Gastroenterol Hepatol 2021;19(12): 2597–605.e4.

90. Chalasani NP, Porter K, Bhattacharya A, et al. Validation of a novel multitarget blood test shows high sensitivity to detect early stage hepatocellular carcinoma. Clin Gastroenterol Hepatol 2022;20(1):173–82.e7.

91. Wolf E, Rich NE, Marrero JA, et al. Utilization of hepatocellular carcinoma surveillance in patients with cirrhosis: a systematic review and meta-analysis. Hepatology 2021;73(2):713–25.

92. Singal AG, Li X, Tiro J, et al. Racial, social, and clinical determinants of hepatocellular carcinoma surveillance. Am J Med 2015;128(1):90.e1–7.

93. Rich NE, Carr C, Yopp AC, et al. Racial and ethnic disparities in survival among patients with hepatocellular carcinoma in the United States: a systematic review and meta-analysis. Clin Gastroenterol Hepatol 2022;20(2):e267–88.

94. Schoenberger H, Rich NE, Jones P, et al. Racial and ethnic disparities in barriers to care in patients with hepatocellular carcinoma. Clin Gastroenterol Hepatol 2023;21(4):1094–6.e2.

95. Wagle NS, Park S, Washburn D, et al. Racial, ethnic, and socioeconomic disparities in curative treatment receipt and survival in hepatocellular carcinoma. Hepatol Commun 2022;6(5):1186–97.

96. Singal AG, Nehra M, Adams-Huet B, et al. Detection of hepatocellular carcinoma at advanced stages among patients in the HALT-C trial: where did surveillance fail? Am J Gastroenterol 2013;108(3):425–32.

97. Singal AG, Yopp AC, Gupta S, et al. Failure rates in the hepatocellular carcinoma surveillance process. Cancer Prev Res 2012;5(9):1124–30.

98. Marquardt P, Liu PH, Immergluck J, et al. Hepatocellular carcinoma screening process failures in patients with cirrhosis. Hepatol Commun 2021;5(9):1481.

99. Parikh ND, Tayob N, Al-Jarrah T, et al. Barriers to surveillance for hepatocellular carcinoma in a multicenter cohort. JAMA Netw Open 2022;5(7):e2223504.

100. Singal AG, Tiro JA, Murphy CC, et al. Patient-reported barriers are associated with receipt of hepatocellular carcinoma surveillance in a multicenter cohort of patients with cirrhosis. Clin Gastroenterol Hepatol 2021;19(5):987–95.e1.

101. Farvardin S, Patel J, Khambaty M, et al. Patient-reported barriers are associated with lower hepatocellular carcinoma surveillance rates in patients with cirrhosis. Hepatology 2017;65(3):875–84.

102. Simmons OL, Feng Y, Parikh ND, et al. Primary care provider practice patterns and barriers to hepatocellular carcinoma surveillance. Clin Gastroenterol Hepatol 2019;17(4):766–73.

103. Beste LA, Ioannou GN, Yang Y, et al. Improved surveillance for hepatocellular carcinoma with a primary care–oriented clinical reminder. Clin Gastroenterol Hepatol 2015;13(1):172–9.

104. Singal AG, Tiro JA, Murphy CC, et al. Mailed outreach invitations significantly improve HCC surveillance rates in patients with cirrhosis: a randomized clinical trial. Hepatology 2019;69(1):121–30.

105. Singal AG, Tiro JA, Marrero JA, et al. Mailed outreach program increases ultrasound screening of patients with cirrhosis for hepatocellular carcinoma. Gastroenterology 2017;152(3):608–15.e4.

106. Singal AG, Reddy S, Radadiya Aka Patel H, et al. Multicenter randomized clinical trial of a mailed outreach strategy for hepatocellular carcinoma surveillance. Clin Gastroenterol Hepatol 2022;20(12):2818–25.e1.

Overview of Current Hepatocellular Carcinoma Staging Systems

Is There an Optimal System?

Mariana Chavez-Villa, MD[a],
Ismael Domínguez-Rosado, MD, MSc[b],*

KEYWORDS

- Hepatocellular carcinoma • Staging systems • Barcelona • AJCC • LI-RADS
- mRECIST • Milan • UCSF

KEY POINTS

- There are multiple staging systems for hepatocellular carcinoma (HCC) that are classified as clinical, pathologic, or radiologic depending on the reason for which they were developed.
- The heterogeneity of patients with HCC, owing to the diversity of treatments and prognosis at the different stages, as well as underlying liver disease, makes it challenging to create a single, optimal staging system.
- Although these models are of great value for standardization and subsequent management and prognosis, individualized and multidisciplinary assessment remains critical for decision making.

INTRODUCTION

There are currently multiple systems for staging patients with hepatocellular carcinoma (HCC), which are used to determine their prognosis and, in some cases, to guide the treatment. Since their creation and clinical use, they have continuously changed to align with the development and improvement of diagnostic tools and new therapeutic alternatives. However, there is yet to be a universally accepted staging system for HCC. On the contrary, a wide variety are used in different geographic areas and in

[a] Department of Surgery, Division of Transplantation, University of Rochester Medical Center, 601 Elmwood Avenue, Rochester, NY 14642, USA; [b] Department of Surgery, Instituto Nacional de Ciencias Médicas y Nutrición Salvador Zubirán, Vasco de Quiroga 15 Tlalpan, Sección XVI, Mexico City C.P. 14000, Mexico
* Corresponding author.
E-mail address: ismaeldominguez83@gmail.com
Twitter: @DraMarianaCh (M.C.-V.); @domcai777 (I.D.-R.)

Surg Oncol Clin N Am 33 (2024) 29–41
https://doi.org/10.1016/j.soc.2023.06.010
1055-3207/24/© 2023 Elsevier Inc. All rights reserved.
surgonc.theclinics.com

diverse scenarios. These can be classified into clinic, pathologic, radiologic, or transplant staging systems, depending on the reason for which they were developed. Overall, some of the most commonly used are Okuda,[1] Cancer of the Liver Italian Program (CLIP),[2] Japan Integrated System (JIS) score,[3] Barcelona Clinic Liver Cancer (BCLC) system,[4] Hong Kong Liver Cancer (HKLC) staging system,[5] American Joint Committee on Cancer (AJCC),[6] Liver Reporting and Data System (LI-RADS),[7] modified Response Evaluation Criteria in Solid Tumors (mRECIST),[8] Milan Criteria,[9] and the University of California San Francisco (UCSF)[10] criteria, respectively.

Although these staging systems propose therapeutic algorithms, clinical decision making must be individualized by multidisciplinary teams responsible for the integration of all available data on each patient. Furthermore, other factors, independent of tumor burden, must be taken into account when evaluating and staging patients. Some of these are underlying liver disease or comorbidities, which may ultimately be as relevant to decision making as tumor burden.

This review aims to describe the most relevant staging systems for HCC in clinical practice and discuss their strengths, limitations, and current controversies.

STAGING SYSTEMS
Clinicopathologic

The Barcelona clinic liver cancer
The BCLC staging system is the most widely used and has been validated in multiple populations. It establishes a prognosis following the 5 stages that are linked to a first-treatment recommendation.[11] It was initially published in 1999 and has been updated since then. The most recent update dates from 2022, following the increase in the armamentarium for treating HCC in recent years. Although substantial changes were made, there are still some pitfalls owing to lack of scientific evidence that preclude the incorporation of some concepts into the algorithm.[4]

Since its inception, it has determined the cancer stage and prognosis based on tumor burden, liver disease severity, and patient performance status. According to the available scientific evidence, the expected outcome is expressed in median survival for each of the 5 tumor stages. The tumor stages are very early stage (BCLC 0), early stage (BCLC A), intermediate stage (BCLC B), advanced stage (BCLC C), and terminal stage (BCLC D). The very early stage includes patients with a solitary less than 2 cm lesion, and the early stage comprises a single lesion or up to 3 nodules less than 3 cm, both with preserved liver function and good performance status. Intermediate-stage patients have large, multinodular tumors without vascular invasion or extrahepatic disease. Patients with advanced stage include tumors with vascular invasion, extrahepatic disease, and intermediate performance status (Eastern Cooperative Oncology Group Performance Status [ECOG-PS] grades 1 to 2). Finally, the terminal stage includes patients with liver dysfunction and bad performance status (ECOG >2). In its original version, potentially curative treatments, such as resection, transplantation, or ablation, were suggested for patients with BCLC 0 and A; patients within BCLC B could be candidates for transarterial chemoembolization (TACE) if the liver function was preserved; patients within BCLC C were advised to undergo systemic treatment with sorafenib; and patients within BCLC D were candidates for supportive treatment only because of their poor prognosis.[12]

After several years of operating in this manner, some limitations that required improvement were recognized. First, it provided limited information on the increasingly important role of liver transplantation (LT) in the treatment of HCC. Second, it did not take into account treatments such as transarterial radioembolization (TARE), which was being increasingly used. Finally, its algorithm did not consider relevant tumor markers, such as alpha-fetoprotein (AFP). In its updated version, although the 5 tumor stages have not changed and continue to be assessed by tumor burden, liver function, and physical status, the way these are measured has undergone a substantial change. Now, AFP concentration is considered independent of the tumor burden. Likewise, liver function should be assessed beyond the conventional Child-Pugh score. Other parameters, like model of end-stage liver disease (MELD) score and albumin-bilirubin (ALBI) score, are suggested to assess and stratify the severity of liver dysfunction. Regarding performance status, in addition to the ECOG scale, other factors, such as age, comorbidities, nutritional status, frailty, socioeconomic status, and support network, should be considered at the time of decision making by a multidisciplinary team. All these factors have relevance in deciding the best treatment option for each patient and lead us to the concept of Treatment Stage Migration, which applies when a specific patient profile induces a modification of the recommendation to the option that would be considered a priority for a more advanced stage.

Another incorporation to the algorithm is patient characterization to decide on an individualized treatment approach (**Fig. 1**). In the case of patients within BCLC 0 and A, the presence or absence of portal hypertension needs to be defined to decide between ablation, resection, or transplantation. Furthermore, individualized clinical decision making in BCLC 0 will determine the best alternative treatment in patients that are not candidates for ablation. In this scenario, TARE has been incorporated as an alternative. Moreover, in intermediate stage patients, in whom previously only TACE was suggested, after patient characterization according to tumor burden and liver function, they may now be candidates for transplantation, TACE, or systemic

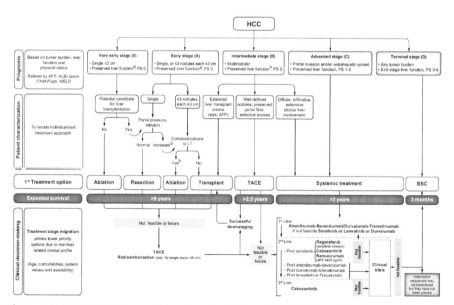

Fig. 1. BCLC staging system and treatments strategy in 2022. [a]Except for those with tumor burden acceptable for transplant. [b]Resection may be considered for single peripheral HCC with adequate remnant liver volume. (*Data from* Reig M, Forner A, Rimola J, et al. BCLC strategy for prognosis prediction and treatment recommendation: The 2022 update. *Journal of Hepatology.* 2022;76(3):681-693.)

therapy. Finally, the patient characterization is also a determinant in BCLC C stages as patients must have preserved liver function and absence of high-bleeding risk to be eligible for treatment with the combination of atezolizumab with bevacizumab, which is currently the treatment of choice.

Regarding LT, although there is more room for it in the 2022 edition, including some of the BCLC B patients as potential candidates with extended criteria, several issues still need to be delineated. As well, although the role of downstaging is briefly mentioned, the inclusion criteria for transplantation after downstaging need to be better specified. Finally, another debated matter is untreatable progression, in which the heterogeneity of progression patterns and individual patient characteristics require a multidisciplinary team discussion to identify the best treatment option. In this regard, a model that stratifies patients according to progression pattern is suggested. Although it does not serve to guide treatment, its value is given by a prognostic stratification.

Okuda

This staging system, developed in Tokyo in 1985, was one of the first to be implemented, following the evaluation of 850 patients with HCC. Patients were classified into three stages according to tumor size, presence or absence of ascites, bilirubin, and serum albumin (**Table 1**). Thus, it assesses tumor burden (tumor size), liver functional reserve (bilirubin, serum albumin), and secondarily, the presence of cirrhosis and portal hypertension (ascites). After the analysis of these 3 groups, the relation between survival and treatment was established, being evident that the prognosis was related to disease staging.[1] This classification was widely used in the decade following its publication; however, it is now considered outdated because it fails to consider several factors (unifocal or multifocal tumors, vascular invasion, or tumors <2 cm in diameter) that are important for prognosis. Thus, with the increasing refinement of diagnostic tools, the system has been insufficient to classify patients in early stages.

American Joint Commission on Cancer

AJCC was one of the most widely used, but, since 2018, there have been relevant changes in this staging system, particularly in the T category, where tumor size is the main prognostic factor in solitary tumors less than 2 cm.[6,13]

1. Solitary lesions ≤2 cm are considered T1a, irrespective of microvascular invasion, whereas in the 7th edition, it was determined if it was a T1 or T2.
2. Solitary lesions greater than 2 cm without vascular invasion are considered T1b.
3. Large lesions greater than 2 cm with vascular invasion or multifocal, none greater than 5 cm, are still considered T2.
4. T3a (multifocal >5 cm) is now T3 on the 8th edition, and T3b (involvement of a primary portal or venous branch) and T4 (direct invasion to adjacent organs) merged into a single T4 category.

Table 1
Okuda staging system

Stage	Tumor Size >50% (+)	(−)	Ascites (+)	(−)	Albumin <3 g/dL (+)	(−)	Bilirubin >3 mg/dL (+)	(−)
I	(−)		(−)		(−)		(−)	
II	1 or 2 (+)							
III	3 or 4 (+)							

The new edition has the advantage of stratifying earlier HCC, in which more treatment options are now available. However, although its external validation shows it to be as adequate as the 7th edition to stage surgically treated patients, some disadvantages might need to be addressed in the following editions:

1. The T2 category includes solitary greater than 2 cm lesions and multifocal less than 5 cm in the same category. On the validation analysis by Kamarajah and colleagues,[14,15] solitary lesions outperformed multifocal in terms of overall survival (OS) in both the surgical cohort (45 vs 39 months) and LT (52 vs 38 months).
2. Although microvascular invasion has no predictive value in the T1 category, on T2 multifocal tumors, median survival is 42 months with microvascular invasion versus 50 months without it. Furthermore, the association between vascular invasion and worse survival persists after stratifying by nodal disease or surgical treatment (resection or transplant).[14,15]

Hong Kong Liver Cancer staging system
Applicability of BCLC staging on Asian patients has been questioned, as the source of validation from BCLC comes from patients with Hepatitis C virus (HCV). Being that Hepatitis B virus (HBV) is more frequent in Asian countries and having less liver dysfunction than HCV, a staging system considering these differences was proposed. The HKLC staging system comprises 4 prognostic factors with relevant roles on the treatment of HCC. These are as follows: liver tumor status, ECOG, Child-Pugh grade, and extrahepatic vascular invasion/metastasis. Liver tumor status comprises the size of the largest tumor, number of tumor nodules, and the presence of intrahepatic vascular invasion. Extrahepatic vascular invasion includes the main portal and inferior vena cava invasion.

The development of this system included 3856 patients treated from 1995 to 2008 at the Queen Mary Hospital in Hong Kong; the majority (79.9%) were hepatitis B carriers. HKLC concordance index was 0.739 versus 0.703 compared with BCLC, having better stratification of intermediate and advanced HCC stages.[5] A comparison between HLKC and AJCC showed better accuracy to differentiate T stages in terms of disease-free survival (DFS) and OS when compared with the AJCC staging system (**Table 2**). This comparison should be taken with care, as all patients underwent surgical treatment, so liver function was preserved, and the population was predominantly HBV positive. It cannot be generalizable to nonsurgical patients or patients with impaired liver function.[16]

Cancer of the Liver Italian Program
This score was derived from 435 patients with HCC treated from 1990 to 1992. It includes Child-Pugh score, tumor morphology, AFP, and portal vein thrombosis[2] (**Table 3**). External validation studies have found that CLIP adequately discriminates against patients with advanced from no advanced HCC, even outperforming AJCC and Okuda staging. Some criticisms are the lack of generalization in Asian patients, with a very broad criteria regarding tumor morphology. In addition, it fails to discriminate prognosis among advanced HCC with CLIP 4 to 6 stages.

Imaging

The following 2 systems were described to standardize the interpretation of diagnostic studies as well as the treatment response (TR). The difference between LI-RADS and mRECIST for HCC is that mRECIST is intended to assess TR at the patient level, and LI-RADS evaluates it on a lesion-by-lesion basis.

Table 2
Descriptions of the different T stages in Hong Kong Liver Cancer staging system and American Joint Committee on Cancer 8th edition

T Stage	HKLC Staging System	AJCC 8th Edition
T1	Single tumor ≤5.0 cm, no microvascular invasion	
T1a		Solitary tumor ≤2 cm with/without vascular invasion
T1b		Solitary tumor >2 cm, no vascular invasion
T2	Single tumor >5.0 cm, no microvascular invasion Or single tumor ≤5.0 cm plus microvascular invasion Or unilobar multiple tumors, no microvascular invasion	Solitary tumor >2 cm plus vascular invasion Or multiple tumors ≤5 cm
T3	Single tumor >5.0 cm plus microvascular invasion	Multiple tumors and >5 cm
T4	Unilobar multiple tumors plus microvascular invasion Or bilobar tumors Or tumor invasion of a branch of the portal or hepatic vein Or tumor invasion of an adjacent organ except the gallbladder or rupture into the peritoneal cavity	Tumor(s) involving a major branch of the portal or hepatic vein with direct invasion of adjacent organ(s) (including the diaphragm) other than the gallbladder or with perforation of visceral peritoneum

Adapted from She WH, Chan ACY, Ma kW, et al. Critical appraisal of TNM versus HKU staging system for postoperative prognostic evaluation of hepatocellular carcinoma. *Ann Transl Med.* 2021;9(11):919-919.

Liver reporting and data system

In order to avoid ambiguities and inconsistencies in the diagnosis of HCC, this system was created with the support of the American College of Radiology with the intention of standardizing the interpretation and reporting of lesions in patients at risk of HCC.[7,17] Initial versions of LI-RADS focused on classifying patients with computed tomography (CT) and MRI; however, recent versions have incorporated the use of ultrasound (US) and contrast-enhanced ultrasound. Like other systems, since the beginning of its use in 2011, it has been updated in accordance with scientific evidence, until its last update in 2018. Over the years, it has become very popular and is now widely used. It has been translated into 14 different languages and has achieved international standardization. Moreover, in 2017, the LI-RADS US and CT/

Table 3
The Cancer of the Liver Italian Program scoring system

	Scores		
Variables	0	1	2
Child-Pugh	A	B	C
Tumor morphology	Uninodular and extension <50%	Multinodular and extension <50%	Massive or extension >50%
AFP (ng/dL)	<400	>400	
Portal vein thrombosis	No	Yes	

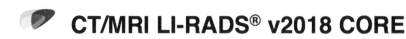

CT/MRI LI-RADS® v2018 CORE

Untreated observation without pathologic proof in <u>patient at high risk for HCC</u>

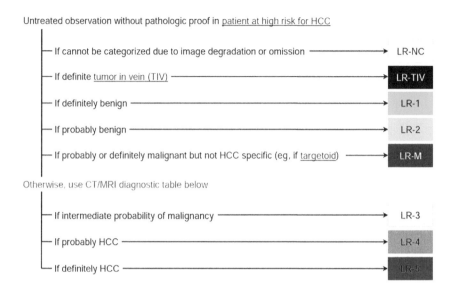

If cannot be categorized due to image degradation or omission	LR-NC
If definite <u>tumor in vein (TIV)</u>	LR-TIV
If definitely benign	LR-1
If probably benign	LR-2
If probably or definitely malignant but not HCC specific (eg, if <u>targetoid</u>)	LR-M

Otherwise, use CT/MRI diagnostic table below

If intermediate probability of malignancy	LR-3
If probably HCC	LR-4
If definitely HCC	LR-5

CT/MRI Diagnostic Table

Arterial phase hyperenhancement (APHE)		No APHE		Nonrim APHE		
Observation size (mm)		< 20	≥ 20	< 10	10-19	≥ 20
Count additional major features:	None	LR-3	LR-3	LR-3	LR-3	LR-4
• Enhancing "capsule" • Nonperipheral "washout"	One	LR-3	LR-4	LR-4	LR-4 / LR-5	LR-5
• Threshold growth	≥ Two	LR-4	LR-4	LR-4	LR-5	LR-5

 Observations in this cell are categorized based on one additional major feature:
 • LR-4 – if enhancing "capsule"
 • LR-5 – if nonperipheral "washout" **OR** threshold growth

Fig. 2. LI-RADS 2018 CT/MRI algorithm. (*Data from* Liver Reporting & Data System | American College of Radiology. Consulted ULR: https://www.acr.org/Clinical-Resources/Reporting-and-Data-Systems/LI-RADS.)

MRI algorithms were incorporated into the American Association for the Study of Liver Diseases (AASLD) guidelines to promote a unified approach to the diagnosis, staging, and treatment of HCC.[18]

CT or MRI for diagnosis and staging is used in patients with high pretest probability. In these, LI-RADS assigns the relative probability that the lesion evaluated is benign, HCC, or other malignancy, assigning them from LR-1 to LR-5 (**Fig. 2**). Finally, LT-tumor in vein (TIV) defines patients with macrovascular invasion. Depending on the classification, patients may or may not require further diagnostic workup. Ultimately, the staging of patients will be determined by the number and size of lesions that are LR-5 and the presence or absence of LR-TIV. Regarding TR, LI-RADS classifies

Treatment Response Algorithm

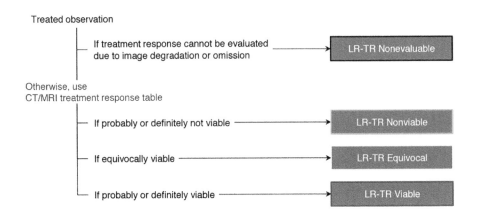

CT/MRI Treatment Response Table

Response Category	Criteria
LR-TR Nonviable	• No lesional enhancement **OR** • Treatment-specific expected enhancement pattern
LR-TR Equivocal	Enhancement atypical for treatment-specific expected enhancement pattern and not meeting criteria for probably or definitely viable
LR-TR Viable	Nodular, masslike, or thick irregular tissue in or along the treated lesion with any of the following: • Arterial phase hyperenhancement **OR** • Washout appearance **OR** • Enhancement similar to pretreatment

Fig. 3. LI-RADS 2017 CT/MRI TR algorithm. BSC, best supportive care; LR-TR, LIRADS treatment response. (*Data from* Liver Reporting & Data System | American College of Radiology. Consulted ULR: https://www.acr.org/Clinical-Resources/Reporting-and-Data-Systems/LI-RADS.)

lesions according to their viability after treatment, dividing them into LR-TR Nonviable, LT-TR Equivocal, or LR-TR Viable (**Fig. 3**).

Whereas this classification has been very useful in standardizing the interpretation of lesions, as well as for the creation of diagnostic and surveillance algorithms, it also has certain limitations. In relation to surveillance and diagnosis, it is only used for patients with cirrhosis or without cirrhosis but with chronic HBV infection, and an increased risk of HCC; however, its usefulness is uncertain in patients with other liver diseases, such as HCV infection and nonalcoholic fatty liver disease, or with precirrhotic patients. On the other hand, the TR classification system is very recent and will require further evaluation and validation.

Modified response evaluation criteria in solid tumors

Developed in 2010, mRECIST was created to address 2 drawbacks of standard RECIST in the context of HCC.[8] First, the lack of tumor shrinkage with effective therapies; and second, the coexistence of cancer and cirrhosis. In this sense, the concept of "viable tumor" was added in order to enable the detection of objective response in patients with no major changes in tumor diameter but substantial intratumoral necrosis secondary to treatment; as well as the addition of factors related to cirrhosis like assessment of lymph nodes, ascites, portal vein thrombosis, and new hepatic nodules. Since then, mRECIST has helped to standardize concepts such as progression-free survival, time-to-progression, and objective response rate, which are used as surrogate endpoints in cancer trials. Consequently, it has been used in clinical research and in major II and III HCC trials.[19] For this reason, the use of RECIST or mRECIST is advocated by European Association of the Study of the Liver–European Organization for Research and Treatment of Cancer, European Society of Medical Oncology, AASLD, and more recently by Korean clinical guidelines to the enrollment of patients with early, intermediate, or advanced HCC.[18,20–24]

Transplant Staging

From an oncologic perspective, LT is considered the best treatment option for selected patients with HCC. On the one hand, it removes potential multifocal tumors not recognized by imaging studies, and on the other hand, it eliminates the possibility of a future HCC in the context of an underlying liver disease. Nonetheless, there is no perfect staging system or eligibility criteria for this either, and multiple criteria have been described, for instance, Milan,[9] UCSF,[10] and Up-to-7.[25] Each has its benefits and drawbacks; however, it should be noted that the more conservative the criteria, the better the overall cancer-related and disease-free survival. Unfortunately, this will be at the cost of substantially reducing the number of patients who could be candidates. Moreover, one aspect that cannot be overlooked is the limited access to transplantation owing to the scarcity of organs and, therefore, the difficulty of their allocation.

It was not until 1996, when Mazzaferro and colleagues[9] demonstrated easily applicable criteria, that LT for HCC became mainstream, demonstrating an excellent 4-year overall and recurrence-free survival rates of 85% and 92%, respectively. After their validation in multiple centers, these have become the worldwide standard for determining eligibility for LT, to the extent that the United Network for Organ Sharing has adopted them as a tool for prioritizing patients on the waiting list. In addition, these were also incorporated into the TNM and BCLC staging systems for HCC. However, although these offer the best survival rates for patients who meet the criteria (single tumor ≤5 cm, or ≤3 tumors each ≤3 cm, and no macrovascular invasion), they are very stringent, thus excluding a large group of patients who could also benefit from LT. As such, the possibility of extending the criteria was soon considered, and in 2001, the group of Yao,[10] at UCSF, showed that patients with a single tumor ≤6.5 cm, or ≤3 nodules with the largest lesion ≤4.5 cm and a total tumor diameter ≤8 cm, had a 1- and 5-year survival rates of 90% and 75%, respectively, compared with a 1-year survival of 50% for patients with tumors exceeding these limits. Based on these observations, it was considered that the criteria could be safely extended without compromising patient survival, and the UCSF criteria were developed. Subsequently, in 2008, the Metroticket Investigator Study Group showed that patients with 7 as the sum of the size of the largest tumor and the number of tumors achieved a 5-year OS of 71.2%, suggesting that more patients could be candidates for LT using the Up-to-seven criteria, with a more precise estimation of survival contouring individual tumor characteristics[25] (**Table 4**).

Name	Transplant Criteria	Overall Survival
Milan	Single tumor ≤5 cm or ≤3 tumors each ≤3 cm, and no macrovascular invasion	4-y OS of 85%
UCSF	Single tumor ≤6.5 cm, or ≤3 nodules with the largest lesion ≤4.5 cm and a total tumor diameter ≤8 cm	5-y OS of 75%
Up-to-7	Seven as the sum of the size of the largest tumor (cm) and the number of tumors	5-y OS of 71%

Table 4
Transplant criteria and survival rates

Improvements in preoperative imaging studies, as well as advances in therapeutic alternatives, including neoadjuvant treatment with immunotherapy and locoregional therapies (LRT), have revolutionized the management of patients with HCC. Such is the case for downstaging, which has served as a surrogate for tumor biology and has allowed a select group of patients with favorable tumor biology to be selected as LT candidates, even if they were initially outside the criteria. The goal is to achieve a similar OS after LT compared with patients who met LT criteria without downstaging. Consequently, standardization of management and TR protocols has been attempted; however, definitions of response to downstaging still need to be evaluated.[26] Despite this, patients with HCC downstaged to Milan criteria undergo LT in many centers, supported by retrospective studies with a moderate level of evidence.[20,21,23] In that sense, the group of Mazzaferro[27] published the first prospective randomized multicenter trial showing that LT after downstaging resulted in improved OS and DFS compared with continuation with nontransplant therapy, with a 5-year OS of 77.5% in the LT group versus 31.2% in the control group. These findings suggest that downstaging and tumor response following downstaging should be included in the proposed extended HCC transplant criteria. Moreover, this may also contribute to prioritizing patients with partial or complete tumor response to LRT. These results should be taken with caution, as the study recruitment was stopped early owing to the restriction to recruit patients in the context of graft allocation policy; however, it is a further step toward optimization of LT in HCC beyond conventional criteria.

DISCUSSION

Since 1985 when Okuda introduced the first staging system for HCC, multiple models have been proposed and incorporated into clinical practice for screening, surveillance, diagnosis, staging, treatment, TR, and prognosis. Despite this, almost 4 decades later, there is not a perfect or comprehensive staging system. The wide clinical and biological heterogeneity in all its stages, as well as its complex management and coexistence with chronic liver diseases make HCC a challenge for universal standardization. Differences in the source of validation data sets make generalization difficult, and it is most likely that different staging systems will continue to be used for distinct populations. Furthermore, in the era of neoadjuvant treatment, the downstaging process remains very heterogeneous, as do the definitions of successful downstaging. Consequently, there are no staging systems that can guide treatment or estimate long-term prognosis. Moreover, the long-term prognostic significance of complete radiologic or pathologic response and how this will guide treatment is still not known.

Thus, 2 of the main challenges for staging systems today are as follows: (1) to incorporate the changes in diagnostic and therapeutic interventions that occur over time, as they are constantly and rapidly changing; and (2) to determine how the newly available medical treatment for advanced disease affects downstaging, thereby affecting subsequent decision making. Ultimately, despite all these ongoing changes, what we cannot fail to consider and highlight is the central role of a multidisciplinary approach to decision making, focused on the particularities of each patient.

SUMMARY

Over the last 4 decades, multiple HCC staging systems have been developed, with the aim of guiding treatment and defining prognosis. Because of the heterogeneity of HCC, as well as rapid advances in diagnostic and therapeutic tools, staging algorithms and eligibility criteria are currently more complex. Recent advances in neoadjuvant therapy, downstaging, and adjuvant therapy have come to change some paradigms; however, this has been accompanied by new questions that need to be answered. To date, there is no perfect or universal staging system; however, as evidence advances, models will continue to be refined. Even so, individualized decision making and a multidisciplinary approach will continue to play a key role.

CLINICS CARE POINTS

- The latest update of Barcelona staging system in 2022 incorporates new concepts in line with recent advances in the armamentarium for treating hepatocellular carcinoma and emphasizes an individualized therapeutic approach.
- The American Joint Committee on Cancer 8th edition has the ability to stratify earlier hepatocellular carcinomas, which is an advantage now that more treatment options are available; however, it has some shortcomings in stratifying T2 tumors that will need to be further addressed.
- The Liver Reporting and Data System and modified Response Evaluation Criteria in Solid Tumors have succeeded in standardizing the interpretation for hepatocellular carcinoma diagnosis as well as for treatment response; however, further efforts are needed to standardize treatment response in the downstaging setting.
- With or without extended criteria, or with or without downstaging, the ultimate goal of liver transplantation models will remain careful patient selection to minimize recurrence and maximize long-term outcomes.

DISCLOSURE

The authors have nothing to disclose.

REFERENCES

1. Okuda K, Ohtsuki T, Obata H, et al. Natural history of hepatocellular carcinoma and prognosis in relation to treatment. Study of 850 patients. Cancer 1985; 56(4):918–28.
2. A new prognostic system for hepatocellular carcinoma: a retrospective study of 435 patients: the Cancer of the Liver Italian Program (CLIP) investigators. Hepatology 1998;28(3):751–5.
3. Kudo M, Chung H, Osaki Y. Prognostic staging system for hepatocellular carcinoma (CLIP score): its value and limitations, and a proposal for a new staging

system, the Japan Integrated Staging Score (JIS score). J Gastroenterol 2003; 38(3):207–15.

4. Reig M, Forner A, Rimola J, et al. BCLC strategy for prognosis prediction and treatment recommendation: The 2022 update. J Hepatol 2022;76(3):681–93.

5. Yau T, Tang VYF, Yao TJ, et al. Development of Hong Kong Liver Cancer staging system with treatment stratification for patients with hepatocellular carcinoma. Gastroenterology 2014;146(7):1691–700.e3.

6. Amin MB, American Joint Committee on Cancer, American Cancer Society, eds AJCC Cancer Staging Manual. Eight edition/editor-in-chief, Mahul B. Amin, MD, FCAP; editors, Stephen B. Edge, MD, FACS (and 16 others); Donna M. Gress, RHIT, CTR-Technical editor ; Laura R. Meyer, CAPM-Managing editor. American Joint Committee on Cancer, Springer; 2017.

7. Liver Reporting & Data System | American College of Radiology. https://www.acr.org/Clinical-Resources/Reporting-and-Data-Systems/LI-RADS. Accessed April 4, 2023.

8. Lencioni R, Llovet JM. Modified RECIST (mRECIST) assessment for hepatocellular carcinoma. Semin Liver Dis 2010;30(1):52–60.

9. Mazzaferro V, Regalia E, Doci R, et al. Liver transplantation for the treatment of small hepatocellular carcinomas in patients with cirrhosis. N Engl J Med 1996; 334(11):693–9.

10. Yao F. Liver transplantation for hepatocellular carcinoma: Expansion of the tumor size limits does not adversely impact survival. Hepatology 2001;33(6):1394–403.

11. Llovet JM, Brú C, Bruix J. Prognosis of hepatocellular carcinoma: the BCLC staging classification. Semin Liver Dis 1999;19(3):329–38.

12. Bruix J, Reig M, Sherman M. Evidence-Based Diagnosis, Staging, and Treatment of Patients With Hepatocellular Carcinoma. Gastroenterology 2016;150(4): 835–53.

13. Edge SB, Byrd DR, Compton CC, et al, editors. AJCC cancer staging handbook: from the AJCC cancer staging manual. 7th edition. Springer; 2010. p. 191–200.

14. Park S, Choi S, Cho YA, et al. Evaluation of the American Joint Committee on Cancer (AJCC) 8th Edition Staging System for Hepatocellular Carcinoma in 1,008 Patients with Curative Resection. Cancer Res Treat 2020;52(4):1145–52.

15. Kamarajah SK, Frankel TL, Sonnenday C, et al. Critical evaluation of the American Joint Commission on Cancer (AJCC) 8th edition staging system for patients with Hepatocellular Carcinoma (HCC): A Surveillance, Epidemiology, End Results (SEER) analysis. J Surg Oncol 2018;117(4):644–50.

16. She WH, Chan ACY, Ma KW, et al. Critical appraisal of TNM versus HKU staging system for postoperative prognostic evaluation of hepatocellular carcinoma. Ann Transl Med 2021;9(11):919.

17. Tang A, Singal AG, Mitchell DG, et al. Introduction to the Liver Imaging Reporting and Data System for Hepatocellular Carcinoma. Clin Gastroenterol Hepatol 2019; 17(7):1228–38.

18. Heimbach JK, Kulik LM, Finn RS, et al. AASLD guidelines for the treatment of hepatocellular carcinoma. Hepatology 2018;67(1):358–80.

19. Llovet JM, Lencioni R. mRECIST for HCC: Performance and novel refinements. J Hepatol 2020;72(2):288–306.

20. European Association for the Study of the Liver. Electronic address: easloffice@easloffice.eu, European Association for the Study of the Liver. EASL Clinical Practice Guidelines: Management of hepatocellular carcinoma. J Hepatol 2018; 69(1):182–236.

21. Marrero JA, Kulik LM, Sirlin CB, et al. Diagnosis, Staging, and Management of Hepatocellular Carcinoma: 2018 Practice Guidance by the American Association for the Study of Liver Diseases. Hepatology 2018;68(2):723–50.
22. Vogel A, Cervantes A, Chau I, et al. Hepatocellular carcinoma: ESMO Clinical Practice Guidelines for diagnosis, treatment and follow-up. Ann Oncol 2019; 30(5):871–3.
23. European Association For The Study Of The Liver, European Organisation For Research And Treatment Of Cancer. EASL-EORTC clinical practice guidelines: management of hepatocellular carcinoma. J Hepatol 2012;56(4):908–43.
24. Liver Cancer Association Korean, National Cancer Center. 2018 Korean Liver Cancer Association-National Cancer Center Korea Practice Guidelines for the Management of Hepatocellular Carcinoma. Gut Liver 2019;13(3):227–99.
25. Mazzaferro V, Llovet JM, Miceli R, et al. Predicting survival after liver transplantation in patients with hepatocellular carcinoma beyond the Milan criteria: a retrospective, exploratory analysis. Lancet Oncol 2009;10(1):35–43.
26. Yao FY, Fidelman N. Reassessing the boundaries of liver transplantation for hepatocellular carcinoma: Where do we stand with tumor down-staging? Hepatology 2016;63(3):1014–25.
27. Mazzaferro V, Citterio D, Bhoori S, et al. Liver transplantation in hepatocellular carcinoma after tumour downstaging (XXL): a randomised, controlled, phase 2b/3 trial. Lancet Oncol 2020;21(7):947–56.

Controversies of Direct-Acting Antivirals in Hepatocellular Carcinoma

Ifrah Fatima, MD[a], Neehar D. Parikh, MD, MSc[b],
Alisa Likhitsup, MD, MPH[b],*

KEYWORDS

- Hepatocellular carcinoma • Hepatitis C virus infection • Direct-acting antivirals

KEY POINTS

- Direct-acting antivirals (DAAs) are highly effective in achieving sustained virological response (SVR) and standard of care for chronic hepatitis C treatment.
- Achieving SVR following hepatitis C treatment has been associated with improvements in liver function, liver fibrosis, liver-related mortality, and transplant-free survival.
- The risk of incident hepatocellular carcinoma (HCC) occurrence was not independently associated with DAAs exposure but rather individual risks including older age, sex, diabetes, hepatitis B coinfection, liver fibrosis, advanced liver disease (Child–Pugh-B/C), and elevated alpha-fetoprotein levels.
- The risk of recurrent HCC after complete response was associated with diabetes, tumor burden (size ≥ 2 cm, multi-focality), prior history of recurrence, palliative intention treatment for HCC, advanced tumor burden, and a short time interval between HCC complete response and DAAs initiation.
- While previous expert opinions have suggested delaying DAAs initiation for at least 4 to 6 months after HCC complete response to allow adequate time for immune surveillance, recent data suggest that earlier treatment in patients with active HCC may allow for better tolerance of HCC therapies and preservation of liver function.

BACKGROUND

Approximately 2.4 million people are affected with chronic hepatitis C virus (HCV) infection in the United States.[1] HCV infection is the leading cause of hepatocellular carcinoma (HCC) and accounts for approximately 25% to 34% of all HCC cases worldwide.[2,3] Direct-acting antivirals (DAAs) treatment has revolutionized the management and treatment of chronic HCV infection. Unlike older HCV treatments that

[a] University of Missouri-Kansas City, 2301 Holmes Street, Kansas City, MO 64108, USA;
[b] University of Michigan, 3912 Taubman Center, 1500 East Medical Center Drive, Ann Arbor, MI 48109, USA
* Corresponding author.
E-mail address: allikhit@med.umich.edu

Surg Oncol Clin N Am 33 (2024) 43–58
https://doi.org/10.1016/j.soc.2023.06.007
1055-3207/24/© 2023 Elsevier Inc. All rights reserved.

surgonc.theclinics.com

relied on interferon and ribavirin, which had limited efficacy and significant side effects, DAAs specifically target key viral enzymes and proteins to block viral replication. DAAs are highly effective in achieving sustained virologic response (SVR) rate more than 95% and several publications have reported achieving SVR following DAAs treatment significantly improved liver dysfunction, portal hypertension, liver fibrosis (regression), as well as liver-related mortality, and transplant-free survival.[4–10] However, soon after the introduction of DAAs, several studies raised concerns about increases in the HCC incidence or recurrence rate following DAAs therapy.[11] In this article, we reviewed current evidence regarding the controversies of HCC incidence and recurrence following DAAs therapy and the most updated practice recommendations for HCC screening or surveillance among HCV populations that received DAA treatment.

DAAs ARE THE STANDARD TREATMENT FOR HCV INFECTION

In 2011, the first DAA approved by the United States Food and Drug Administration (FDA) was boceprevir, followed shortly by telaprevir. Since then, many other DAAs have been approved for the treatment of HCV, including sofosbuvir, daclatasvir, ledipasvir, and others. SVR is defined as undetectable HCV RNA in the blood 12 weeks after the end of treatment, and it is considered a cure for HCV infection. DAA therapy targets vital HCV RNA replication proteins. Combination of *non-structural protein 5B* (NS5B) RNA polymerase inhibitor with *non-structural protein 5A* (NS5A) inhibitor or non-structural protein 3/4A (NS3/4A) protease inhibitor is highly effective in achieving greater than 95% SVR rate.[4] The drug profile is considered safe and well-tolerated with minimal side effects. DAAs are now the first line of treatment for all HCV infections in all populations.[10]

HCV INFECTION AND RISK OF HCC

Hepatitis C is an RNA virus from the *Flaviridae* group that primarily affects hepatocytes. Only about a quarter of patients can eliminate HCV from their bodies. The necroinflammatory damage, regeneration, and repair lead to tissue fibrosis or cirrhosis.[12] HCC development in patients with HCV usually occurs in the background of established cirrhosis; however, approximately 20% of HCC develops in non-cirrhotic liver. The estimated lifetime incidence of HCC among chronic HCV infections is 1% to 3% over 30 years of infection, and the annual rate of HCC is 2% to 4% once cirrhosis is established.[13]

The risk factors associated with HCC development among chronic HCV infections include the duration and severity of the infection, male sex, hepatitis B virus or human immunodeficiency virus-coinfection, diabetes, obesity, smoking, alcohol consumption, and the degree of liver fibrosis.[13,14]

The mechanisms involved in the development of HCC can be broadly classified into direct, indirect, and bystander mechanisms. Many pathways directly involve in HCV-induced HCC such as β1-catenin accumulation, P53 tumor suppressor gene degradation, Rb gene mutation, receptor tyrosine kinase activation, and telomerase reverse transcriptase activation.[12,15] The sterile inflammation as a result of chronic injury from both viral and non-viral agents leads to cellular stress, increases inflammatory cytokines expressions such as tumor necrosis factor-α, *interleukin-1β*, interleukin-23, and interleukin-6, and are associated with HCC development.[12] It is theorized that HCV infection creates a tumorigenic environment that promotes uninfected hepatocytes transformation similar to other microorganisms exerting a bystander effect like *Fusobacterium* in colorectal cancer and *Helicobacter pylori* in gastric cancer.[16]

DAA TREATMENT AND INCIDENCE OF HCC

Elimination of HCV by attaining SVR has been shown to significantly reduce mortality, decompensation, and risk of HCC. This was seen with interferon (IFN) therapy as well. Early concerns about the incidence of HCC following DAAs treatment were raised by Conti and colleagues and they reported that the incidence rate of HCC was 3.16% following DAAs therapy.[17] This was a retrospective study and lacked a control group. It has been hypothesized that HCC occurrence after DAA therapy may be linked to the cohort of patients who are already at a higher risk of HCC including older and decompensated cirrhosis. Kanwal and colleagues reported in patients who achieved SVR following DAAs treatment were associated with a 76% reduction in risk of HCC when compared with patients who did not achieve SVR.[18] Ioannou and colleagues reported data from a large veterans cohort of HCV patients who received DAAs treatment; the HCC incidence was 0.92% among SVR versus 5.19% among non-SVR with a mean follow-up time of 1.5 years.[19] Since then, numerous other studies have revealed a substantially lower risk of HCC occurrence approximately 1% to 5%, and summarized in **Table 1**.[17–38]

A recent large retrospective study with 92,567 patients (32% cirrhosis) showed a cumulative incidence of HCC following DAAs treatment of 2%, 3.87%, and 5.4% at 1, 2, and 3 years, respectively.[36] Similar results after 5-year follow-up of 1494 patients (23.9% cirrhosis) reported the incidence of HCC 1.1% at 1 year to 5.6% at 5 years.[37] These studies suggest an underlying risk of HCC might linger for years even after attaining SVR. There was also an association seen between the incidence of HCC with the liver fibrosis stage, and compensation level [Child–Turcotte–Pugh (CTP) status].[26,27,31,33–36,38] Overall, the incidence of HCC is approximately 0.2% to 0.8% in non-cirrhotic patients, and 2% to 5% in cirrhotic patients during 2 to 5 years of follow-up after achieved SVR following DAAs.[33,34,36–38]

DAAs TREATMENT AND RECURRENCE OF HCC

In 2016, studies reported a substantial rise in HCC recurrence at 27% to 28% at 3 to 6 months after treatment with DAAs.[17,39] Since then, multiple studies reported a wide range of HCC recurrence rates from 0% to 50%, which are summarized in **Table 2**.[17,28,29,32,39–62]

El Kassas and colleagues reported DAAs increased HCC recurrence with a recurrence rate ratio 3.61 (95% CI 1.84–7.11).[53] However, several other studies demonstrated DAAs decreased HCC recurrence (HR 0.24 and HR 0.35).[46,48] Another study demonstrated HCC cumulative recurrence rate at 1 and 2 years was 21.1% and 29.0% in the DAAs-treated group compared to 30.5% and 61% in the control group.[40] DAAs treatment was associated with improved overall survival (HR 0.39, 95% CI 0.17–0.91).[45] A large retrospective cohort from North America demonstrated SVR following DAAs treatment was associated with a significant reduction in risk of death (HR 0.29, 95% CI 0.18–0.47) but not in non-SVR (HR 0.29, 95% CI 0.55–2.33).[63] When liver transplant patients were evaluated for HCC recurrence, patients who received DAAs prior to transplantation showed a trend toward a higher risk of HCC recurrence when compared to the risk in untreated patients (27.8% vs 9.5%), although it was not statistically insignificant.[64]

In the past 10 years, a few significant meta-analyses have been conducted to assess the risk of HCC recurrence following therapy with DAAs. It remains a hotly contested topic as it explores the answer to the question if patients with a history of HCC should be treated with DAAs or not. The drawback of these meta-analyses included the unavailability of individual data. This places limitations on the analysis of HCC

Table 1
Incidence of HCC following DAA treatment

Author, year	Country	Study Design	Patients (N)	HCC (n)	Mean Follow-up	Incidence Rate
Conti et al,[17] 2016	Italy	Retrospective	285, cirrhosis	9	6 mo	3.16%
Cheung et al,[20] 2016	UK	Prospective	406, decompensated cirrhosis	17	6 mo	4%
Akuta et al,[21] 2016	Japan	Retrospective	958, all stages	14	13 mo	0.74%
Ravi et al,[22] 2017	US	Retrospective	66, cirrhosis	6	6 mo	9%
Calleja et al,[23] 2017	Spain	Retrospective	3233, 46.7% cirrhosis	30	18 mo	0.93%
Kanwal et al,[18] 2017	US	Retrospective	22,500, 29.7% cirrhosis	271	22,963 PY	1.18%, overall 0.9% in SVR 3.45% in non-SVR
Ioannou et al,[19] 2017	US	Retrospective	21,948, 23.8% cirrhosis	445	18 mo	0.92% in SVR 5.19% in non-SVR
Innes et al,[24] 2017	UK	Retrospective	272, cirrhosis	12	475 PY	2.5%
Li et al,[25] 2018	US	Retrospective	5834, 19.9% cirrhosis	50	13 mo	0.86%
Romano et al,[26] 2018	Italy	Prospective	3917, F3-4	55	18 mo	0.46% in F3 1.49% in CTP-A 3.61% in CTP-B
Calvaruso et al,[27] 2018	Italy	Prospective	2249, cirrhosis	78	14 mo	2.1% in CTP-A 7.8% in CTP-B
Masetti et al,[28] 2018	Italy	Prospective	943, cirrhosis	54	17.3 mo	5.7%
Lleo et al,[29] 2019	Italy	Prospective	1766, cirrhosis	50	12 mo	2.4%
Marino et al,[30] 2019	Spain	Retrospective	1123, cirrhosis	72	10 mo	3.73%
Shiha et al,[31] 2020	Egypt	Prospective	2372, advanced fibrosis/cirrhosis	109	24 mo	2.34%, overall 0.66%, advanced fibrosis 2.92%, cirrhosis
Sangiovanni et al,[32] 2020	Italy	Prospective	1161, cirrhosis	48	17 mo	3.1%

Study	Country	Design	N, cirrhosis	Cases	Follow-up	Incidence
Kanwal et al,[33] 2020	US	Retrospective	18,076, 38.4% cirrhosis	544	34.8 mo	Cumulative incidence at 1,2,3 y; 1.1%, 1.9%, 2.8%, overall; 2.2%, 3.8%, 5.6%, cirrhosis
Kumada et al,[34] 2021	Japan	Retrospective	567, 38.1% cirrhosis	18	43.8 mo	Cumulative incidence at 2, 4 y; 0, 4.6%, MRE<4.5 kPa; 0.6%, 14.2%, MRE>4.5 kPa
Tahata et al,[35] 2022	Japan	Retrospective	224, cirrhosis	15	9.5 mo	Cumulative incidence at 1 y; 4.1%, CTP-A; 8.2%, CTP-B; 21.2%, CTP-C
Kramer et al,[36] 2022	US	Retrospective	92,567, 32% cirrhosis	3247	30 mo	Cumulative incidence at 1, 2, 3 y; 2%, 3.8%, 5.4%, cirrhosis; 0.2%, 0.5%, 0.8%, non-cirrhosis
Mawatari et al,[37] 2022	Japan	Prospective	1494, 23.9% cirrhosis	60	47.6 mo	Cumulative Incidence at 1, 2, 3, 4, 5 y; 1.1%, 1.8%, 3.5%, 4.7%, 5.6%
Leal et al,[38] 2023	Brazil	Prospective	1075, all stages	51	40 mo	1.46/100 PY, overall; 2.31/100 PY, F4; 0.45/100 PY, F3; 0.2/100 PY, F2

Abbreviations: CTP, Child–Turcotte–Pugh; kPA, kilopascal; MRE, magnetic resonance elastography; PY, person-year; SVR, sustained virological response.

Table 2
Recurrence of HCC following DAA treatment

Author, year	Country	Study Design	Patients (N)	HCC (n)	Recurrence Rate	HCC to DAA Initiation	Follow-up Duration	Factors Associated
Conti et al,[17] 2016	Italy	Retrospective	59, cirrhosis	17	28.81%	53.7 wk	6 mo	
Reig et al,[39] 2016	Spain	Retrospective	58, cirrhosis	16	27.3%	44.8 wk	8.2 mo	
Rinaldi et al,[40] 2016	Italy	Not reported	15, cirrhosis	1	7.7%, DAA 47%, non DAA	49 wk	3 mo	
ANRS,[41] 2016	France	Prospective	189, 80% cirrhosis	24	12.7%	1.8 y (0.7–4.4)	20.2 mo	
ANRS,[41] 2016	France	Prospective	13, cirrhosis	1	20.5%	Not reported	21.3 mo	
Torres et al,[42] 2016	US	Prospective	8, 88% cirrhosis	0	0	30 mo	12 mo	
Zeng et al,[43] 2016	China	Prospective	10, cirrhosis	0	0	Not reported	15 mo	
Bielen et al,[44] 2017	Belgium	Retrospective	41, 98% cirrhosis	6	15%	52 wk	33 mo	
Cabibbo et al,[45] 2017	Italy	Prospective	143, cirrhosis	24	20.3%	44 wk	8.7 mo	Tumor size >2.5 cm (HR 2.73), prior recurrence (HR 2.22)
Ikeda et al,[46] 2017	Japan	Retrospective	177, cirrhosis	61	34.5%	42.8 wk	20.7 mo	DAA reduced HCC recurrence HR 0.35 Multiple tumors HR 2.18 AFP > 41 mg/L HR 1.75
Nagata et al,[47] 2017	Japan	Retrospective	83, 33% advanced fibrosis(>F3)	22	29%	Not reported	27.6 mo	Post-treatment AFP >5.5 ng/mL (p 0.002), WFA + M2BP > 2.2 COI (p 0.004)

Study	Country	Type			Outcome			Finding
Virlogeux et al,[48] 2017	France	Retrospective	23, cirrhosis	11	47.8% 1.7/100 PY treated 4.2/100 PY untreated	29 wk	35.7 mo	DAAs reduce HCC recurrence HR 0.24 (95% CI 0.1–0.55).
Minami et al,[49] 2017	Japan	Retrospective	27, cirrhosis	8	Cumulative recurrence at 1, 2 y 21.1%, 29.8% DAA 26.3%, 52.9%, IFN 30.5%, 61%, control	23.2 wk	15.6 mo	Multiple tumors (HR 1.33) Tumor size >2 cm (HR 1.46) Pre Rx AFP ≥100 ng/mL (HR 1.41) CTP-A (HR 0.79)
Zavaglia et al,[50] 2017	Italy	Retrospective	31, cirrhosis	1	3.2%	77.2 wk	8 mo	Longer interval between complete HCC treatment and DAA initiation
Kolly et al,[51] 2017	Europe	Retrospective	47	20	42%	48 wk	12 mo	Longer time between HCC treatment and start DAA therapy (HR 0.89)
Huang et al,[52] 2018	US	Retrospective	62, cirrhosis	29	Cumulative incidence at 1 y 47% DAA 49.8% no DAA	33 wk	12 mo	Single HCC treatment (HR 0.20)
El Kassas et al,[53] 2018	Egypt	Prospective	53	20	37.7% DAA 25.4% no DAA	32 wk	16 mo	DAA increase recurrence rate ratio 3.61 (95% CI 1.84–7.11)

(continued on next page)

Table 2
(continued)

Author, year	Country	Study Design	Patients (N)	HCC (n)	Recurrence Rate	HCC to DAA Initiation	Follow-up Duration	Factors Associated
Masetti et al,[28] 2018	Italy	Not reported	102, cirrhosis	41	39%	Not reported	17.3 mo	Previous HCC (OR 10.76, 5.9–19.3) No reduction of AFP (OR 2.98, 1.6–5.54)
Lleo et al,[29] 2019	Italy	Prospective	161, cirrhosis	38	23%	HCC diagnosis to DAA initiation ≥12 mo vs <12 mo (HR 2.09, 0.94–4.61, $P = .07$)	12 mo	Lack of SVR (HR 5.21, 1.75–15.5) AFP ≥10 ng/dL (HR 6.19, 1.81–21.2)
Degasperi et al,[54] 2019	Italy	Retrospective	60, cirrhosis	20	33%	48 wk	25 mo	Diabetes (HR 4.12, 1.55–10.93)
Cabibbo et al,[55] 2019	Italy	Prospective	102, cirrhosis	28	27.5%	8 wk	21.4 mo	DAA improved overall survival (HR 0.39, 0.17–0.91) and hepatic decompensation (HR 0.32, 0.13–0.84)
Lin et al,[56] 2020	Taiwan	Retrospective	60, cirrhosis	22	37.1% DAA vs 45.8% no DAA Recurrence-free survival at 1, 2, 3 y 85%, 73%, 40.7% DAA 83%, 78%, 61% no DAA ($P = .278$)	Not reported	20 mo	

Study	Country	Type	N, cirrhosis	Recurrence n	Recurrence %	Duration	Follow-up	Risk factors
Kuo et al,[57] 2020	Taiwan	Retrospective	112, cirrhosis	22	26.8% DAA vs 56.8% IFN vs 58.8% untreated	Up to 122 wk	8–17 mo	
Sangiovanni et al,[32] 2020	Italy	Prospective	124, cirrhosis	40	32%	76 wk	16 mo	Alcohol abuse HR 2.10 (1.08–4.09 history of recurrent HR 2.87(1.35–6.39)
Chi et al,[58] 202	Taiwan	Prospective	107, 76% cirrhosis	33	30.8%	32 wk	26.9 mo	No SVR status HR 2.16 1.15–4.07
Ahn et al,[59] 2021	Korea	Retrospective	100, cirrhosis	37	37% Cumulative recurrence at 1, 2 y 28.4%, 61.3%		15.8 mo	Short last HCC Rx < 12 mo (HR 2.89, 1.27–6.59)
Ochi et al,[60] 2021	Japan	Retrospective	56	20	36.7% DAA vs 68.7% no DAA	26 wk	48 mo	Tumor size >30 mm (HR 1.91 1.61–3.16) Received DAA (HR 0.46 0.27–0.77)
Elbaz et al,[61] 2021	Egypt	Retrospective	523	105	20.1%	159 wk	40 mo	Non-SVR ($P<.01$)
Ogawa et al,[62] 2022	Japan	Retrospective	326, cirrhosis	171	52.4%	62 wk	32.4 mo	Cirrhosis HR 1.85, ≥2 HCC nodules HR 1.52, previous palliative HCC treatment HR 1.71

Abbreviations: DAA, direct-acting antiviral agents; HCC, hepatocellular carcinoma; HR, hazard ratio; IFN, interferon; SVR, sustained virological response.

recurrence as a time-dependent variable. The time-to-event outcomes are also affected by the variability in the duration of follow-up of individual studies. These restrictions are especially important when the follow-up times between studies vary. Most of these studies also did not document the presence of complications from cirrhosis so it remains unclear if overall survival was driven by HCC recurrence and tumor progression alone or hepatic decompensation.

Meta-analysis for HCC recurrence following therapy with DAAs reported pooled HCC recurrence of 21.9% (95% CI 16.2%–28.3%).[65] Another recent meta-analysis analyzed the individual data level of 977 patients from 21 studies and concluded pooled HCC recurrence rate of 20 per 100 person-years, and there was no significant difference between DAAs-exposed and DAAs-unexposed groups in propensity score–matched patients.[66] However, the underlying patient heterogeneity and variations in the length of follow-up were the major factors contributing to the nonconclusiveness of the study. The assessment of complete response by imaging after palliative therapies, such as transarterial chemoembolization (TACE), may miss viable tumor cells that could have disseminated and contributed to cancer recurrence. Liu and colleagues concluded that DAAs therapy prevents recurrence and improves the overall survival of patients receiving non-transplantation treatment for HCV-related HCC.[67]

FACTORS ASSOCIATED WITH HCC OCCURRENCE

Several publications have demonstrated that achieving SVR following DAA treatment decreased the incidence of HCC.[18,19,25,27] Among patients without cirrhosis, underlying hypertension (HR 1.59, 95% CI 1.65–1.74), diabetes (HR 2.14, 95% CI 1.11–4.12), increased fibrosis-4 (FIB)-4 greater than 3.25 (HR 4.58, 95% CI 1.81–11.6), and alcohol abuse (HR 2.93, 95% CI 1.38–6.21) have all been associated with HCC occurrence.[18,36] Kanwal and colleagues demonstrated the presence of cirrhosis was associated with HCC development (HR 4.73, 95% CI 3.34–6.68), and similar results were reported from several studies.[17,18,27,31,36,37] Older age, male sex, diabetes, hepatitis B virus coinfection (HBsAg reactive), and hepatitis C treatment experience were associated with HCC occurrence.[24,26,31,37,54] Alcohol abuse was also associated with HCC incidence with HR 1.56, 95% CI 1.11–2.18.[18] Low albumin level, low platelet, and aspartate aminotransferase to platelet ratio index (APRI) score greater than 2.5, higher liver stiffness by transient elastography or MR elastography greater than 4.5 kPa, and CTP-B/C were associated with HCC occurrence.[17,24,26,27,34,37,54] Kramer and colleagues demonstrated that the change of FIB-4 score from less than 3.25 at baseline to greater than 3.25 overtime was associated with HCC occurrence with HR 3.12, 95% CI 2.12–4.60.[36] Several studies evaluated alpha-fetoprotein (AFP) levels, and pretreatment AFP greater than 20 ng/mL and end-of-treatment AFP greater than or equal to 5.3 ng/mL were associated with HCC occurrence.[25,31,37] When interpreting the data on increased risk of HCC in patients treated with DAAs, one must consider the spectrum bias of patients treated early on with DAAs, many of whom report more advanced liver disease and other high-risk characteristics for incident HCC.

FACTORS ASSOCIATED WITH HCC RECURRENCE

Lack of SVR contributed to increased HCC recurrence.[29,58,61] The presence of diabetes, liver cirrhosis, and decompensated/advanced liver disease (CTP-B/C) were associated with HCC recurrence.[54,62] History of alcohol abuse was rarely measured and documented in the described studies but was reported to have an increased association with HCC recurrence in one study.[32]

T2 HCC lesions were also associated with HCC recurrence; tumor size $\geq$2 cm (HR 1.46, P <.001), $\geq$2.5 cm (HR 2.73, 95% CI 1.23–6.06), and $\geq$3 cm (HR 1.91, 95% CI 1.61–3.16)[49,55,60] Multifocal HCC tumors were associated with HCC recurrence with HR range between 1.33 and 2.18, P <.05.[46,49,62] Prior history of HCC recurrence was associated with repeat recurrences.[32,45] This can be due to incomplete eradication and the tendency of malignant cells and tumor mutations to persist.

AFP levels were evaluated variably among studies. Pretreatment AFP $\geq$10 ng/mL was associated with HCC recurrence with HR 6.19, 95% CI 1.81–21.2, while another study reported pretreatment AFP greater than 40 mg/L was associated with HCC recurrence with HR 1.75 95% CI 1.08–2.86, and pretreatment AFP $\geq$100 ng/mL was associated with early HCC recurrence HR 1.41, P = .001.[29,46,49] Post-treatment AFP elevation greater than 5.5 ng/mL or persistent AFP elevation after treatment was also associated with HCC recurrence.[28,47] An AFP greater than 7 ng/mL at 12 weeks after initiation of DAAs was associated with early HCC recurrence (defined as within 6 months after SVR).[62] Palliative treatment intention for HCC which includes TACE, TACE with radiofrequency ablation (RFA), TACE with resection, particle radiotherapy, or percutaneous ethanol injection were associated with late recurrence (over 6 months after SVR) with HR 1.71, 95% CI 1.13–2.60 when compared with curative treatment modalities including resection, RFA, or combined RFA and resection.[62]

Several studies have demonstrated shorter interval from HCC complete response to DAA initiation (<1 year) was associated with HCC recurrence.[50,51,59,62] Ogawa and colleagues reported the shorter time from HCC complete response to DAA initiation (<1 year) was associated with both early HCC recurrence HR 2.39, 95% CI 1.07–5.35 and late HCC recurrence HR 1.70, 95% CI 1.16–2.97.[62]

CONTROVERSIES OF THE TIMING OF DAA THERAPY INITIATION FOLLOWING HCC TREATMENT

There are no clear data to support the association between treatment with DAAs and newly diagnosed or recurrent HCC. DAAs are highly effective and well-tolerated; more than 90% of patients with cirrhosis achieved SVR. The purported mechanism behind DAA treatment and increased risk of HCC centers around the role of the immune system in cancer surveillance. Rapid viral elimination due to DAAs eliminates the virus-associated immune surveillance and reduces immune cancer surveillance and promotes HCC development.[68] IFN-based regimens had slower viral suppression and inflammatory signal reduction occurred not as abruptly when compared to the DAAs regimen. Furthermore, the use of IFN may have secured the immune cancer-control benefits induced by IFN with its known antiproliferative effect and regulate immune cell activity including macrophages, dendritic cells, B cells, T cells, and innate lymphocytes and creating a well-orchestrated immune response against cancer cells.[39] It is important to note that this mechanism is largely speculative without strong translational data to support this as a means by which HCC recurrence could be higher in patients with treated HCC. While expert opinion is mixed on the timing of DAA initiation in patients with a history of HCC, given the lack of strong data supporting recurrence risk, and the benefits of DAAs on HCV-related necroinflammation, an early treatment paradigm may be reasonable.[63] Achieving SVR following DAAs treatment promotes fibrosis regression, improved liver function, portal hypertension, overall survival, and transplant-free survival. Furthermore, achieving SVR among HCV-related patients with active HCC decreased risks of hepatic decompensation compared to viremic patients.[69] Thus, in clinical practice, many have opted to treat all patients with HCV with DAAs, even concomitantly with active HCC.

CURRENT GAPS IN KNOWLEDGE

When analyzing studies on HCC occurrence and recurrence, one must consider the heterogeneity in study design (retrospective and prospective), inception points, lack of proper control groups, and the impact of competitive risk factors on survival. Additionally, studies on HCC recurrence exhibit heterogeneity in baseline patient and tumor characteristics, as well as in the type of curative treatments and radiological response assessment. There are also differences in the definition of HCC recurrence and the schedules of follow-up after treatment. In summary, although observational studies are useful for investigating the effectiveness and safety of medical treatments in real-world scenarios, they have several limitations such as confounding and extensive heterogeneity. DAAs have been shown to be useful in achieving SVR and improving survival. Given the mixed data and lack of clear mechanism behind the negative effects of DAAs, earlier treatment and eradication of HCV is a rationale approach at this time, even in patients with active HCC, in order to improve or maintain liver functions and alter the risk of de novo HCC development.

SUMMARY

Chronic hepatitis C infection remains one of the leading causes of hepatocellular carcinoma. This risk is even higher in patients with cirrhosis. The treatment of hepatitis C with DAAs has prevented its horizontal transmission, transformed the epidemiology of the disease, and furthered the goals of viral hepatitis elimination in the coming decade. DAAs have been shown to achieve SVR with clinically significant improvement in liver function, morbidity, mortality, and transplant-free survival. Early after the introduction of DAAs, concerns were raised regarding the increased risk of incident and recurrent HCC. However, these data were most likely a result of the spectrum bias, poorly designed cohort studies without adequate comparator groups, and lack of prospective studies.

Variable results have been described in the literature, but more recent studies have concluded that DAAs reduce the risk of HCC in SVR patients, when compared to untreated and unsuccessfully treated patients. DAA therapy overall decreases the risk of both occurrence and recurrence of HCC but does not annul it, probably due to an underlying pro-angiogenic environment and/or decreased immune surveillance after treatment. Further, prospective data as to the safety and benefits of HCV treatment in patients with active HCC would be useful in clinical practice. In the absence of these data, and the limitations of the data on risks of DAAs, it is reasonable practice to treat all patients with HCV with DAAs regardless of their HCC status in order to realize the benefits of viral elimination for all patients.

DISCLOSURE

A. Likhitsup and I. Fatima have nothing to disclose. N.D. Parikh has served on advisory boards for Gilead, Fujifilm, Exelixis, Eisai, and Genentech.

REFERENCES

1. Hofmeister MG, Rosenthal EM, Barker LK, et al. Estimating Prevalence of Hepatitis C Virus Infection in the United States, 2013-2016. Hepatology 2019;69(3): 1020–31.
2. Perz JF, Armstrong GL, Farrington LA, et al. The contributions of hepatitis B virus and hepatitis C virus infections to cirrhosis and primary liver cancer worldwide. J Hepatol 2006;45(4):529–38.

3. de Martel C, Maucort-Boulch D, Plummer M, et al. World-wide relative contribution of hepatitis B and C viruses in hepatocellular carcinoma. Hepatology 2015; 62(4):1190–200.
4. Reddy KR, Lim JK, Kuo A, et al. All-oral direct-acting antiviral therapy in HCV-advanced liver disease is effective in real-world practice: observations through HCV-TARGET database. Aliment Pharmacol Ther 2017;45(1):115–26.
5. McDonald SA, Pollock KG, Barclay ST, et al. Real-world impact following initiation of interferon-free hepatitis C regimens on liver-related outcomes and all-cause mortality among patients with compensated cirrhosis. J Viral Hepat 2020;27(3): 270–80.
6. Kaldindi Y, Jung J, Feldman R, et al. Association of Direct-Acting Antiviral Treatment With Mortality Among Medicare Beneficiaries With Hepatitis C. JAMA Netw Open 2020;3(7):e2011055.
7. Verna EC, Morelli G, Terrault NA, et al. DAA therapy and long-term hepatic function in advanced/decompensated cirrhosis: Real-world experience from HCV-TARGET cohort. J Hepatol 2020;73(3):540–8.
8. Sahakyan Y, Lee-Kim V, Bremner KE, et al. Impact of direct-acting antiviral regimens on mortality and morbidity outcomes in patients with chronic hepatitis c: Systematic review and meta-analysis. J Viral Hepat 2021;28(5):739–54.
9. Meunier L, Belkacemi M, Pageaux GP, et al. Patients Treated for HCV Infection and Listed for Liver Transplantation in a French Multicenter Study: What Happens at Five Years? Viruses 2022;15(1):137.
10. Ghany MG, Morgan TR. AASLD-IDSA Hepatitis C Guidance Panel. Hepatitis C Guidance 2019 Update: American Association for the Study of Liver Diseases-Infectious Diseases Society of America Recommendations for Testing, Managing, and Treating Hepatitis C Virus Infection. Hepatology 2020;71(2):686–721.
11. Singal AG, Lim JK, Kanwal F. AGA Clinical Practice Update on Interaction Between Oral Direct-Acting Antivirals for Chronic Hepatitis C Infection and Hepatocellular Carcinoma: Expert Review. Gastroenterology 2019;156(8):2149–57.
12. Kanda T, Goto T, Hirotsu Y, et al. Molecular Mechanisms Driving Progression of Liver Cirrhosis towards Hepatocellular Carcinoma in Chronic Hepatitis B and C Infections: A Review. Int J Mol Sci 2019;20(6):1358.
13. El-Serag HB, Kanwal F. Epidemiology of hepatocellular carcinoma in the United States: where are we? Where do we go? Hepatology 2014;60(5):1767–75.
14. Desai A, Sandhu S, Lai JP, et al. Hepatocellular carcinoma in non-cirrhotic liver: A comprehensive review. World J Hepatol 2019;11(1):1–18.
15. Pezzuto F, Buonaguro L, Buonaguro FM, et al. Frequency and geographic distribution of TERT promoter mutations in primary hepatocellular carcinoma. Infect Agent Cancer 2017;12:27.
16. McGivern DR, Lemon SM. Tumor suppressors, chromosomal instability, and hepatitis C virus-associated liver cancer. Annu Rev Pathol 2009;4:399–415.
17. Conti F, Buonfiglioli F, Scuteri A, et al. Early occurrence and recurrence of hepatocellular carcinoma in HCV-related cirrhosis treated with direct-acting antivirals. J Hepatol 2016;65(4):727–33.
18. Kanwal F, Kramer J, Asch SM, et al. Risk of Hepatocellular Cancer in HCV Patients Treated With Direct-Acting Antiviral Agents. Gastroenterology 2017; 153(4):996–1005.e1.
19. Ioannou GN, Green PK, Berry K. HCV eradication induced by direct-acting antiviral agents reduces the risk of hepatocellular carcinoma. J Hepatol 2017. https://doi.org/10.1016/j.jhep.2017.08.030. S0168-8278(17)32273-0.

20. Cheung MCM, Walker AJ, Hudson BE, et al. Outcomes after successful direct-acting antiviral therapy for patients with chronic hepatitis C and decompensated cirrhosis. J Hepatol 2016;65(4):741–7.

21. Akuta N, Kobayashi M, Suzuki F, et al. Liver Fibrosis and Body Mass Index Predict Hepatocarcinogenesis following Eradication of Hepatitis C Virus RNA by Direct-Acting Antivirals. Oncology 2016;91(6):341–7.

22. Ravi S, Axley P, Jones D, et al. Unusually High Rates of Hepatocellular Carcinoma After Treatment With Direct-Acting Antiviral Therapy for Hepatitis C Related Cirrhosis. Gastroenterology 2017;152(4):911–2.

23. Calleja JL, Crespo J, Rincón D, et al. Effectiveness, safety and clinical outcomes of direct-acting antiviral therapy in HCV genotype 1 infection: Results from a Spanish real-world cohort. J Hepatol 2017;66(6):1138–48.

24. Innes H, Barclay ST, Hayes PC, et al. The risk of hepatocellular carcinoma in cirrhotic patients with hepatitis C and sustained viral response: Role of the treatment regimen. J Hepatol 2018;68(4):646–54.

25. Li DK, Ren Y, Fierer DS, et al. The short-term incidence of hepatocellular carcinoma is not increased after hepatitis C treatment with direct-acting antivirals: An ERCHIVES study. Hepatology 2018;67(6):2244–53.

26. Romano A, Angeli P, Piovesan S, et al. Newly diagnosed hepatocellular carcinoma in patients with advanced hepatitis C treated with DAAs: A prospective population study. J Hepatol 2018;69(2):345–52.

27. Calvaruso V, Cabibbo G, Cacciola I, et al. Incidence of Hepatocellular Carcinoma in Patients With HCV-Associated Cirrhosis Treated With Direct-Acting Antiviral Agents. Gastroenterology 2018;155(2):411–21.e4.

28. Masetti C, Lionetti R, Lupo M, et al. Lack of reduction in serum alpha-fetoprotein during treatment with direct antiviral agents predicts hepatocellular carcinoma development in a large cohort of patients with hepatitis C virus-related cirrhosis. J Viral Hepat 2018;25(12):1493–500.

29. Lleo A, Aglitti A, Aghemo A, et al. Predictors of hepatocellular carcinoma in HCV cirrhotic patients treated with direct acting antivirals. Dig Liver Dis 2019;51(2):310–7.

30. Mariño Z, Darnell A, Lens S, et al. Time association between hepatitis C therapy and hepatocellular carcinoma emergence in cirrhosis: Relevance of non-characterized nodules. J Hepatol 2019;70(5):874–84 [Erratum in: J Hepatol. 2021;74(2):491].

31. Shiha G, Mousa N, Soliman R, et al. Incidence of HCC in chronic hepatitis C patients with advanced hepatic fibrosis who achieved SVR following DAAs: A prospective study. J Viral Hepat 2020;27(7):671–9.

32. Sangiovanni A, Alimenti E, Gattai R, et al. Undefined/non-malignant hepatic nodules are associated with early occurrence of HCC in DAA-treated patients with HCV-related cirrhosis. J Hepatol 2020;73(3):593–602.

33. Kanwal F, Kramer JR, Asch SM, et al. Long-Term Risk of Hepatocellular Carcinoma in HCV Patients Treated With Direct Acting Antiviral Agents. Hepatology 2020;71(1):44–55.

34. Kumada T, Toyoda H, Yasuda S, et al. Prediction of Hepatocellular Carcinoma by Liver Stiffness Measurements Using Magnetic Resonance Elastography After Eradicating Hepatitis C Virus. Clin Transl Gastroenterol 2021;12(4):e00337.

35. Tahata Y, Hikita H, Mochida S, et al. Liver-related events after direct-acting antiviral therapy in patients with hepatitis C virus-associated cirrhosis. J Gastroenterol 2022;57(2):120–32.

36. Kramer JR, Cao Y, Li L, et al. Longitudinal Associations of Risk Factors and Hepatocellular Carcinoma in Patients With Cured Hepatitis C Virus Infection. Am J Gastroenterol 2022;117(11):1834–44.

37. Mawatari S, Kumagai K, Oda K, et al. Features of patients who developed hepatocellular carcinoma after direct-acting antiviral treatment for hepatitis C Virus. PLoS One 2022;17(1):e0262267.
38. Leal C, Strogoff-de-Matos J, Theodoro C, et al. Incidence and Risk Factors of Hepatocellular Carcinoma in Patients with Chronic Hepatitis C Treated with Direct-Acting Antivirals. Viruses 2023;15(1):221.
39. Reig M, Mariño Z, Perelló C, et al. Unexpected high rate of early tumor recurrence in patients with HCV-related HCC undergoing interferon-free therapy. J Hepatol 2016;65(4):719–26.
40. Rinaldi L, Di Francia R, Coppola N, et al. Hepatocellular carcinoma in HCV cirrhosis after viral clearance with direct acting antiviral therapy: preliminary evidence and possible meanings. World Cancer Research Journal 2016;3:e748.
41. ANRS collaborative study group on hepatocellular carcinoma (ANRS CO22 HEPATHER, CO12 CirVir and CO23 CUPILT cohorts). Electronic address: stanislas.pol@aphp.fr. Lack of evidence of an effect of direct-acting antivirals on the recurrence of hepatocellular carcinoma: Data from three ANRS cohorts. J Hepatol 2016;65(4):734–40.
42. Torres HA, Vauthey JN, Economides MP, et al. Hepatocellular carcinoma recurrence after treatment with direct-acting antivirals: First, do no harm by withdrawing treatment. J Hepatol 2016;65(4):862–4.
43. Zeng QL, Li ZQ, Liang HX, et al. Unexpected high incidence of hepatocellular carcinoma in patients with hepatitis C in the era of DAAs: Too alarming? J Hepatol 2016;65(5):1068–9.
44. Bielen R, Moreno C, Van Vlierberghe H, et al. The risk of early occurrence and recurrence of hepatocellular carcinoma in hepatitis C-infected patients treated with direct-acting antivirals with and without pegylated interferon: A Belgian experience. J Viral Hepat 2017;24(11):976–81.
45. Cabibbo G, Petta S, Calvaruso V, et al. Is early recurrence of hepatocellular carcinoma in HCV cirrhotic patients affected by treatment with direct-acting antivirals? A prospective multicentre study. Aliment Pharmacol Ther 2017;46(7):688–95.
46. Ikeda K, Kawamura Y, Kobayashi M, et al. Direct-Acting Antivirals Decreased Tumor Recurrence After Initial Treatment of Hepatitis C Virus-Related Hepatocellular Carcinoma. Dig Dis Sci 2017;62(10):2932–42.
47. Nagata H, Nakagawa M, Asahina Y, et al. Effect of interferon-based and -free therapy on early occurrence and recurrence of hepatocellular carcinoma in chronic hepatitis C. J Hepatol 2017;67(5):933–9.
48. Virlogeux V, Pradat P, Hartig-Lavie K, et al. Direct-acting antiviral therapy decreases hepatocellular carcinoma recurrence rate in cirrhotic patients with chronic hepatitis C. Liver Int 2017;37(8):1122–7.
49. Minami T, Tateishi R, Nakagomi R, et al. The impact of direct-acting antivirals on early tumor recurrence after radiofrequency ablation in hepatitis C-related hepatocellular carcinoma. J Hepatol 2016;65(6):1272–3.
50. Zavaglia C, Okolicsanyi S, Cesarini L, et al. Is the risk of neoplastic recurrence increased after prescribing direct-acting antivirals for HCV patients whose HCC was previously cured? J Hepatol 2017;66(1):236–7.
51. Kolly P, Waidmann O, Vermehren J, et al. Hepatocellular carcinoma recurrence after direct antiviral agent treatment: A European multicentre study. J Hepatol 2017;67(4):876–8.
52. Huang AC, Mehta N, Dodge JL, et al. Direct-acting antivirals do not increase the risk of hepatocellular carcinoma recurrence after local-regional therapy or liver transplant waitlist dropout. Hepatology 2018;68(2):449–61.

53. El Kassas M, Funk AL, Salaheldin M, et al. Increased recurrence rates of hepatocellular carcinoma after DAA therapy in a hepatitis C-infected Egyptian cohort: A comparative analysis. J Viral Hepat 2018;25(6):623–30.
54. Degasperi E, D'Ambrosio R, Iavarone M, et al. Factors Associated With Increased Risk of De Novo or Recurrent Hepatocellular Carcinoma in Patients With Cirrhosis Treated With Direct-Acting Antivirals for HCV Infection. Clin Gastroenterol Hepatol 2019;17(6):1183–91.e7.
55. Cabibbo G, Celsa C, Calvaruso V, et al. Direct-acting antivirals after successful treatment of early hepatocellular carcinoma improve survival in HCV-cirrhotic patients. J Hepatol 2019;71(2):265–73.
56. Lin WC, Lin YS, Chang CW, et al. Impact of direct-acting antiviral therapy for hepatitis C-related hepatocellular carcinoma. PLoS One 2020;15(5):e0233212.
57. Kuo YH, Wang JH, Chang KC, et al. The influence of direct-acting antivirals in hepatitis C virus related hepatocellular carcinoma after curative treatment. Invest New Drugs 2020;38(1):202–10.
58. Chi CT, Chen CY, Su CW, et al. Direct-acting antivirals for patients with chronic hepatitis C and hepatocellular carcinoma in Taiwan. J Microbiol Immunol Infect 2021;54(3):385–95.
59. Ahn YH, Lee H, Kim DY, et al. Independent Risk Factors for Hepatocellular Carcinoma Recurrence after Direct-Acting Antiviral Therapy in Patients with Chronic Hepatitis C. Gut Liver 2021;15(3):410–9.
60. Ochi H, Hiraoka A, Hirooka M, et al. Direct-acting antivirals improve survival and recurrence rates after treatment of hepatocellular carcinoma within the Milan criteria. J Gastroenterol 2021;56(1):90–100.
61. Elbaz T, Waked I, El-Akel W, et al. Impact of successful HCV treatment using direct acting antivirals on recurrence of well ablated hepatocellular carcinoma. Expert Rev Anti Infect Ther 2022;20(2):307–14.
62. Ogawa E, Nakamuta M, Furusyo N, et al. Long-term assessment of recurrence of hepatocellular carcinoma in patients with chronic hepatitis C after viral cure by direct-acting antivirals. J Gastroenterol Hepatol 2022;37(1):190–9.
63. Singal AG, Rich NE, Mehta N, et al. Direct-Acting Antiviral Therapy for Hepatitis C Virus Infection Is Associated With Increased Survival in Patients With a History of Hepatocellular Carcinoma. Gastroenterology 2019;157(5):1253–63.e2.
64. Yang JD, Aqel BA, Pungpapong S, et al. Direct acting antiviral therapy and tumor recurrence after liver transplantation for hepatitis C-associated hepatocellular carcinoma. J Hepatol 2016;65(4):859–60.
65. Saraiya N, Yopp AC, Rich NE, et al. Systematic review with meta-analysis: recurrence of hepatocellular carcinoma following direct-acting antiviral therapy. Aliment Pharmacol Ther 2018;48(2):127–37.
66. Sapena V, Enea M, Torres F, et al. Hepatocellular carcinoma recurrence after direct-acting antiviral therapy: an individual patient data meta-analysis. Gut 2022;71(3):593–604.
67. Liu H, Yang XL, Dong ZR, et al. Clinical benefits of direct-acting antivirals therapy in hepatitis C virus patients with hepatocellular carcinoma: A systematic review and meta-analysis. J Gastroenterol Hepatol 2022;37(9):1654–65.
68. Nault JC, Colombo M. Hepatocellular carcinoma and direct acting antiviral treatments: Controversy after the revolution. J Hepatol 2016;65(4):663–5.
69. Parikh ND, Mehta N, Hoteit MA, et al. Association between sustained virological response and clinical outcomes in patients with hepatitis C infection and hepatocellular carcinoma. Cancer 2022;128(19):3470–8.

Up-to-Date Role of Liver Imaging Reporting and Data System in Hepatocellular Carcinoma

Victoria Chernyak, MD, MS

KEYWORDS

- Hepatocellular carcinoma • Liver imaging reporting and data system • LI-RADS
- HCC • Imaging • Diagnosis

KEY POINTS

- Liver Imaging Reporting and Data System (LI-RADS) has 4 algorithms for hepatocellular carcinoma (HCC) surveillance, diagnosis, and treatment response assessment.
- Diagnostic algorithms provide criteria for ordinal categories, each of which reflects a discrete probability of HCC and guides patient management in a reproducible and standardized manner.
- The LR-5 (definite HCC) category has greater than or equal to 95% positive predictive value for diagnosis of HCC, obviating biopsy confirmation before treatment.
- Ultrasound LI-RADS algorithm, in addition to assessment categories, includes visualization scores, which is the first standardized approach for defining and reporting image quality surveillance ultrasound.

BACKGROUND

In 2020, primary liver cancer was the sixth most commonly diagnosed cancer worldwide and the third leading cause of cancer-related mortality.[1] Hepatocellular carcinoma (HCC) comprises 75% to 85% of all primary liver cancers.[1] Liver Imaging Reporting and Data System (LI-RADS, LR), endorsed by the American College of Radiology, is a standardized, comprehensive system for imaging, interpretation, and reporting findings in patients at high risk for HCC.[2] Since the initial release in 2011, LI-RADS has grown to include 4 algorithms used for HCC surveillance with ultrasound (US LI-RADS), HCC diagnosis with computed tomography (CT) or MRI (CT/MRI LI-RADS) and contrast-enhanced ultrasound (CEUS LI-RADS), and treatment response assessment (LI-RADS TRA) following locoregional therapy using CT or MRI.[2] The

Department of Radiology, Memorial Sloan Kettering Cancer Center, New York City, NY, USA
E-mail address: vichka17@hotmail.com
Twitter: @VChernyakMD (V.C.)

Surg Oncol Clin N Am 33 (2024) 59–72
https://doi.org/10.1016/j.soc.2023.06.006
1055-3207/24/© 2023 Elsevier Inc. All rights reserved.

surgonc.theclinics.com

latest versions of CT/MRI diagnostic LI-RADS (v2018) and US LI-RADS were incorporated by the American Association for Study of Liver Diseases (AASLD) HCC Practice Guidance since 2018.[3] In 2022, the use of LI-RADS for interpretation of imaging studies in patients at risk for HCC was included in a set of quality measures in HCC care by the Practice Metrics Committee of the AASLD, confirming its use as a current standard of care.[4] Finally, in 2023, the Organ Procurement and Transplantation Network updated its criteria for definite HCC to fully align with the LI-RADS v2018.[5]

HEPATOCELLULAR SURVEILLANCE

The LI-RADS US algorithm, released in 2017, provides a standardized approach to performance, interpretation, and reporting of ultrasound done for HCC surveillance. The algorithm includes 3 categories, applied at the examination level, which then guide patient management (**Table 1**).[6]

Multicenter studies demonstrated that US-1 examinations are seen in 87% to 90% of patients undergoing HCC surveillance, US-2 in 5% to 7% of patients, and US-3 in 5% to 6% of patients.[7,8] On follow-up, 50% of US-2 examination have no imaging correlate and 10% correspond to benign observations.[9] For US-3 examinations, there was no correlate on diagnostic CT or MRI in 41%, 33% corresponded to benign observations, and 6% to observations with intermediate probability of malignancy.[10] The positive predictive value (PPV) of US-3 for probably or definitely malignant categories is 15% in all patients and 26% in patients with cirrhosis.[11]

Despite being the main tool for HCC surveillance across the world, the quality of ultrasound may substantially limit the sensitivity for HCC in 20%.[12] The US LI-RADS was the first system to standardize assessment of the image quality by including a visualization score (A–C), in addition to assessment categories[6].

- A: no or minimal limitations, unlikely to meaningfully affect the sensitivity
- B: moderate limitations, which may obscure small masses
- C: severe limitations, which significantly lower sensitivity for focal liver lesions

Visualization score C impairs sensitivity, with nearly 8 times higher odds for a false-negative examination, compared with examinations with scores A or B.[13] However, only 42% of patients with visualization score C also have score C on a follow-up, warranting at least one repeat ultrasound before switching to alternate surveillance strategies in most patients.[14]

Table 1
US LI-RADS categories

Category	Definition	Management[a]
US-1 (negative)	Either no observations or only definitely benign observations	Return to the routine surveillance schedule
US-2 (subthreshold)	Observation < 10 mm, not definitely benign	3–6 mo surveillance
US-3 (positive)	Either observation ≥ 10 mm, not definitely benign, or new thrombus in vein	Further characterization with multiphase contrast-enhanced imaging (CT, MRI, or CEUS)

[a] Based on US LI-RADS® Category. Retrieved from: https://www.acr.org/-/media/ACR/Files/RADS/LI-RADS/LI-RADS-US-Algorithm-Portrait-2017.pdf.

Table 2 LI-RADS diagnostic categories on computed tomography, MRI, and contrast-enhanced ultrasound		
Category	Definition	Pooled Percentage of HCC[a]
LR-NC	Not categorizable due to image quality or omission of required phases	N/A
LR-1	Definitely benign	CT/MRI: 0; CEUS: 0
LR-2	Probably benign	CT/MRI: 3 (1–6); CEUS: 1 (0–6)
LR-3	Intermediate probability of malignancy	CT/MRI: 38 (27–49); CEUS: 21 (13–31)
LR-4	Probable HCC	CT/MRI: 73 (65–82); CEUS: 75 (61–85)
LR-5	Definite HCC	CT/MRI: 96 (95–97); CEUS: 96 (94–98)
LR-M	Probably or definitely malignant, not HCC specific	CT/MRI: 33 (26–40); CEUS: 56 (44–69)
LR-TIV	Definite tumor in vein	CT/MRI: 80 (71–89); CEUS: 97 (77–100)

[a] Percentages are given based on meta-analytic data in references[15] (CT/MRI) and[16] (CEUS); ranges in parentheses reflect 95% confidence intervals.

DIAGNOSTIC ALGORITHMS
Overview

Following US-3 examination or detection of an indeterminate lesion in a high-risk patient on either noncontrast or single-phase CT or MRI, a diagnostic multiphase study is performed for further characterization. The diagnostic LI-RADS includes 2 algorithms: CT/MRI LI-RADS, applicable to CT and MRI, and CEUS LI-RADS, applicable to CEUS. Although some differences between algorithms exist due to inherent differences between the modalities, the overall approach is the same. Both algorithms include 8 diagnostic categories, where each category reflects a probability of HCC or benign disease. The probability of HCC increases linearly from LR-1 to LR-5 categories (**Table 2**).[15,16] Observations meeting criteria for LR-5, LR-M, and LR-TIV categories are nearly always malignant, with the pooled probabilities of overall malignancy being 99%, 97%, and 95%, respectively, on CEUS and 100% in each on CT/MRI.[15,17]

Both CT/MRI and CEUS algorithms use diagnostic tables to assign LR-3, LR-4, and LR-5 categories based on various combinations of major features. Major features on CT/MRI include nonrim arterial phase hyperenhancement (APHE), nonperipheral washout, enhancing capsule, size, and threshold growth.[2] Major features on CEUS include nonrim APHE, late and mild washout, and size. Although CEUS algorithm is validated in multiple studies, including meta-analyses,[16,17] CEUS is not yet as widely adopted in clinical practice as is CT/MRI. Therefore, the concepts discussed later are based on CT/MRI LI-RADS. However, it is important to note that these concepts, with some modality-specific modifications, are equally relevant to CEUS LI-RADS.

HCC is a unique solid organ malignancy, as it can be definitively diagnosed based on imaging, without the need for pathologic confirmation.[3,18] Meta-analysis based on nearly 10,000 patients with more than 11,500 observations demonstrated that the proportion of HCC in LR-5 category is the same (95%–96%) on CT, MRI with extracellular contrast agents, and MRI with hepatobiliary contrast agents (**Fig. 1**).[15] As a result, the patients with observations meeting criteria for LR-5 category are referred for management without histologic confirmation.[3,19] Near-perfect PPV of LR-5 category for the diagnosis of HCC is achieved at the expense of only modest sensitivity (48%–61%)[20] and is guarded by following important rules:

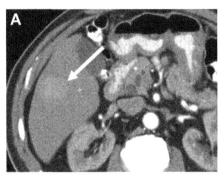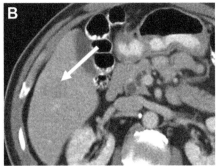

Fig. 1. LR-5 (definite HCC) observation in a 47-year-old man with alcoholic cirrhosis. Axial CT in arterial (*A*) and portal venous (*B*) phases demonstrates a 33-mm observation with nonrim arterial phase hyperenhancement (*arrow, A*) and washout (*arrow, B*), which meets criteria for LR-5. The lesion was confirmed to be moderately differentiated HCC on resection.

- *LI-RADS patient population*: the LI-RADS diagnostic algorithms are applicable only to patients who have at least one of the following:
  - ○ Cirrhosis
  - ○ Chronic hepatitis B viral infection, with or without cirrhosis
  - ○ Personal history of HCC (including after receipt of liver transplantation)

LI-RADS does not apply to patients who are younger than 18 years or who have vascular causes of cirrhosis (eg, Fontan-associated liver disease), as patients with these conditions have a propensity to develop hypervascularized benign nodules mimicking HCC.

Application of LI-RADS in appropriate patient population is crucial for maintaining the required high PPV of LR-5, as, based on Bayes theorem, the posttest probability of HCC depends on pretest conditional pretest probability of HCC (ie, pretest probability of HCC once a solid lesion is detected on imaging).[21] Assuming positive likelihood ratio of LR-5 category to be 17,[22] a pretest probability of greater than or equal to 53% is required to achieve posttest probability of greater than or equal to 95%.[23] Although it is difficult to establish pretest probability experimentally, we can extrapolate that in high-risk patients, the pretest probability is sufficiently high, as the PPVs of LR-5 criteria in this population reaches the desired 95% mark or greater.[15] Conversely, a lesion with imaging characteristics same as an LR-5 observation in a healthy individual with a low conditional pretest probability of HCC of 1% would result in posttest probability of HCC of no more than 14.5%.[23]

- *LR-5 criteria include major features only:* LI-RADS diagnostic algorithms assign LR-3, LR-4, and LR-5 categories based on the combination of major features. Although CT/MRI LI-RADS recognizes multiple ancillary features, it prohibits

---

Box 1
LI-RADS v2018 criteria for LR-5 (definite HCC) category on computed tomography/MRI

Nonrim APHE *AND* size ≥ 10 mm *AND*:
- Nonperipheral washout only
- Threshold growth only
- ≥ 2 additional major features (nonperipheral washout, threshold growth, enhancing capsule)

Nonrim APHE *AND* size ≥ 20 mm *AND* enhancing capsule only

upcategorizing LR-4 category to LR-5 based on ancillary features of malignancy, that is, LR-5 is assigned based on one of the defined combinations of major features (**Box 1**).[2] Although allowing application of ancillary features to upcategorize some of LR-4 observations could potentially improve sensitivity of LR-5 category, the sacrifice in specificity would lead to a drop in the PPV less than the desired 95% threshold.[24]

- *LR-5 required features*: although several combinations of major features result in LR-5 categorization, all of them require the presence of 2 features: nonrim APHE and size greater than or equal to 10 mm.

During hepatocarcinogenesis, sinusoidal capillarization and recruitment of unpaired arterioles result in relative increase of arterial blood flow, leading to an appearance of APHE, a hallmark imaging feature of HCC.[25] However, early HCCs tend to have sparse zones of sinusoidal capillarization and small numbers of unpaired arteries, reflecting relatively undeveloped neoangiogenesis, and therefore lack APHE.[25] Although 18% of all HCCs less than 30 mm are hypovascular, differentiation between early HCCs and high-grade dysplastic nodules is challenging, both pathologically and radiologically.[25–27] Consequently, the PPV of imaging for HCC in observations that lack APHE is only 56%.[28] As a result, LR-5 category can only be applied to observations with nonrim APHE. Similarly, size greater than or equal to 10 mm is required for LR-5, as the probability of HCC in small lesions is insufficiently high: the annual rate of HCC development in subcentimeter lesions is approximately 5%.[29] Furthermore, only 73.5% of all subcentimeter LR-4 observations with nonrim APHE are HCC.[28]

- *Uncertainty rules:* currently, 3 of 5 major features on CT and MRI are assessed qualitatively, by comparing the observation with the background liver. Given commonly present heterogeneity of both liver lesions and background parenchyma, the interreader agreement for qualitative features of LI-RADS is substantial (with kappa values ranging from 0.65 to 0.72).[30,31] Recognizing the importance of maximizing reproducibility, LI-RADS rules state if there is any doubt whether a feature is present, the feature should be assessed as absent.[32] This rule also helps to ensure that only observations that unequivocally have the required combination of features are categorized LR-5. In addition, the rules state that if there is uncertainty between a targetoid feature versus major feature (eg, rim vs nonrim APHE), the feature should be characterized as targetoid. This rule results in preferential assignment of LR-M category to any lesions where a targetoid morphology may be present, ensuring that a potential non-HCC malignancy is assigned LR-M category rather than LR-5 (**Fig. 2**).

- *Tie-breaking rules:* occasionally, even after application of the algorithm, a radiologist may be deciding between 2 categories. For example, a rounded 9-mm observation with nonrim APHE and no other major features meets criteria for LR-3 category. On the other hand, cirrhotic livers are prone to developing areas of perfusional abnormalities as a result of reduced portal vein perfusion and compensatory hepatic artery perfusion.[33] Such vascular pseudolesions are seen as areas of increased enhancement on the arterial and, when rounded, may be difficult to distinguish from true lesions. As a result, a radiologist may be uncertain whether the aforementioned observation should be assigned LR-3 or LR-2 category. According to the LI-RADS tie-breaking rules, the category that conveys a lower certainty (of benignity, malignancy, or hepatocellular origin) should be selected. Thus, in this example, the radiologist should assign LR-3 category, as it reflects a lower certainty of benignity. As a result of tie-breaking rule, any indecision in LR-5 category should result in assignment of either LR-4

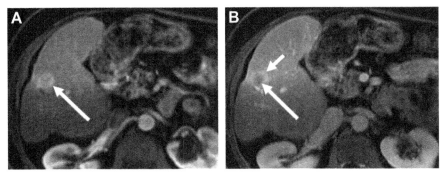

Fig. 2. Use of uncertainty rules. Axial T1-weighted MR images in arterial (*A*) and portal venous (*B*) phases in a 52-year-old man with history of resected HCC demonstrate a 20 mm observation. The observation has arterial phase hyperenhancement (APHE) (*arrow, A*), washout (*long arrow, B*), and enhancing capsule (*short arrow, B*). There is uncertainty whether the morphology of APHE is rim (most pronounced at the observation periphery) or nonrim (*not* most pronounced at the observation periphery). When deciding between targetoid (rim APHE) and major (nonrim APHE), LI-RADS instructs to choose targetoid. This observation was reported as having rim APHE and categorized LR-M. Biopsy revealed intrahepatic cholangiocarcinoma.

(lower certainty of malignancy) or LR-M (lower certainty of hepatocellular origin) categories.

The aforementioned stringent rules help achieve near-perfect posttest probability and eliminate the need for histologic confirmation. On the flip side, only approximately 50% to 70% of pathologically proven HCC meet criteria for LR-5 category.[34,35] It is important to remember that assigning HCC to a category other than LR-5 is *not* a system error, whereas assigning LR-5 category to a non-HCC entity is a false-positive result.

Management Implications of Liver Imaging Reporting and Data System Categories

The LI-RADS categories themselves are not discrete pathologic lesions: aside from LR-5, where most of the observations are HCC, every other category is composed of a group of pathologic entities (**Fig. 3**). Rather, the LI-RADS categories provide a distinct probability that a given observation is an HCC (see **Table 1**), and these probabilities guide patient management (**Fig. 4**).[32]

Because nearly all observations in LR-5, LR-TIV, and LR-M categories are malignant, the patients are referred for multidisciplinary discussion, and an individualized management plan is established. Because a substantial proportion of LR-M and LR-TIV observations represents non-HCC malignancies, such as intrahepatic cholangiocarcinoma,[15,16] a biopsy of LR-M and LR-TIV observations is usually performed to establish a diagnosis before treatment.[19] Similarly, the management of patients without observations or only with definitely benign (LR-1) or probably benign observation (LR-2) is relatively straightforward: because the probability of HCC in these patients is nearly nil, they return to routine surveillance. The patients with LR-3 observations get close imaging monitoring every 3 to 6 months, and LR-4 observations can be either closely monitored, biopsied for definitive diagnosis, or treated presumptively as HCC.[19]

The management of LR-3 and LR-4 observations presents a challenge in clinical practice, as the probability of malignancy in these categories is neither insufficiently

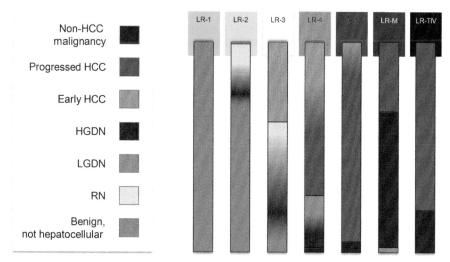

Fig. 3. Distribution of various pathologic entities in each LI-RADS categories. HCC, hepatocellular carcinoma; HGDN, high-grade dysplastic nodule; LGDN, low-grade dysplastic nodule; RN, regenerative nodule. Examples of benign nonhepatocellular entities: cyst, hemangioma, focal fibrosis. Examples of non-HCC malignancies: intrahepatic cholangiocarcinoma, metastases, combined HCC-cholangiocarcinoma.

low for return to routine surveillance nor insufficiently high for immediate treatment. Furthermore, natural history of LR-3 and LR-4 observations is heterogeneous. Of all LR-3 observations, 23% to 60% remain LR-3, 15% to 68% decrease to LR-1/2%, 2% to 5% progress to LR-4, and 7% to 24% progress to LR-5/M.[36–39] Of all LR-4 observations, in 6 to 12 months, 44% remain LR-4 and 33% to 38% progress to LR-5/M, and an important minority decreases in category to LR-3 (13%) or LR1/2 (3%).[38,40] The

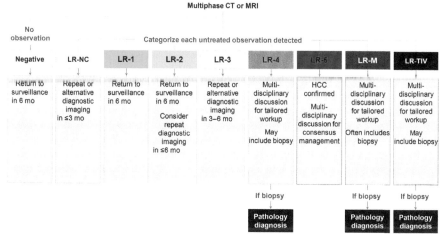

Fig. 4. Summary of management options for LI-RADS categories. (CT/MRI LI-RADS®-Based Management: Suggested Imaging Workup Options & Time Intervals. Retrieved from: https://www.acr.org/-/media/ACR/Files/RADS/LI-RADS/LI-RADS-2018-Core.pdf?la=en).

cumulative incidence of malignancy in LR-3 observations is approximately 25% by year 3 and 65% by year 4.[41] Thus, 75% of patients with LR-3 observations would undergo imaging study every 3 to 6 months for 3 years and would not develop frank malignancy. One can imagine that if such patients could be identified accurately, they could return to routine surveillance for at least first 3 years, potentially resulting in substantial health care cost reduction. Although some studies identified various independent predictors of progression to HCC,[40,42–47] so far there is no reliable method to accurately identify those LR-3 and LR-4 observations that will remain stable or decrease in category.

Advantages of Liver Imaging Reporting and Data System

- *Granular categorization across the entire spectrum of liver observations:* CT/MRI LI-RADS is one of the many systems used for imaging diagnosis of HCC that exist in the world.[48] What sets the LI-RADS apart is the fact that it provides diagnostic criteria for the entire spectrum of observations found in high-risk patients. Conversely, other imaging diagnostic systems only define criteria for observations that can be conclusively diagnosed as HCC on imaging.[48] These systems rely on radiologists' prior knowledge of typical imaging appearance of benign entities and offer no guidance on diagnosis of a group of indeterminate observations that neither meet imaging criteria for definite HCC nor have typical appearance of benign lesions. Such indeterminate lesions are common and include a wide variety of benign, malignant, and premalignant lesions. Given the broad range of biological aggressiveness in this group of lesions, a reliable approach to risk stratification is crucial to ensure that management is driven by a reproducible set of rules rather than by subjective assessment of interpreting radiologist and by local institutional practices. Some guidelines recommend biopsy for all indeterminate liver lesions, whenever possible.[49] However, a biopsy is not feasible in half of the indeterminate lesions.[50] Furthermore, in those lesions that can be biopsied, the false-negative rate is 3% to 11%.[51] Finally, there is no scientific evidence that biopsy-all approach is either cost-effective or improves patient outcomes.

- *Improved performance of less experienced radiologists:* LI-RADS was created to standardize image acquisition, interpretation, and reporting of observations in patients at high risk of HCC. The long-term goal of LI-RADS is universal adoption in clinical practice, both in academic setting and private practice, by liver imaging novices and experts alike. Before development of standardized criteria, the level of radiologist's training and experience played an important role in determining the accuracy of interpretation. LI-RADS may level the playing field between novices and experts by providing explicit criteria and rules for interpretation. In a study by Wang and colleagues, inexperienced radiologists interpreted liver observations on CEUS as either benign or malignant using conventional criteria and then, after training, using CEUS LI-RADS criteria.[52] The performance was then compared with that of experienced radiologists using conventional criteria. Not surprisingly, the experienced readers outperformed inexperienced ones across all performance parameters (ie, sensitivity, specificity, positive and negative predictive values) using conventional criteria.[52] For example, PPVs of conventional criteria for inexperienced and experienced readers were 64% to 66% and 82% to 88%, respectively.[52] Compared with conventional criteria, the use of LI-RADS resulted in significant increase of all performance parameters of inexperienced readers.[52] More importantly, the performance of inexperienced readers increased to levels equal and even surpassing those of experienced readers: for instance, the PPVs of inexperienced readers using LI-RADS were 91% to 94%, as compared with 82% to 88% in experienced ones.[52]

- *Improved clarity of communication:* in addition to providing a set of rules for category assignment, LI-RADS includes a comprehensive lexicon, defining a set of terms used for liver imaging.[53] Adoption of universal lexicon and terminology has a potential to improve patient care by reducing variability between reports.[54] Furthermore, the use of clearly defined descriptors for each category (eg, "definite HCC") instead of nonstandardized descriptors (eg, "suspicious for HCC") in radiology reports allows for clearer and more consistent communication between radiologists and clinicians.[55] For example, in a study by Corwin and colleagues, on direct review of imaging, 55% of lesions reported as "consistent with HCC" were LR-5, 25% were LR-4, 15% were LR-TIV, and 5% were LR-3.[55] Thus, when clinician receives a report that describes a lesion "consistent with HCC," it could represent an aggressive cancer with macrovascular invasion (LR-TIV) or a lesion with only 33% probability of being an HCC (LR-3), and clinicians have no way of knowing which of these the patient has.
- *Scientific impact:* to date, PubMed lists more than 650 publications on LI-RADS, of which 39 performed systematic review and/or meta-analysis, focusing on diagnostic performance of categories and imaging features, interreader reliability, and intermodality comparison of various algorithms. In addition, LI-RADS had a positive effect on scientific literature dealing with the diagnosis of primary liver cancers. In the period of 2017 to 2019, 57% of published scientific studies investigating diagnosis of HCC on MRI used LI-RADS lexicon and 61% used LI-RADS diagnostic criteria.[56] Since release of LI-RADS, there has been decrease in use of study-specific definitions for major features from 80% in 2011 to 2013 to 25% in 2017 to 2019, as well as decrease in use of study-specific imaging diagnostic criteria for HCC from 69% in 2011 to 2013 to 12% in 2017 to 2019, leading to a substantially improved consistency of study design.[56]

TREATMENT RESPONSE ASSESSMENT

LI-RADS TRA algorithm, released in 2017, provides lesion-level response assessment on CT or MRI following locoregional treatment with ablative or embolic therapies. The algorithm includes 3 categories: LR-TR Nonviable, LR-TR Equivocal, and LR-TR Viable (**Table 3**) (**Fig. 5**). Recent meta-analyses reported that LR-TR Viable category has pooled sensitivity and specificity for incomplete necrosis of 56% to 63% and 91% to 90%, respectively.[57,58] Expanding the definition of viable disease to include

Table 3	
Computed tomography/MRI LI-RADS treatment response assessment categories	
Category	**Definition**
LR-TR Nonviable	No lesional enhancement OR treatment-specific expected enhancement pattern
LR-TR Equivocal	Enhancement atypical for treatment-specific expected enhancement pattern and not meeting criteria for LR-TR Viable
LR-TR Viable	Nodular, masslike, or thick irregular tissue in or along the treated lesion with any of the following: • Arterial phase hyperenhancement OR • Washout OR • Enhancement similar to pretreatment

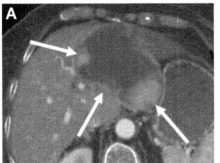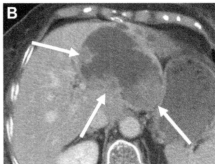

Fig. 5. LR-TR Viable in an 88-year-old woman following transarterial embolization of biopsy-proven HCC. Axial CT in arterial (*A*) and portal venous (*B*) phases demonstrates several masslike areas (*arrows*) along observation periphery, with arterial phase hyperenhancement (*A*) and washout (*B*), corresponding to viable tumor.

both LR-TR Viable and Equivocal categories improved sensitivity to 71% to 73%, with decrease of specificity to 82% to 87%.[57,58] One of the challenges in TRA validation is the fact that most studies do not distinguish between microscopic and macroscopic viable disease. As expected, imaging may not be able to accurately detect microscopic disease; this is supported by a recent study reporting that of pathologically viable tumors with size less than 10 mm, only 10% are categorized LR-TR Viable, as opposed to 67% of pathologically viable tumors measuring greater than or equal to 10 mm.[59]

FUTURE DIRECTIONS

As it did in the past 12 years, LI-RADS continues to grow and improve in response to scientific evidence and user feedback. In 2023, the LI-RADS will update to the current ultrasound surveillance and CT/MRI TRA algorithms and release a new CEUS TRA algorithm for ablative and embolic therapies and a new CT/MRI TRA algorithm for radiation-based therapies. More distant goals include expansion of the applicable population, developing guidance on surveillance with abbreviated MRI, incorporating novel prognostic features,[60] simplifying the algorithms, improving their performance, and developing tools to assist with standardized reporting and lesion tracking over time. The ultimate goal is to transform LI-RADS from a purely diagnostic system to a system that provides diagnostic, prognostic, and predictive information to allow for more individualized patient management.[61]

SUMMARY

Since 2011, LI-RADS had established a broad influence both in clinical care and scientific arena by standardizing imaging, interpretation, and reporting in high-risk patients undergoing surveillance for HCC, diagnosis of potential HCC, and following locoregional treatment with ablative and embolization therapies.

DISCLOSURE

The author has nothing to disclose.

CLINICS CARE POINTS

- LI-RADS algorithms are applicable only to patients with cirrhosis, chronic hepatiis B infection or personal history of HCC.

- LI-RADS ultrasound algorithm includes both diagnostic category and a visualization score reflecting the quality of the study.

- LR-5 category (Definite HCC) has >95% PPV for the diagnosis of HCC, allowing nonsinvasive diagnosis.- 99% of LR-M (probably or definitely malignant not HCC specific) observations are malignant, and approxmately 33% are HCC; therefore, LR-M observations require a biopsy in most cases.

- LR-TR Viable category has 91-96% specificity for viable disease following locoregiomal treatment.

REFERENCES

1. Sung H, Ferlay J, Siegel RL, et al. Global Cancer Statistics 2020: GLOBOCAN Estimates of Incidence and Mortality Worldwide for 36 Cancers in 185 Countries. CA Cancer J Clin 2021;71(3):209–49.
2. Chernyak V, Fowler KJ, Kamaya A, et al. Liver Imaging Reporting and Data System (LI-RADS) Version 2018: Imaging of Hepatocellular Carcinoma in At-Risk Patients. Radiology 2018;289(3):816–30.
3. Marrero JA, Kulik LM, Sirlin CB, et al. Diagnosis, Staging, and Management of Hepatocellular Carcinoma: 2018 Practice Guidance by the American Association for the Study of Liver Diseases. Hepatology 2018;68(2):723–50.
4. Asrani SK, Ghabril MS, Kuo A, et al. Quality measures in HCC care by the Practice Metrics Committee of the American Association for the Study of Liver Diseases. Hepatology 2022;75(5):1289–99.
5. Kierans AS, Chernyak V, Mendiratta-Lala M, et al. The Organ Procurement and Transplantation Network hepatocellular carcinoma classification: Alignment with Liver Imaging Reporting and Data System, current gaps, and future direction. Liver Transpl 2023;29(2):206–16.
6. Available at: https://www.acr.org/-/media/ACR/Files/RADS/LI-RADS/LI-RADS-US-Algorithm-Portrait-2017.pdf: ACR. Accessed July 20, 2023.
7. Fetzer DT, Browning T, Xi Y, et al. Associations of Ultrasound LI-RADS Visualization Score With Examination, Sonographer, and Radiologist Factors: Retrospective Assessment In Over 10,000 Examinations. AJR American Journal of roentgenology 2022;218(6):1010–20.
8. Millet JD, Kamaya A, Choi HH, et al. ACR Ultrasound Liver Reporting and Data System: Multicenter Assessment of Clinical Performance at One Year. J Am Coll Radiol 2019;16(12):1656–62.
9. Tse JR, Shen L, Bird KN, et al. Outcomes of LI-RADS US-2 Subthreshold Observations Detected on Surveillance Ultrasound. AJR American journal of roentgenology 2022;219(5):774 83.
10. Sevco TJ, Masch WR, Maturen KE, et al. Ultrasound (US) LI-RADS: Outcomes of Category US-3 Observations. AJR American journal of roentgenology 2021;217(3):644–50.
11. Tse JR, Shen L, Tiyarattanachai T, et al. Positive predictive value of LI-RADS US-3 observations: multivariable analysis of clinical and imaging features. Abdom Radiol (NY) 2023;48(1):271–81.

12. Simmons O, Fetzer DT, Yokoo T, et al. Predictors of adequate ultrasound quality for hepatocellular carcinoma surveillance in patients with cirrhosis. Alimentary pharmacology & therapeutics 2017;45(1):169–77.
13. Chong N, Schoenberger H, Yekkaluri S, et al. Association between ultrasound quality and test performance for HCC surveillance in patients with cirrhosis: a retrospective cohort study. Aliment Pharmacol Ther 2022;55(6):683–90.
14. Tiyarattanachai T, Fetzer DT, Kamaya A. Multicenter Study of ACR Ultrasound LI-RADS Visualization Scores on Serial Examinations: Implications for Surveillance Strategies. AJR American journal of roentgenology 2022;219(3):445–52.
15. Lee S, Kim YY, Shin J, et al. Percentages of Hepatocellular Carcinoma in LI-RADS Categories with CT and MRI: A Systematic Review and Meta-Analysis. Radiology 2023;307(1):e220646.
16. Zhou Y, Qin Z, Ding J, et al. Risk Stratification and Distribution of Hepatocellular Carcinomas in CEUS and CT/MRI LI-RADS: A Meta-Analysis. Front Oncol 2022; 12:873913.
17. Qin Z, Zhou Y, Ding J, et al. Risk stratification for hepatocellular carcinoma of contrast-enhanced ultrasound Liver Imaging Reporting and Data System (LI-RADS) and the diagnostic performance of LR-5 and LR-M: a systematic review and meta-analysis. Clin Radiol 2022;77(4):e280–6.
18. Mueller C, Waldburger N, Stampfl U, et al. Non-invasive diagnosis of hepatocellular carcinoma revisited. Gut 2018;67(5):991–3.
19. Mitchell DG, Bruix J, Sherman M, et al. LI-RADS (Liver Imaging Reporting and Data System): summary, discussion, and consensus of the LI-RADS Management Working Group and future directions. Hepatology 2015;61(3):1056–65.
20. Kim YY, Lee S, Shin J, et al. Diagnostic performance of CT versus MRI Liver Imaging Reporting and Data System category 5 for hepatocellular carcinoma: a systematic review and meta-analysis of comparative studies. Eur Radiol 2022; 32(10):6723–9.
21. Medow MA, Lucey CR. A qualitative approach to Bayes' theorem. Evid Based Med 2011;16(6):163–7.
22. Ren AH, Zhao PF, Yang DW, et al. Diagnostic performance of MR for hepatocellular carcinoma based on LI-RADS v2018, compared with v2017. J Magn Reson Imaging 2019;50(3):746–55.
23. Safari S, Baratloo A, Elfil M, et al. Evidence Based Emergency Medicine; Part 4: Pre-test and Post-test Probabilities and Fagan's nomogram. Emerg (Tehran) 2016;4(1):48–51.
24. Kang JH, Choi SH, Byun JH, et al. Ancillary features in the Liver Imaging Reporting and Data System: how to improve diagnosis of hepatocellular carcinoma ≤ 3 cm on magnetic resonance imaging. Eur Radiol 2020;30(5):2881–9.
25. Park HJ, Choi BI, Lee ES, et al. How to Differentiate Borderline Hepatic Nodules in Hepatocarcinogenesis: Emphasis on Imaging Diagnosis. Liver Cancer 2017;6(3): 189–203.
26. Takayasu K, Arii S, Sakamoto M, et al. Clinical implication of hypovascular hepatocellular carcinoma studied in 4,474 patients with solitary tumour equal or less than 3 cm. Liver Int 2013;33(5):762–70.
27. Aggarwal A, Horwitz JK, Dolan D, et al. Hypo-vascular hepatocellular carcinoma and liver transplantation: Morphological characteristics and implications on outcomes. J Surg Oncol 2019;120(7):1112–8.
28. Tang Q, Ma C. Performance of Gd-EOB-DTPA-enhanced MRI for the diagnosis of LI-RADS 4 category hepatocellular carcinoma nodules with different diameters. Oncol Lett 2018;16(2):2725–31.

29. Min YW, Gwak GY, Lee MW, et al. Clinical course of sub-centimeter-sized nodules detected during surveillance for hepatocellular carcinoma. World J Gastroenterol : WJG 2012;18(21):2654–60.

30. Kang JH, Choi SH, Lee JS, et al. Inter-reader reliability of CT Liver Imaging Reporting and Data System according to imaging analysis methodology: a systematic review and meta-analysis. Eur Radiol 2021;31(9):6856–67.

31. Kang JH, Choi SH, Lee JS, et al. Interreader Agreement of Liver Imaging Reporting and Data System on MRI: A Systematic Review and Meta-Analysis. J Magn Reson Imaging 2020;52(3):795–804.

32. Available at: https://www.acr.org/-/media/ACR/Files/RADS/LI-RADS/LI-RADS-2018-Core.pdf?la=en. The American College of Radiology LI-RADS v2018 Core. 2018. Accessed July 20, 2023.

33. Cao QY, Zou ZM, Wang Q, et al. MRI manifestations of hepatic perfusion disorders. Exp Ther Med 2018;15(6):5199–204.

34. Ehman EC, Behr SC, Umetsu SE, et al. Rate of observation and inter-observer agreement for LI-RADS major features at CT and MRI in 184 pathology proven hepatocellular carcinomas. Abdom Radiol (NY) 2016;41(5):963–9.

35. Basha MAA, AlAzzazy MZ, Ahmed AF, et al. Does a combined CT and MRI protocol enhance the diagnostic efficacy of LI-RADS in the categorization of hepatic observations? A prospective comparative study. Eur Radiol 2018;28(6):2592–603.

36. Arvind A, Joshi S, Zaki T, et al. Risk of Hepatocellular Carcinoma in Patients With Indeterminate (LI-RADS 3) Liver Observations. Clin Gastroenterol Hepatol 2021;21(4):1091–3.e3.

37. Shropshire E, Mamidipalli A, Wolfson T, et al. LI-RADS ancillary feature prediction of longitudinal category changes in LR-3 observations: an exploratory study. Abdom Radiol (NY) 2020;45(10):3092–102.

38. Tanabe M, Kanki A, Wolfson T, et al. Imaging Outcomes of Liver Imaging Reporting and Data System Version 2014 Category 2, 3, and 4 Observations Detected at CT and MR Imaging. Radiology 2016;281(1):129–39.

39. Hong CW, Park CC, Mamidipalli A, et al. Longitudinal evolution of CT and MRI LI-RADS v2014 category 1, 2, 3, and 4 observations. Eur Radiol 2019;29(9):5073–81.

40. Sofue K, Burke LMB, Nilmini V, et al. Liver imaging reporting and data system category 4 observations in MRI: Risk factors predicting upgrade to category 5. J Magn Reson Imaging 2017;46(3):783–92.

41. Kim YY, Choi JY, Kim SU, et al. MRI Ancillary Features for LI-RADS Category 3 and 4 Observations: Improved Categorization to Indicate the Risk of Hepatic Malignancy. AJR American journal of roentgenology 2020;215(6):1354–62.

42. Yang HJ, Song JS, Choi EJ, et al. Hypovascular hypointense nodules in hepatobiliary phase without T2 hyperintensity: long-term outcomes and added value of DWI in predicting hypervascular transformation. Clin Imag 2018;50:123–9.

43. Saitoh T, Sato S, Yazaki T, et al. Progression of Hepatic Hypovascular Nodules with Hypointensity in the Hepatobiliary Phase of Gd-EOB-DTPA-enhanced MRI in Hepatocellular Carcinoma Cases. Internal medicine (Tokyo, Japan) 2018;57(2):165–71.

44. Hwang JA, Kang TW, Kim YK, et al. Association between non-hypervascular hypointense nodules on gadoxetic acid-enhanced MRI and liver stiffness or hepatocellular carcinoma. European journal of radiology 2017;95:362–9.

45. Cho YK, Kim JW, Kim MY, et al. Non-hypervascular Hypointense Nodules on Hepatocyte Phase Gadoxetic Acid-Enhanced MR Images: Transformation of MR

Hepatobiliary Hypointense Nodules into Hypervascular Hepatocellular Carcinomas. Gut and liver 2018;12(1):79–85.

46. Rosenkrantz AB, Pinnamaneni N, Kierans AS, et al. Hypovascular hepatic nodules at gadoxetic acid-enhanced MRI: whole-lesion hepatobiliary phase histogram metrics for prediction of progression to arterial-enhancing hepatocellular carcinoma. Abdom Radiol (NY) 2016;41(1):63–70.

47. Kim YS, Song JS, Lee HK, et al. Hypovascular hypointense nodules on hepatobiliary phase without T2 hyperintensity on gadoxetic acid-enhanced MR images in patients with chronic liver disease: long-term outcomes and risk factors for hypervascular transformation. Eur Radiol 2016;26(10):3728–36.

48. Tang A, Cruite I, Mitchell DG, et al. Hepatocellular carcinoma imaging systems: why they exist, how they have evolved, and how they differ. Abdom Radiol (NY) 2018;43(1):3–12.

49. EASL Clinical Practice Guidelines. Management of hepatocellular carcinoma. J Hepatol 2018;69(1):182–236.

50. Renzulli M, Pecorelli A, Brandi N, et al. The Feasibility of Liver Biopsy for Undefined Nodules in Patients under Surveillance for Hepatocellular Carcinoma: Is Biopsy Really a Useful Tool? J Clin Med 2022;11(15).

51. Suo L, Chang R, Padmanabhan V, et al. For diagnosis of liver masses, fine-needle aspiration versus needle core biopsy: which is better? J Am Soc Cytopathol 2018; 7(1):46–9.

52. Wang JY, Feng SY, Xu JW, et al. Usefulness of the Contrast-Enhanced Ultrasound Liver Imaging Reporting and Data System in Diagnosing Focal Liver Lesions by Inexperienced Radiologists. J Ultrasound Med 2020;39(8):1537–46.

53. Fowler KJ, Bashir MR, Fetzer DT, et al. Universal Liver Imaging Lexicon: Imaging Atlas for Research and Clinical Practice. Radiographics 2023;43(1):e220066.

54. Chernyak V, Tang A, Do RKG, et al. Liver imaging: it is time to adopt standardized terminology. Eur Radiol 2022;32(9):6291–301.

55. Corwin MT, Lee AY, Fananapazir G, et al. Nonstandardized Terminology to Describe Focal Liver Lesions in Patients at Risk for Hepatocellular Carcinoma: Implications Regarding Clinical Communication. AJR American journal of roentgenology 2018;210(1):85–90.

56. Ahn Y, Choi SH, Jang JK, et al. Impact of the Liver Imaging Reporting and Data System on Research Studies of Diagnosing Hepatocellular Carcinoma Using MRI. Korean J Radiol 2022;23(5):529–38.

57. Kim TH, Woo S, Joo I, et al. LI-RADS treatment response algorithm for detecting incomplete necrosis in hepatocellular carcinoma after locoregional treatment: a systematic review and meta-analysis using individual patient data. Abdom Radiol (NY) 2021;46(8):3717–28.

58. Youn SY, Kim DH, Choi SH, et al. Diagnostic performance of Liver Imaging Reporting and Data System treatment response algorithm: a systematic review and meta-analysis. Eur Radiol 2021;31(7):4785–93.

59. Kim YY, Kim MJ, Yoon JK, et al. Incorporation of Ancillary MRI Features Into the LI-RADS Treatment Response Algorithm: Impact on Diagnostic Performance After Locoregional Treatment of Hepatocellular Carcinoma. AJR American journal of roentgenology 2022;218(3):484–93.

60. Fowler KJ, Burgoyne A, Fraum TJ, et al. Pathologic, Molecular, and Prognostic Radiologic Features of Hepatocellular Carcinoma. Radiographics 2021;41(6): 1611–31.

61. Chernyak V, Fowler KJ, Do RKG, et al. LI-RADS: Looking Back, Looking Forward. Radiology 2023;307(1):e222801.

Evolution of Systemic Therapy in Advanced Hepatocellular Carcinoma

Anthony Bejjani, MD[a], Richard S. Finn, MD[b],*

KEYWORDS

- Hepatocellular carcinoma • HCC • Systemic therapy • Immunotherapy • Treatment

KEY POINTS

- This clinical activity of systemic therapies has significantly improved over time with modern immunotherapy doublets being the standard of care with significant improvements in overall survival and favorable side effect profiles.
- With the large number of approved drugs to treat HCC, the appropriate transition to systemic treatment is critical to maximize the benefit of these drugs and to sequence treatments at progression.
- Moving systemic therapy to earlier stages of HCC is appropriate, recognizing that patients with large, multifocal, and/ or infiltrative HCC are less likely to benefit from loco-regional approaches and are better served with systemic therapy.
- There is now positive phase 3 date for the use of systemic therapy (atezolizumab and bevacizumab) in the adjuvant setting post-curative resection and other studies are ongoing in this setting and in combination with TACE.

INTRODUCTION

The recognition that hepatocellular carcinoma (HCC) is a rising problem globally dates back decades; however, the development of effective medical treatment for the disease has only led to robust improvements in patient outcomes in the recent past. Despite multiple efforts to demonstrate that medical therapy can improve survival in advanced HCC, only in 2008 was the oral multikinase inhibitor sorafenib shown to improve outcomes versus placebo/best supportive care.[1] Key to its success was the definition of appropriate candidates for systemic therapy and clinical trial enrollment. To that end, the development, validation, and deployment of the Barcelona Clinic Liver Cancer (BCLC) staging system for patient stratification was key,[2]

[a] Hematology/Oncology, VA Greater Los Angeles Health System, 11301 Wilshire Boulevard, Los Angeles, CA 90073, USA; [b] Department of Medicine, Division of Hematology/ Oncology, Geffen School of Medicine at UCLA, 2825 Santa Monica Boulevard, Suite 200, Santa Monica, CA 90404, USA
* Corresponding author.
E-mail address: rfinn@mednet.ucla.edu

Surg Oncol Clin N Am 33 (2024) 73–85
https://doi.org/10.1016/j.soc.2023.06.003

recognizing important prognostic factors for outcomes in HCC including performance status, liver function/Child-Pugh, and tumor characteristics including vascular invasion. With the approval of sorafenib, it was recognized that a disease once viewed as impossible for novel drug development became a crowded space for clinical trials that have resulted in several approved agents that are significantly improving survival for patients (**Fig. 1**). These have been a springboard to development in earlier-stage disease, with studies now showing a role for adjuvant therapy after curative resection. As knowledge evolves and regimens are proven to be more active, the importance of multidisciplinary management in patients with all stages of HCC will become more important to optimize patient outcomes. Key to optimizing patient outcomes is an understanding of the evolution and current role of these therapies in the HCC landscape.

SORAFENIB, MULTITARGETED TYROSINE KINASE INHIBITORS, AND VASCULAR ENDOTHELIAL GROWTH FACTOR TARGETING

Sorafenib, a multikinase inhibitor targeting vascular endothelial growth factor (VEGF) receptors 1-3 (VEGFR1-3), platelet-derived growth factor receptor-β (PDGFR-β), and rapidly accelerated fibrosarcoma (RAF), proceeded through clinical development given its dual targeting of angiogenesis and growth pathways.[1] The overall survival (OS) benefit in the phase III SHARP trial, later complemented by a similarly designed phase III trial in the Asia Pacific region, led to its approval by the US Food and Drug Administration (FDA) in 2007.[1,3] Careful selection of patients in the design of these trials, namely limiting recruitment to patients with well compensated cirrhosis (Child Pugh A), likely contributed to successfully capturing the benefit of sorafenib. Although objective response rates were not high (2%), improvements in OS, progression-free survival (PFS), and time to progression (TTP) all favored sorafenib, suggesting that preservation of liver function by halting progression of HCC may have contributed to the overall survival benefit.[1]

Similar multikinase inhibitors with slightly different kinase profiles though still with antiangiogenesis components were selected for further development, balancing efficacy and safety in a group of patients with cancer and underlying liver disease. Tyrosine kinase inhibitors (TKIs) with more potent inhibition of VEGF, such as sunitnib,[4] brivanib (specific for VEGFR and fibroblast growth factor receptors [FGFR]), and linifanib (specific for all VEGFR and PDGFR isoforms), all failed to show either noninferiority (linifanib) or superiority (sunitinib, linifanib, and brivanib) to sorafenib for overall

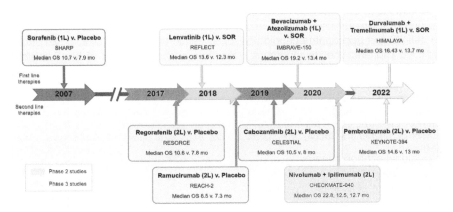

Fig. 1. Evolution of systemic therapy in advanced hepatocellular carcinoma.

survival.[4–6] Brivanib, the first molecule to move into the newly found second-line setting for advanced HCC, also failed to improve overall survival in patients who already progressed on sorafenib (BRISK-PS).[7]

In the front-line setting, lenvatinib, an inhibitor of VEGFR 1-3, FGFR1-4, PDGFRα, RET, and KIT, demonstrated noninferiority to sorafenib for initial treatment of advanced HCC in the REFLECT trial[8] leading to global approval. Although median survival for lenvatinib was longer at 13.6 months vs 12.3 months for sorafenib, the hazard ratio (HR) 0.92 (95% confidence interval [CI] 0.79–1.06) only met the criteria for noninferiority. Key secondary endpoints favored lenvatinib, including an objective response rate (ORR) of 18.8%, and progression-free survival (PFS) of 7.4 months versus 3.7 months. Lenvatinib was associated with more and higher-grade hypertension and proteinuria, whereas the reverse was true for sorafenib in regards to hand-foot skin reaction. Donafenib, a deuterated form of sorafenib, with similar kinase activity, showed improved overall survival (OS) in Chinese patients with advanced HCC over sorafenib.[9]

Alongside TKI development came trials looking at monoclonal antibodies towards VEGF signaling.[10] Bevacizumab, a monoclonal antibody towards a ligand, VEGF-A, was originally evaluated as a single agent[11] and in combination with TACE[12] but did not move into full development in HCC until a decade later. Initial concerns about bleeding risk with bevacizumab were eventually mitigated by refining inclusion criteria and the requirement of a screening endoscopy. Ramucirumab, a monoclonal antibody towards VEGFR-2, had an acceptable safety profile but limited efficacy in all patients with advanced HCC in the initial phase 3 REACH trial looking at its use after sorafenib progression.[13] A preplanned analysis of the AFP high subgroup, however, identified a treatment effect and subsequently led to the phase 3 REACH-2 trial, in which ramucirumab improved overall survival compared with placebo, in patients with AFP of at least 400 ng/mL.[14] This remains the only biomarker approved therapy for HCC.

The second-line setting was a long felt unmet need as there were no drugs shown to improve outcomes for patients intolerant to, or with progression on sorafenib. Approved TKIs in second-line all inhibited VEGF receptor but also targeted other pathways critical for growth and survival such as rearranged during transfection (RET), MET (hepatocyte growth factor receptor), and RAF. Regorafenib, which retains sorafenib's structure with the exception of fluorination in 1 position, has a broader kinase profile including inhibition of VEGFR, PDGFR, RET, KIT, FGFR1, and TIE-2.[15] The phase III RESORCE trial selected patients with advanced HCC and documented progression (versus discontinuing for intolerance) on sorafenib, who had stayed on drug for a minimum period of time, and remained as compensated CP A cirrhosis.[15] The addition of regorafenib led to an improvement in median OS by 2.8 months with a HR of 0.63 compared with placebo.[15] Cabozantinib, an inhibitor of VEGFR1-3, MET, and AXL, improved median OS by 2.2 months compared with placebo after progression on sorafenib in the CELESTIAL trial.[16] Uniquely, this trial also had about 25% of patients who were third-line. Key results from front-line and second-line phase 3 studies are in **Table 1**.

THE CHECKPOINT INHIBITOR REVOLUTION

Monoclonal antibodies targeting 2 immune checkpoints, CTLA-4/B27 and PD-1/PD-L1, have impacted the care of patients with most solid tumors in some way. These agents restore anticancer immunity and by doing so stimulate an immune response to the tumor. This antitumor effect is balanced against the potential for immune-related adverse events that can affect almost any organ. For safety reasons, early

Table 1
Phase III studies

	Trial Name	Active Arm	Control	OS Benefit	ORR
Front-line	SHARP	Sorafenib	Placebo	10.7 vs 7.9 months HR 0.69; 95% CI, 0.55-0.87; P<.001	2%
	REFLECT	Lenvatinib	Sorafenib	13.6 vs 12.3 months HR 0.92; 95% CI, 0.79–1.06, noninferior	18.8%
	IMbrave150	Atezolizumab/ bevacizumab	Sorafenib	19.2 vs 13.4 months HR 0.58; 95% CI, 0.42–0.79, P<.001	30%
Second-line	HIMALAYA	Durvalumab/ tremlimumab	Sorafenib	16.43 vs 13.77 months HR 0.78; 96.02% CI, 0.65–0.93, P=.0035	20%
	RESORCE	Regorafenib	Placebo	10.6 vs 7.8 months HR 0.63; 95% CI 0.50–0.79, P<.0001	7%
	CELESTIAL[a]	Cabozantinib	Placebo	10.2 vs 8.0 months HR, 0.76; 95% CI 0.63-0.92; P=.005	7%
	REACH-2	Ramucirumab	Placebo	8.5 vs 7.3 months HR 0.71; 95% CI 0.531–0.949; P=.0199	5%
	KEYNOTE 240	Pembrolizumab	Placebo	13.8 vs 10.6 months HR 0.781; 95% CI, 0.611–0.998; P=.0238	18.3%
	CHECKMATE 040 (Phase 1b/2)	Nivolumab/ ipilimumab	Single-arm	mOS 22.8 months (95% CI 9.4-NE)	32%

Abbreviation: ORR, objective response rate by RECIST 1.1.
[a] Also included third-line.

clinical trials with these agents excluded patients with cirrhosis and/or active viral hepatitis. This led to a paucity of data about the safety of these medications in patients with chronic liver disease, a critical deficiency given that more than 90% of patients with HCC have underlying cirrhosis.[17] Initial landmark studies with single-agent checkpoint inhibitors were the single-arm phase I/II Checkmate 040 trial and single-arm phase II Keynote 224 trial, evaluating nivolumab and pembrolizumab, respectively, in patients previously treated with sorafenib.[18,19] Both agents had objective response rates (ORR) of approximately 15-20% and were well tolerated in mostly Child Pugh A cirrhosis patients, leading to accelerated approval by the FDA.[18,19] Data from case series and another cohort of Checkmate 040 showed that Child Pugh B7/8 patients with HCC had comparable safety profiles to Child Pugh A patients, although with OS only in range of 5.9 to 8.6 months.[20–22] Nivolumab and pembrolizumab were then evaluated in randomized phase III trials – Checkmate 459 for nivolumab and KEYNOTE 240 (worldwide)/KEYNOTE 394 (Asia) for pembrolizumab.[23–25] Nivolumab was evaluated in the front-line setting versus sorafenib with the primary endpoint of improving OS. The phase III study recapitulated the single-agent activity of nivolumab that supported its accelerated approval and the favorable safety profile but failed to meet the primary endpoint of improving OS. Survival was 16.4 months with nivolumab and 14.7 months with sorafenib (HR 0.85 [95% CI 0.72–1.02];

P=.075).[25] Interestingly, the upper limit of the CI here was 1.02, less than the 1.08 used in other trials to declare noninferiority; however, the study was designed as a superiority trial. Two phase III trials evaluated pembrolizumab versus placebo in the second-line setting. Again, the safety and single-agent response rates were confirmed, but in KEYNOTE 240 overall survival narrowly missed this coprimary endpoint, whereas in KEYNOTE 394, it did meet its survival endpoint.[23,24] More recently, the results of the RATIONALE-301 study evaluating the single-agent PD-1 inhibitor tislelizumab versus sorafenib in the front-line setting were presented.[26] This study met its noninferiority endpoint with similar results as CHECKMATE 459 with an HR for OS 0.85 (95% CI 0.712–1.019; P=.0398) and an ORR of 14.3% and a long median duration of response of 36.1 months, no %. Adverse events with single-agent checkpoint inhibitors in HCC patients are similar to other malignancies and most commonly include fatigue, hypothyroidism, and rash.[27] The predominant difference is how to manage immune-related hepatitis, accounting for a difference in baseline liver function.[27]

The results of studies with single-agent checkpoint inhibitors suggested that strategies to improve response rates may yield significant improvements in OS. Despite efforts, no single biomarker has been validated to help select patients who may benefit from these agents. In addition, there are no clinical criteria that identify patients who respond better or worse to these agents. Preclinical studies demonstrated that targeting VEGF induces changes in the tumor microenvironment and provided rationale to evaluate anti-VEGF/checkpoint inhibitor combinations in clinical trials.[28] Atezolizumab, a PD-L1 inhibitor, and bevacizumab, were explored initially in a phase Ib trial that demonstrated a strong signal of antitumor efficacy with an ORR of 36% and really no new safety signals as compared with single-agent PD-1 therapies.[29] This led to IMbrave150, a global Phase III randomized study comparing atezolizumab and bevacizumab to sorafenib as initial treatment for patients with advanced HCC.[30] The study mandated endoscopy within 6 months of trial enrollment to minimize the risk of variceal bleeding seen in the first studies of single-agent bevacizumab HCC studies.[11,30] The study accrued a global population of patients with high-risk characteristics including main portal vein invasion. The study met its coprimary endpoints of improving PFS and OS, with mature results showing median OS of 19.2 months with atezolizumab and bevacizumab compared to 13.4 months with sorafenib (HR, 0.66 [95% CI, 0.52, 0.85]; P=.0009).[31] In addition, ORR was 30% with combination. Again, there were no new safety signals with the combination, which was better tolerated than sorafenib. Notably, the combination had higher grade and frequency of hypertension and proteinuria, but was otherwise better tolerated than sorafenib with improved quality of life. With these data, atezolizumab and bevacizumab defined a new standard for front-line HCC. The anti-VEGF antibody and checkpoint inhibitor approach was further supported by a phase III study in China comparing the combination of sintilimab (anti PD-1 antibody) and IBI305 (bevacizumab biosimilar) to sorafenib with a HR of 0.57 (95% CI, 0.43 to 0.75; P<.0001) for OS favoring the combination in its first interim analysis.[32]

A similar effort was underway to combine anti-VEGF TKIs and checkpoint inhibitors. Pembrolizumab, combined with lenvatinib, demonstrated safety with a response rate of 36% and median OS of 22 months in a single-arm phase Ib study.[33] This led to the global randomized phase III LEAP-002 study comparing pembrolizumab and lenvatinib to lenvatinib alone. Of note, this was the first phase III study in advanced HCC using lenvatinib, instead of sorafenib, as a control arm. It was also one of the few placebo-controlled and double-blind studies, whereas other phase 3 studies were open-label since their designs compared an intravenous to oral regimen. Despite an

ORR of 26.1%, and an OS of 21.2 months, the combination did not statistically improve OS versus 19.0 months with lenvatinib (HR = 0.840; P=.0227), missing the statistical threshold of P=.0185.[34] The OS of the lenvatinib arm of 19 months was un-expected given the survival time 13.4 months for lenvatinib in the reflect study. These data represent the improvement in survival in HCC that has occurred over time with improved access after progression on first-line therapy to active drugs approved in HCC. Atezolizumab and cabozantinib similarly missed its endpoint of OS in initial treatment of patients with HCC, compared with sorafenib, in the Phase III COSMIC-312 study, with a median OS of 15.4 months in the combination group versus 15.5 months in the sorafenib group (HR 0.90, 96% CI 0.69–1·18; P=.44).[35] The objective response rates and PFS were lower than expected for the combination arm.[35] Unlike the 2 trials previously mentioned, a recently presented study using the PD-1 inhibitor camrelizumab and the VEGFR2-TKI rivoceranib did meet both its primary endpoints in a phase III study versus sorafenib.[36] PFS was improved from 3.7 to 5.6 months (HR 0.5, 95% CI 0.41–0.65; P<.000) and OS from 15.2 to 22.1 months (HR, 0.62, 95% CI 0.49–0.80; P<.0001). The study accrued over 80% of the patients from Asia and as a result over 70% of the patients had hepatitis B virus (HBV)-related liver cancer. The confirmed ORR for the combination was 25.4%. The regimen was associated with a higher than expected side effect profile, with over 80% of patients having grade 3/4 treatment-related adverse events. Although most of the adverse events are similar to other VEGFR targeted TKIs, rivoceranib uniquely is associated with reactive cutaneous capillary endothelial proliferation. Approval of this regimen is pending.

The success of dual checkpoint inhibition (CTLA-4 and PD-(L)-1) in other solid tumors led to exploring their use in patients with HCC. The Checkmate 040 trial included multiple dosing schedules of nivolumab and the CTLA4 antibody ipilimumab in patients after prior sorafenib.[37] The nivolumab/ipilimumab arm with nivolumab dosed at 1 mg/kg and ipilimumab at 3 mg/kg (4 total doses) followed by nivolumab 240 mg every 2 weeks received accelerated approval given ORR 33% and the highest median OS of the combinations (22.8 months [9.4 to NE]).[37] Tremelimumab, a CTLA-4 inhibitor, had shown some clinical activity in patients with HCC coinfected with hepatitis C, but had not yet been approved for any indication in other cancers.[38] A phase I/II study established using a 1-time dose of tremelimumab 300 mg along with durvalumab 1500 mg as what would be recommended to proceed in a phase III study.[39] In the phase III HIMALAYA trial, the combination arm (STRIDE) and durvalumab monotherapy arm were individually compared with sorafenib for superiority in overall survival and noninferiority for overall survival, respectively.[40] The primary endpoint of the study being the combination arm versus sorafenib. The median OS was 16.43 months with STRIDE (HR 0.78, P=.0035), 16.56 months with durvalumab (HR 0.86, 95.67% CI 0.73-1.03; noninferiority margin 1.08).[40] Neither regimen improved PFS, but the ORR with the combination was 20.1%. These regimens are generally well-tolerated, but consistent with both of these PD-1/CTLA-4 combinations, there is an increase in immune-mediated adverse events compared with regimens that contain only a PD-(L)-1 antibody.

BRINGING SYSTEMIC THERAPY TO EARLIER-STAGE DISEASE

Before there were effective systemic therapies, the use of local-regional approaches such as TACE expanded to fill a void. Now, with more active regimens that have double-digit response rates and improve survival, there is increased recognition that some patients with intermediate-stage (BCLC B) HCC may be better served with systemic therapy. The phase III studies discussed previously consistently have 15% to 20% of patients who are BCLC B and felt not to be appropriate for locoregional therapy (LRT) or have progressed after LRT. There is increased recognition that BCLC stage B patients still represent a large unmet need given the heterogeneity of the group, with some patients presenting with multiple large lesions having the same prognosis as those with advanced BCLC C stage.[41] In an updated BCLC strategy, it is recognized that some patients, such as those with diffuse, infiltrating tumors, may be better served with systemic therapy.[42]

In the context of a clinical trial, there is strong rationale to combine systemic treatment with LRT. From a clinical standpoint, LRT is not curative, and although it has been shown to improve survival, patients eventually become refractory or develop contraindications such as migration to an advanced stage. Therefore, a systemic treatment that can improve tumor control and delay progression would be of value. Scientifically, ischemia induced by TACE leads to an increase in angiogenic factors like VEGF, which may potentially be exploited by the various anti-VEGF therapies approved for treatment in HCC. After its approval, sorafenib was evaluated with TACE in numerous trials that were largely negative.[43,44] In a phase III open-label study from China, lenvatinib significantly improved OS (17.8 versus 11.5 months; HR, 0.45; $P<.001$) when added to TACE in a phase III trial compared with lenvatinib monotherapy.[45] This trial accrued patients with mostly HBV-related HCC and included a diverse population of patients including those with macrovascular invasion and extrahepatic spread. The applicability to a Western population is not entirely clear; however, the trial demonstrated that combining newer active agents with TACE may be safe and effective. In addition, tumor necrosis induced by LRT may stimulate antigen release and modify the tumor microenvironment, which in combination with immunotherapy, can augment an antitumor response with checkpoint inhibitors.[46] There are several ongoing studies assessing the efficacy of this approach (**Table 2**), and if positive, it could establish a new standard of care for intermediate HCC.

HCC is a curable disease when found early. Resection and ablation have been shown to curative in select patients, but the recurrence rate is high.[47,48] Recurrence in HCC follows a bimodal pattern, with early recurrences felt to be secondary to the primary tumor, whereas a later recurrence is felt to be a result of de novo HCC occurring in a diseased organ. Some patients with BCLC stage A also may have a high risk of recurrence and prognosis similar to stage B patients based on tumor characteristics.[49] Management strategies may overlap for those with BCLC stage A and B, where resection may be feasible for some staged as B without portal hypertension, and be at high risk for recurrence. Examples may include resection of a primary tumor greater than 5 cm in diameter or resection of multifocal disease with microvascular invasion. Adjuvant studies with sorafenib after curative resection in patients at high risk for recurrence did not show any benefit. There are several ongoing phase III studies using checkpoint inhibitor-based therapies in this setting (**Table 3**). Data from the IMbrave050 phase III trial were recently presented.[50] The study evaluated the ability of atezolizumab and bevacizumab to delay recurrence following curative resection or ablation in patients at high risk of recurrence (**Table 4**). Patients were randomized in an open-label study to receive 1 year of atezolizumab and bevacizumab every 3 weeks or active surveillance. The primary endpoint was recurrence free-survival (RFS). With a median follow-up of 17.4 months, there was a significant decrease in the risk of recurrence with atezolizumab and bevacizumab; HR = 0.72 (95% CI: 0.56, 0.93, $P=.012$). The median RFS was not reached in either arm. The benefit was consistent across subgroups, and the safety profile of the combination was as expected based on prior studies. Given this is an adjuvant study with tissue readily

Table 2
Phase III trials for concurrent/adjuvant treatment after locoregional treatment for hepatocellular carcinoma

Systemic Therapy Used	Locoregional Treatment Used	Comparator Group	Disease Setting	Target Number of Patients	Name of Trial	NCT Identifier
Lenvatinib and camrelizumab	TACE	Lenvatinib	BCLC stage C	168	LEN-TAC	NCT05738616
Lenvatinib and sintilimab	TACE	Lenvatinib	BCLC stage C	427	N/A	NCT05608200
Lenvatinib and pembrolizumab	TACE	TACE + placebo	BCLC stage A or B not amenable to curative ablation or resection	450	LEAP-012	NCT04246177
Lenvatinib with TACE	TACE	Lenvatinib after progression after TACE	BCLC stage C	299	N/A	NCT05220020
Durvalumab/tremelimumab or Durvalumab/tremelimumab/ lenvatinib	TACE	TACE alone	BCLC stage A or B not amenable to curative ablation or resection	525	EMERALD-3	NCT05301842
Durvalumab/bevacizumab or durvalumab	TACE	TACE + placebo	BCLC stage A or B not amenable to curative ablation or resection	724	EMERALD-1	NCT03778957
Nivolumab/ipilimumab or nivolumab	TACE	Active surveillance after TACE	BCLC stage A or B not amenable to curative ablation or resection	N/A	CheckMate 74W	NCT04340193
Nivolumab	TACE	Active surveillance after TACE	BCLC stage A or B not amenable to curative ablation or resection	522	TACE-3	NCT04268888

Table 3
Adjuvant phase III trials in early hepatocellular carcinoma

Checkpoint Regimen	Treatment	Control Arm	N	Title	Trial Number
Pembrolizumab	Resection or ablation	Placebo	950	KEYNOTE-937	NCT03867084
Nivolumab	Resection or ablation	Placebo	545	CheckMate 9DX	NCT03383458
Durvalumab/ bevacizumab or durvalumab	Resection or ablation	Placebo	908	EMERALD-2	NCT03847428
Atezolizumab/ bevacizumab	Resection or ablation	Active surveillance	668	IMbrave050	NCT04102098

available, biomarker studies to help identify patients who may get a greater benefit are awaited. The study data were too immature to assess effects on OS. Taken together, these data hold promise that systemic therapy will be an option for patients after resection or ablation to help reduce the risk of recurrence. Results from single-agent immunotherapy trials and other combinations are awaited.

FUTURE DIRECTIONS

The therapeutic options for patients with HCC is changing rapidly. Survival for patients with advanced disease has markedly improved with the introduction of checkpoint inhibitors in the front-line setting. How to optimally sequence the available drugs is not known, but as in other malignancies, exposing patients to sequential active agents may continue to improve survival. Already, there are numerous early phase studies evaluating novel combination to approach to new clinical scenarios:

What to do for patients who do not benefit from front-line IO (de novo resistance)
How best to treat patients who originally benefit from IO but then progress (acquired resistance)

Molecular studies have identified several potential targets for therapy, and results are awaited.[48] In addition, the safety of newer regimens has been established, and their use in the presurgical/neoadjuvant setting is yielding important biomarker insights and higher response rates than have been seen with their use in the advanced

Table 4
Definition of high-risk of recurrence used in the IMBRAVE 050 study

Curative Treatment	Criteria for High Risk of HCC Recurrence
Resection	• ≤3 tumors, with largest tumor >5 cm regardless of vascular invasion[a] or poor tumor differentiation (grade 3 or 4) • ≥4 tumors, with largest tumor ≤5 cm regardless of vascular invasion[a] or poor tumor differentiation (grade 3 or 4) • ≤3 tumors, with largest tumor ≤5 cm with vascular invasion[a] and/or poor tumor differentiation (grade 3 or 4)
Ablation	• 1 tumor >2 cm but ≤5 cm • Multiple tumors (≤4 tumors), all ≤ 5 cm

[a] Microvascular invasion or minor macrovascular portal vein invasion of the portal vein—Vp1/Vp2.

setting.[51–54] The use of this approach to assess novel regimens and incorporating pathologic response rates as an endpoint will soon occur. Taken together, this is an exciting time for clinicians in the HCC space, as research efforts are being translated into better outcomes for patients.

CLINICS CARE POINTS

- Systemic therapy improves survival in patients with advanced HCC and those with intermediate disease that are unsuitable for locoregional therapies.
- Atezolizumab and bevacizumab is the most acitve systmeic therapy available based on its magnitude of benefit in OS and PFS and ORR.
- For patients that cannot receive bevacizumab, durvalumab and tremelimumab is an acceptable option.
- At progression on an IO regimen, sequencing other approved drugs is an appropriate options.
- Systemic therapy is active in early stage disease as seen in the IMBRAVE 050 study in the adjuvant seeting.

REFERENCES

1. Llovet JM, Ricci S, Mazzaferro V, et al. Sorafenib in advanced hepatocellular carcinoma. N Engl J Med 2008;359:378–90.
2. Llovet JM, Bru C, Bruix J. Prognosis of hepatocellular carcinoma: the BCLC staging classification. Semin Liver Dis 1999;19:329–38.
3. Cheng AL, Kang YK, Chen Z, et al. Efficacy and safety of sorafenib in patients in the Asia-Pacific region with advanced hepatocellular carcinoma: a phase III randomised, double-blind, placebo-controlled trial. Lancet Oncol 2009;10:25–34.
4. Cheng AL, Kang YK, Lin DY, et al. Sunitinib versus sorafenib in advanced hepatocellular cancer: results of a randomized phase III trial. J Clin Oncol 2013;31:4067–75.
5. Johnson PJ, Qin S, Park J-W, et al. Brivanib versus sorafenib as first-line therapy in patients with unresectable, advanced hepatocellular carcinoma: results from the randomized phase III BRISK-FL study. J Clin Oncol 2013;31:3517–24.
6. Cainap C, Qin S, Huang W-T, et al. Linifanib versus sorafenib in patients with advanced hepatocellular carcinoma: results of a randomized phase III trial. J Clin Oncol 2015;;33:172–9.
7. Llovet JM, Decaens T, Raoul JL, et al. Brivanib in patients with advanced hepatocellular carcinoma who were intolerant to sorafenib or for whom sorafenib failed: results from the randomized phase III BRISK-PS study. J Clin Oncol 2013;31:3509–16.
8. Kudo M, Finn RS, Qin S, et al. Lenvatinib versus sorafenib in first-line treatment of patients with unresectable hepatocellular carcinoma: a randomised phase 3 non-inferiority trial. Lancet 2018;391:1163–73.
9. Qin S, Bi F, Gu S, et al. Donafenib versus sorafenib in first-line treatment of unresectable or metastatic hepatocellular carcinoma: a randomized, open-label, parallel-controlled phase II-III trial. J Clin Oncol 2021;39:3002–11.
10. Finn RS, Bentley G, Britten CD, et al. Targeting vascular endothelial growth factor with the monoclonal antibody bevacizumab inhibits human hepatocellular carcinoma cells growing in an orthotopic mouse model. Liver Int 2009;29:284–90.

11. Siegel AB, Cohen EI, Ocean A, et al. Phase II trial evaluating the clinical and biologic effects of bevacizumab in unresectable hepatocellular carcinoma. J Clin Oncol 2008;26:2992–8.
12. Britten CD, Gomes AS, Wainberg ZA, et al. Transarterial chemoembolization plus or minus intravenous bevacizumab in the treatment of hepatocellular cancer: a pilot study. BMC Cancer 2012;12:16.
13. Zhu AX, Park JO, Ryoo BY, et al. Ramucirumab versus placebo as second-line treatment in patients with advanced hepatocellular carcinoma following first-line therapy with sorafenib (REACH): a randomised, double-blind, multicentre, phase 3 trial. Lancet Oncol 2015;16:859–70.
14. Zhu AX, Kang Y-K, Yen C-J, et al. REACH-2: a randomized, double-blind, placebo-controlled phase 3 study of ramucirumab versus placebo as second-line treatment in patients with advanced hepatocellular carcinoma (HCC) and elevated baseline alpha-fetoprotein (AFP) following first-line sorafenib. J Clin Oncol 2018;36:4003.
15. Bruix J, Qin S, Merle P, et al. Regorafenib for patients with hepatocellular carcinoma who progressed on sorafenib treatment (RESORCE): a randomised, double-blind, placebo-controlled, phase 3 trial. Lancet 2017;389:56–66.
16. Abou-Alfa GK, Meyer T, Cheng AL, et al. Cabozantinib in patients with advanced and progressing hepatocellular carcinoma. N Engl J Med 2018;379:54–63.
17. Llovet JM, Montal R, Sia D, et al. Molecular therapies and precision medicine for hepatocellular carcinoma. Nat Rev Clin Oncol 2018;15:599–616.
18. El-Khoueiry AB, Sangro B, Yau T, et al. Nivolumab in patients with advanced hepatocellular carcinoma (CheckMate 040): an open-label, non-comparative, phase 1/2 dose escalation and expansion trial. Lancet 2017;389:2492–502.
19. Zhu AX, Finn RS, Edeline J, et al. Pembrolizumab in patients with advanced hepatocellular carcinoma previously treated with sorafenib (KEYNOTE-224): a non-randomised, open-label phase 2 trial. Lancet Oncol 2018;19:940–52.
20. Kambhampati S, Bauer KE, Bracci PM, et al. Nivolumab in patients with advanced hepatocellular carcinoma and Child-Pugh class B cirrhosis: safety and clinical outcomes in a retrospective case series. Cancer 2019;125:3234–41.
21. Scheiner B, Kirstein MM, Hucke F, et al. Programmed cell death protein-1 (PD-1)-targeted immunotherapy in advanced hepatocellular carcinoma: efficacy and safety data from an international multicentre real-world cohort. Aliment Pharmacol Ther 2019;49:1323–33.
22. Kudo M, Matilla A, Santoro A, et al. Checkmate-040: Nivolumab (NIVO) in patients (pts) with advanced hepatocellular carcinoma (aHCC) and Child-Pugh B (CPB) status. J Clin Oncol 2019;37:327.
23. Finn RS, Ryoo BY, Merle P, et al. Pembrolizumab as second-line therapy in patients with advanced hepatocellular carcinoma in KEYNOTE-240: a randomized, double-blind, phase III trial. J Clin Oncol 2020;38:193–202.
24. Qin S, Chen Z, Fang W, et al. Pembrolizumab versus placebo as second-line therapy in patients from asia with advanced hepatocellular carcinoma: a randomized, double-blind, Phase III Trial. J Clin Oncol 2023;41:1434–43.
25. Yau T, Park JW, Finn RS, et al. Nivolumab versus sorafenib in advanced hepatocellular carcinoma (CheckMate 459): a randomised, multicentre, open-label, phase 3 trial. Lancet Oncol 2022;23:77–90.
26. Qin S, Kudo M, Meyer T, et al. Final analysis of RATIONALE-301: randomized, phase 3 study of tislelizumab versus sorafenib as first-line treatment for unresectable hepatocellular carcinoma. Presented at the ESMO Annual Meeting, Paris (France), 2022.

27. Bejjani A, Finn RS. Current state of immunotherapy for HCC—supporting data and toxicity management. Current Hepatology Reports 2018;17(4):434–43.

28. Chen DS, Mellman I. Oncology meets immunology: the cancer-immunity cycle. Immunity 2013;39:1–10.

29. Lee MS, Ryoo BY, Hsu CH, et al. Atezolizumab with or without bevacizumab in unresectable hepatocellular carcinoma (GO30140): an open-label, multicentre, phase 1b study. Lancet Oncol 2020;21:808–20.

30. Finn RS, Qin S, Ikeda M, et al. Atezolizumab plus bevacizumab in unresectable hepatocellular carcinoma. N Engl J Med 2020;382:1894–905.

31. Finn RS, Qin S, Ikeda M, et al. IMbrave150: updated overall survival (OS) data from a global, randomized, open-label phase III study of atezolizumab (atezo) + bevacizumab (bev) versus sorafenib (sor) in patients (pts) with unresectable hepatocellular carcinoma (HCC). J Clin Oncol 2021;39:267.

32. Ren Z, Xu J, Bai Y, et al. Sintilimab plus a bevacizumab biosimilar (IBI305) versus sorafenib in unresectable hepatocellular carcinoma (ORIENT-32): a randomised, open-label, phase 2-3 study. Lancet Oncol 2021;22:977–90.

33. Finn RS, Ikeda M, Zhu AX, et al. Phase Ib study of lenvatinib plus pembrolizumab in patients with unresectable hepatocellular carcinoma. J Clin Oncol 2020;38:2960–70.

34. Finn RS, Kudo M, Merle P, et al. LBA34 - Primary results from the phase III LEAP-002 study: lenvatinib plus pembrolizumab versus lenvatinib as first-line (1L) therapy for advanced hepatocellular carcinoma (aHCC). Ann Oncol 2022; 33(suppl_7):S808–69.

35. Kelley RK, Rimassa L, Cheng AL, et al. Cabozantinib plus atezolizumab versus sorafenib for advanced hepatocellular carcinoma (COSMIC-312): a multicentre, open-label, randomised, phase 3 trial. Lancet Oncol 2022;23:995–1008.

36. Qin S, Chan LS, Gu S, et al. Camrelizumab (C) plus rivoceranib (R) vs. sorafenib (S) as first-line therapy for unresectable hepatocellular carcinoma (uHCC): a randomized, phase III trial. Presented at the ESMO, Paris (France), 2022.

37. Yau T, Kang YK, Kim TY, et al. Efficacy and safety of nivolumab plus ipilimumab in patients with advanced hepatocellular carcinoma previously treated with sorafenib: the CheckMate 040 randomized clinical trial. JAMA Oncol 2020;6:e204564.

38. Sangro B, Gomez-Martin C, de la Mata M, et al. A clinical trial of CTLA-4 blockade with tremelimumab in patients with hepatocellular carcinoma and chronic hepatitis C. J Hepatol 2013;59:81–8.

39. Kelley RK, Sangro B, Harris W, et al. Safety, efficacy, and pharmacodynamics of tremelimumab plus durvalumab for patients with unresectable hepatocellular carcinoma: randomized expansion of a phase I/II study. J Clin Oncol 2021;39:2991–3001.

40. Abou-Alfa GK, Lau G, Kudo M, et al. Tremelimumab plus durvalumab in unresectable hepatocellular carcinoma. NEJM Evidence 2022;1. EVIDoa2100070.

41. Biolato M, Gallusi G, Iavarone M, et al. Prognostic ability of BCLC-B subclassification in patients with hepatocellular carcinoma undergoing transarterial chemoembolization. Ann Hepatol 2018;17:110–8.

42. Reig M, Forner A, Rimola J, et al. BCLC strategy for prognosis prediction and treatment recommendation: the 2022 update. J Hepatol 2022;76:681–93.

43. Lencioni R, Llovet JM, Han G, et al. Sorafenib or placebo plus TACE with doxorubicin-eluting beads for intermediate stage HCC: the SPACE trial. J Hepatol 2016;64:1090–8.

44. Meyer T, Fox R, Ma YT, et al. Sorafenib in combination with transarterial chemoembolisation in patients with unresectable hepatocellular carcinoma (TACE 2): a randomised placebo-controlled, double-blind, phase 3 trial. Lancet Gastroenterol Hepatol 2017;2:565–75.

45. Peng Z, Fan W, Zhu B, et al. Lenvatinib combined with transarterial chemoembolization as first-line treatment for advanced hepatocellular carcinoma: a phase III, randomized clinical trial (LAUNCH). J Clin Oncol 2023;41:117–27.
46. Greten TF, Mauda-Havakuk M, Heinrich B, et al. Combined locoregional-immunotherapy for liver cancer. J Hepatol 2019;70:999–1007.
47. Chan AWH, Zhong J, Berhane S, et al. Development of pre and post-operative models to predict early recurrence of hepatocellular carcinoma after surgical resection. J Hepatol 2018;69:1284–93.
48. Llovet JM, Kelley RK, Villanueva A, et al. Hepatocellular carcinoma. Nat Rev Dis Primers 2021;7:6.
49. Wan L, Dong DH, Wu XN, et al. Single large nodule (>5 cm) prognosis in hepatocellular carcinoma: kinship with Barcelona Clinic Liver Cancer (BCLC) stage A or B? Med Sci Monit 2020;26:e926797.
50. Chow P CM, Cheng AL, et al. IMbrave050: Phase 3 study of adjuvant atezolizumab + bevacizumab versus active surveillance in patients with hepatocellular carcinoma at high risk of disease recurrence following resection or ablation. AACR Annual Meeting Abstract CT003, 2023.
51. Marron TU, Galsky MD, Taouli B, et al. Neoadjuvant clinical trials provide a window of opportunity for cancer drug discovery. Nat Med 2022;28:626–9.
52. Marron TU, Schwartz M, Corbett V, et al. Neoadjuvant immunotherapy for hepatocellular carcinoma. J Hepatocell Carcinoma 2022;9:571–81.
53. Ho WJ, Zhu Q, Durham J, et al. Neoadjuvant cabozantinib and nivolumab converts locally advanced HCC into resectable disease with enhanced antitumor immunity. Nat Cancer 2021;2:891–903.
54. Kaseb AO, Hasanov E, Cao HST, et al. Perioperative nivolumab monotherapy versus nivolumab plus ipilimumab in resectable hepatocellular carcinoma: a randomised, open-label, phase 2 trial. Lancet Gastroenterol Hepatol 2022;7:208–18.

Role of Neoadjuvant Therapy Prior to Curative Resection in Hepatocellular Carcinoma

Zachary Whitham, MD[a], David Hsiehchen, MD[b],*

KEYWORDS

- Immune checkpoint inhibitors • Hepatocellular carcinoma
- Neoadjuvant systemic therapy • Immunotherapy

KEY POINTS

- Neoadjuvant therapy possesses several potential advantages for the treatment of solid tumors.
- Neoadjuvant immune checkpoint inhibitor (ICI) therapy in hepatocellular carcinoma has demonstrated promising preliminary results with limited toxicity and no evidence of delaying surgery in patients with early-stage, resectable disease.
- Neoadjuvant space lacks biomarkers needed to guide decisions about which patients would have the most benefit from neoadjuvant ICI therapy.

INTRODUCTION

Liver cancer has the sixth highest incidence and third highest mortality amongst cancer types worldwide with hepatocellular carcinoma (HCC) being the most frequent type of primary liver tumor.[1] Widespread public health measures to control viral hepatitis in the United States have led to a decline in HCC incidence; however, the continued sharp rise of non-alcoholic fatty liver disease may threaten to reverse this trend.[2] HCC typically arises in a background of cirrhosis leading to recommendations for screening programs from organizations such as the American Association of Study of Liver Disease (AASLD).[3] Despite measures to capture patients with early-stage disease, only a small portion of patients present with adequate liver function and future liver remnant for curative resection or ablation.[4] For the few patients that undergo curative intent resection or ablation, 5-year recurrence rates remain as high as 70%.[5,6]

Support: T32 DK007745 (Z. Whitham).

[a] Department of Surgery, Division of Surgical Oncology, University of Texas Southwestern Medical Center, 5323 Harry Hines Boulevard, Dallas, TX 75390, USA; [b] Department of Medicine, Division of Hematology/Oncology, University of Texas Southwestern Medical Center, 5323 Harry Hines Boulevard, Dallas, TX 75390, USA

* Corresponding author.

E-mail address: David.hsieh@utsouthwestern.edu

Surg Oncol Clin N Am 33 (2024) 87–97
https://doi.org/10.1016/j.soc.2023.07.003
1055-3207/24/© 2023 Elsevier Inc. All rights reserved.

Following resection or ablation there is a bimodal pattern of intrahepatic recurrence with early emergence of disease attributed to residual micrometastases,[6–8] whereas late recurrence is most likely secondary to carcinogenesis of the field defect within the liver itself.[9] Given the high rates of recurrence following curative treatment and the few patients eligible for curative treatment at HCC diagnosis, it is crucial that treatment strategies be implemented to reduce recurrence and downstage patients to curative treatments.

Neoadjuvant therapy possesses several potential advantages for the treatment of solid tumors. In HCC, neoadjuvant therapy offers an opportunity for tumor downstaging as well as the prevention of early recurrence.[10] As many patients present with impaired liver function at baseline, preservation of future liver remnant by downsizing tumors may expand the patient population eligible for surgery or ablation.[11] This concept expands to liver transplantation as it may downstage patients into Milan or expanded transplant criteria.[12] Neoadjuvant therapy may eliminate these occult cancer cells which are left following resection and also offer a measure to test the biology of the HCC tumor. For instance, pathologic response to neoadjuvant therapy may offer prognostic information and help guide the selection of adjuvant treatment regimens.[10]

This review will provide an overview of immune checkpoint inhibitors (ICIs) as neoadjuvant therapy for HCC. We will begin by summarizing the mechanisms of action of neoadjuvant ICIs, followed by a review of recent results from neoadjuvant trials in resectable and locally advanced HCC, and then give an overview of ongoing clinical trials and future directions for the field.

IMMUNOLOGIC MECHANISMS OF NEOADJUVANT IMMUNE CHECKPOINT INHIBITORS

Immune checkpoints are cell surface receptors that help to regulate the activity of the adaptive immune system to permit peripheral tolerance.[8,13] Programmed death receptor 1 (PD-1) is a transmembrane protein present on activated CD8 T cells, natural killer cells, B cells, and antigen-presenting cells.[14] This receptor protein interacts with its ligand, programmed death-ligand 1 (PD-L1), to induce exhaustion in CD8 T cells preventing autoimmunity. Malignant tumors may upregulate PD-L1 to reduce the adaptive immune response through tumor evasion leading to tumor growth and metastasis.[8,14,15] ICIs disrupt PD-1 and PD-L1 interactions which allow effector CD8 T cells to continue immune surveillance and destruction of tumoral cells. While some tumor responses to ICIs may be delayed, administration of even a single dose has been shown to bolster CD8 T cell activity and increase anti-tumoral responses.[16] This suggests that even short exposures to ICIs may trigger potent and possibly durable anti-tumor effects, supporting the utility of ICIs in a defined neoadjuvant treatment window.

Immunotherapy has been studied throughout all phases of cancer treatment. New clinical data are now showing the advantages of neoadjuvant ICI administration in breast and colon cancers.[17,18] Liu and colleagues studied neoadjuvant versus adjuvant immunotherapy in a murine breast cancer model demonstrating greater therapeutic efficacy in the neoadjuvant setting.[19] When the tumor remains in vivo during immunotherapy, a wide range of neoantigens are released allowing for a robust T-cell response. Administering immunotherapy in the adjuvant setting failed to demonstrate the same level of clonal expansion. Creating the sustained response desired for cancer therapy requires neoantigen abundance.[20] Tumor-draining lymph nodes may also play a significant role in T-cell activation.[21] In theory, removal of neoantigens within the tumor during surgery may also limit the robustness of the T-cell response in the adjuvant setting. Additionally, neoadjuvant immunotherapy with clonal T-cell expansion has been shown to create a "vaccine effect," where primed T cells circulate with active tumor surveillance.[19,22] A recent trial in stage III and IV melanoma patients undergoing planned surgical resection demonstrated that neoadjuvant plus adjuvant pembrolizumab (PD-1) therapy offered greater event-free survival compared to adjuvant pembrolizumab alone. This trial serves as a proof-of-principle for the rationale of neoadjuvant therapy in tumor subtypes including HCC with high tumor immunogenicity.[23]

NEOADJUVANT SYSTEMIC THERAPY TRIALS IN HEPATOCELLULAR CARCINOMA

Since the approval of sorafenib, a non-specific inhibitor of vascular endothelial growth factor receptor (VEGFR) and tyrosine kinase (TKI), in patients with advanced HCC in 2007, systemic therapy options have evolved dramatically in the treatment of HCC. In 2018, lenvatinib, a VEGFR and TKI inhibitor, demonstrated noninferiority to sorafenib in overall survival with a superior objective response rate, 19% versus 6%, compared to sorafenib.[24] Regorafenib and cabozantinib (VEGFR inhibitors) were both approved as second-line therapies in the advanced HCC setting, both with response rates under 10%.[25,26] Given the relatively low objective response rates seen with TKIs with or without VEGFR inhibition, it is not surprising to see the lack of efficacy of these agents in the neoadjuvant HCC setting. In 2020, the landscape of systemic therapy for HCC changed dramatically as the IMbrave150 clinical trial demonstrated that the combination of atezolizumab (anti-PD-L1 ICI) and bevacizumab (anti-vascular endothelial growth factor [VEGF] antibody) was superior to sorafenib in the treatment of advanced HCC with respect to overall survival.[27] Perhaps the most encouraging result from the IMbrave150 trial was the objective response rates of nearly 30% in the combination ICI arm. The significant improvement of response rates seen with modern immune checkpoint inhibition compared to the low response rates observed with anti-angiogenic TKI and VEGF inhibitors for the first time has offered promise not only for the treatment of advanced HCC, but also in the neoadjuvant and adjuvant setting (which is discussed elsewhere in this issue).

Kaseb and colleagues compared the safety and effectiveness of perioperative monotherapy with nivolumab (anti-PD-1 antibody) and nivolumab plus ipilimumab (anti-cytotoxic T lymphocyte–associated antigen-4 antibody) in 27 patients with resectable HCC.[28] Each patient (n = 13) in this randomized, open-label phase 2 trial received 3 doses of nivolumab alone in 2-week intervals prior to surgical resection with adjuvant therapy administered for up to years following surgery. Patients (n = 14) selected for combination therapy received a single dose of ipilimumab with the first cycle of neoadjuvant nivolumab and up to 4 doses of ipilimumab every 6 weeks in the adjuvant setting. Grade 3 to 4 adverse events were higher with nivolumab plus ipilimumab (43%) than with nivolumab alone (23%). In both arms there was no delay in receipt of curative surgical resection due to complications of treatment. Of the 20 patients who underwent surgical resection, there was no significant difference in significant pathologic response, defined as greater than 70% tumor rate of necrosis (3 of 9, 33% in nivolumab group vs 3 of 11, 27% in nivolumab and ipilimumab group). The estimated median progression-free survival was 9.4 months (95% confidence interval [CI] 1.47–not estimable) in the nivolumab group and 19.5 months (95% CI 8–not estimable) with combination therapy. The estimated 2-year progression-free survival was 42% (95% CI 21–81) with nivolumab alone compared to 26% (95% CI 8–78) with combination therapy. The pathologic response rate was associated with increased T-cell infiltrate within the tumor microenvironment in both cohorts. Importantly, only 75% of patients with a priori identified "resectable" disease underwent surgical resection calling into question both the efficacy of the neoadjuvant therapy regimen and the definition of resectable disease that needs to be clarified in future neoadjuvant and window of opportunity trials.

Marron and colleagues performed an open-label, phase-2 trial evaluating perioperative cemiplimab, an anti-PD-1 antibody, for resectable HCC.[29] All 21 patients enrolled in this trial received 2 cycles of cemiplimab 3 weeks apart prior to definitive surgical resection within 22 days of initiation of therapy. In the adjuvant setting, patients received up to an additional 8 cycles of therapy every 3 weeks. The primary endpoint of the study was significant pathologic tumor necrosis, defined as greater than 70% on the resected specimen. Similar to the previous study, treatment was well tolerated with only 1 patient having a delay in surgical resection of 2 weeks due to pneumonitis requiring treatment with steroids. This study evaluated the safety and tolerability of this medication in the neoadjuvant setting with 20 (95%) patients reporting an adverse event, including 7 (21%) patients developing grade 3 adverse events. Of the 20 patients who received surgery, 4 (20%) demonstrated significant tumor necrosis, while 3 (15%) patients achieved complete pathologic response. Three additional patients had between 50% and 70% necrosis of the resected tumor, while the remaining 13 patients had 30% or less necrosis. Only 3 (15%) patients had a radiographic response prior to surgery by response evaluation criteria in solid tumors (RECIST) criteria without statistically significant correlation to pathologic results. Similar to the previous trial by Kaseb and colleagues, pre-treatment tumor biopsies and blood collection were mandated enabling comparisons between pre-treatment and post-treatment tissue. Patients demonstrating pathologic response of at least 50% had increased tumor cell infiltrate with clonal expansion of intratumoral $CXCL13^+$ T helper cells and granzyme K^+PD-1^+ effector-like $CD8^+$ T cell.[30] As data collection continues with ongoing adjuvant therapy, we eagerly await further results showing the efficacy of cemiplimab with regards to survival outcome measures.

In the previously described 2 clinical trials, patients were enrolled based on being eligible for surgical resection prior to therapy. Ho and colleagues performed a phase 1b study of neoadjuvant cabozantinib (TKI) and nivolumab in patients with HCC.[11] Each of the 15 patients enrolled in this trial had locally advanced or borderline resectable HCC that would not have been candidates for upfront surgery due to high-risk features including multifocal disease, portal vein invasion, or tumor diameter greater than 10 cm. Every patient received 8 weeks of cabozantinib and 4 cycles of nivolumab every 2 weeks starting after 2 weeks lead in the period of cabozantinib monotherapy. No patients experienced treatment-related adverse events that delayed surgical resection; 1 death occurred before surgery due to biliary sepsis. Fourteen patients (93.3%) experienced a treatment-related adverse event. Two (13.3%) patients experienced a grade 3 or higher adverse events, both of which were immune related attributed to nivolumab. Twelve of the 14 patients who completed the neoadjuvant regimen became eligible for surgery and underwent complete resection. Twelve patients achieved an R0 resection with pathology demonstrating major pathologic response (>90% tumor necrosis) in 5 (42%) patients, including 1 complete pathologic response. Based on RECIST criteria, only 1 (7%) patient had a radiographic response with the remainder showing stable disease. With a median follow-up of 1 year, 5 of the 12 patients who underwent surgical resection had recurred. Overall survival at the time of analysis was not mature. Similar to the previous 2 studies, mandatory pre-therapy tumor biopsies allowed an in-depth profiling of tumor tissue to examine the effect of ICI therapy. Immune profiling demonstrated an enrichment in T effector cells, as well as tertiary lymphoid structures, CD138+ plasma cells, and a distinct spatial arrangement of B cells in responders as compared to non-responders, indicating an orchestrated

B-cell contribution to antitumor immunity in HCC. Again, the lack of radiographic response coupled with the definition of "resectability" calls into question whether this trial truly demonstrated downstaging of patients outside of resection criteria and whether neoadjuvant therapy can be a successful downstaging strategy.

Xia and colleagues studied the efficacy of perioperative camrelizumab (PD-1 inhibitor) and apatinib (VEGF-2 inhibitor) for patients with resectable HCC in a phase 2 trial.[31] Each patient received 3 cycles of neoadjuvant camrelizumab 2 weeks apart while taking a daily dose of oral apatinib for the first 21 days of treatment. Adjuvant therapy was initiated within 4 weeks of surgery consisting of 8 cycles of camrelizumab in 3-week intervals and oral apatinib. Twenty patients were enrolled with 17 patients ultimately undergoing surgical resection; 2 patients withdrew their consent prior to completion and 1 patient experienced progression prohibiting surgical resection. Of these patients, 3 (18%) achieved a major pathologic response, defined as at least 90% tissue necrosis on final histology, and an additional patient (6%) experienced a complete pathologic response. Three (17%) achieved a radiographic response based on RECIST criteria and 6 (33%) patients based on modified RECIST criteria. For the 18 patients who completed neoadjuvant therapy, 16 (89%) experienced an adverse event with 3 (17%) grade 3 or higher adverse events. One (5.6%) patient required initial dose adjustment of apatinib due to hypertension. Two (11.1%) required treatment with steroids for severe liver function injury or severe skin rash prior to surgery. In the perioperative period, 7 (38.8%) patients experienced posthepatectomy grade A liver failure as per International Study Group of Liver Surgery criteria, 3 (16.7%) experienced postoperative biliary leakage, 2 (11.1%) patients required blood transfusions, and 1 (5.6%) patient experienced chest tightness. Adjuvant therapy was given to 13 patients. Although the high degree of pathologic response on the resected specimen was promising, the relatively high rate of postoperative complications calls into the question the future role of combination of camrelizumab and apatinib therapy in the neoadjuvant setting.

UNANSWERED QUESTIONS AND CHALLENGE TRIALS IN THE NEOADJUVANT HEPATOCELLULAR CARCINOMA SETTING

The 4 previously mentioned trials highlight both the promise of ICI therapy in the neoadjuvant setting and the issues that need further clarification prior to widespread adaptation of neoadjuvant therapy for HCC. Perhaps the most pertinent issue in trial design for neoadjuvant studies using ICIs is the appropriate validated endpoint. Pathologic endpoints such as pathologic complete response or objective response rates have been validated in neoadjuvant trials using ICIs in both breast and colon cancer, but thus far no similar endpoint in HCC neoadjuvant trials has been validated. The AASLD consensus guidelines have recommended either pathologic response or 1-year recurrence as appropriate endpoints, but this is based on a paucity of evidence.[32] As such, in all 4 aforementioned neoadjuvant trials disparate endpoints, other than safety and tolerability, were used. Whether pathologic response rates are associated with overall survival in HCC similar to breast and colon cancer remains unclear and future maturation of the previously described trials coupled with readouts from currently accruing trials might offer more insight into the selection of appropriate endpoints.

The second unanswered question in neoadjuvant HCC clinical trial design is the optimal duration of therapy. Since the aim of ICI therapy in a neoadjuvant setting is not primarily through a tumor-killing mechanism, but more so priming of the immune system against micrometastatic disease in an attempt to reduce early recurrences, a briefer duration of ICI therapy may be warranted and decrease the potential of immune-related adverse events (irAEs) delaying or preventing curative therapy.

Table 1
Actively accruing clinical trials for neoadjuvant immunotherapy in hepatocellular carcinoma.

NCT Identifier	Study Design	Inclusion Criteria	Intervention	Primary Endpoint	N
PRIMER-1/NCT05185739	Phase II Multi-arm	Resectable HCC	Pembrolizumab every 3 wk for 2 cycles Lenvatinib 8 or 12 mg PO daily for 6 wk Pembrolizumab every 3 wk for 2 cycles and lenvatinib daily	Major pathologic response (>90% tumor necrosis)	60
DYNAMIC/NCT04954339	Phase II Single arm	Potentially resectable BCLC stage B/C HCC High-risk resectable HCC	Atezolizumab and bevacizumab for 2 cycles preoperatively, then 4 additional cycles postoperatively	Pathologic complete response rate Immunophenotypes of tumor-infiltrating immune cells	45
NCT04658147	Phase I Multi-arm	Resectable HCC	Nivolumab every 4 wk for 2 cycles preoperatively, then every 4 wk for 10 cycles postoperatively Nivolumab with relatlimab every 4 wk for 2 cycles preoperatively, then every 4 wk for 10 cycles postoperatively	Number of patients who complete treatment and proceed to surgery	20
NCT03510871	Phase II Single arm	Resectable HCC with high risk for recurrence	Nivolumab and ipilimumab every 3 wk for 2–4 cycles prior to surgery	Tumor shrinkage >10% by RECIST criteria	40
NCT04123379	Phase II Multi-arm	Resectable HCC	Cohorts A, B are for non-small cell lung cancer Cohort C: nivolumab every 4 wk for 2 cycles preoperatively, then 3 cycles postoperatively Cohort D: nivolumab every 4 wk for 2 cycles preoperatively with BMS-813160 orally twice daily for 28 d, then nivolumab for 3 cycles postoperatively Cohort E: nivolumab every 4 wk for 2 cycles preoperatively with BMS-986253 once, then nivolumab for 3 cycles postoperatively	Major pathologic response (>90% tumor necrosis) Significant tumor necrosis (>70% necrosis)	50

Trial	Phase/Design	Condition	Intervention	Primary Endpoint	N
NCT03867370	Phase Ib/II Multi-arm	Resectable HCC	Toripalimab single preoperative dose, then every 3 wk for up to 48 wk postoperatively Toripalimab single dose with lenvatinib orally daily, then toripalimab every 3 wk with daily lenvatinib for up to 48 wk Toripalimab single dose with lenvatinib orally daily, then toripalimab alone every 3 wk for up to 48 wk	Pathologic response rate	40
NCT05194293	Phase II Single arm	Resectable HCC	Regorafenib orally daily for 21 d with durvalumab IV on day 1, cycle repeats every 28 d for up to 2 y until decision to proceed to surgery, disease progression, excessive toxicity, or patient withdrawal	Objective response rate by RECIST criteria	30
CAPT/NCT04930315	Phase II Multi-arm	Resectable HCC	Perioperative camrelizumab every 2 wk for 4 cycles with apatinib orally daily for 6 wk, then camrelizumab every 2 wk for additional 8 cycles Adjuvant camrelizumab every 2 wk for up to 12 cycles	1-y tumor recurrence-free rate	78
NCT03916627	Phase II	Resectable HCC, Non-Small Cell Lung Cancer, Head and Neck Squamous Cell Cancer	Cohort A is non-small cell lung cancer Cohort B1: perioperative cemiplimab Cohort B2: perioperative cemiplimab with preoperative SBRT Cohort B3: perioperative cemiplimab and fianlimab Cohort C is head and neck squamous cell cancer	Significant tumor necrosis	73
NeoLeap-HCC/NCT05389527	Phase II Single arm	Resectable HCC	Pembrolizumab every 3 wk for 3 cycles with lenvatinib orally daily for 9 wk, then resume combination therapy for up to 1 y	Major pathologic response ($\geq$50% necrosis)	43

(continued on next page)

Table 1
(continued)

NCT Identifier	Study Design	Inclusion Criteria	Intervention	Primary Endpoint	N
NCT04721132	Phase II Single Arm	Resectable HCC	Atezolizumab and bevacizumab every 3 wk for 3 cycles preoperatively	Pathologic complete response rate Incidence of adverse events	30
PRIME-HCC/NCT03682276	Phase I/II Single arm	Resectable HCC; ECOG 0–1; CP-A	Ipilimumab once with nivolumab every 3 wk for 2 cycles	Delay to surgery Treatment-related adverse events	32

Abbreviations: BCLC, Barcelona Clinic Liver Cancer; HCC, hepatocellular carcinoma; RECIST, response evaluation criteria in solid tumors; SBRT, stereotactic body radiation therapy.

Unless otherwise stated, all trials were open-label and inclusion criteria required patients to be deemed adequate surgical candidates with Eastern Cooperative Oncology Group performance status of 0–1 and Child-Pugh class A.

Previous research has demonstrated a cumulative effect of ICI therapy and related irAEs with toxicities occurring more often after a month or longer of therapy. Given that the selection of patients is based on resectable disease and the rationale for ICI neoadjuvant therapy is based on a priming mechanism it seems evident that a shorter duration of therapy is reasonable.

The final challenge in the neoadjuvant space is the lack of biomarkers needed to guide decisions about which patients would have the most benefit from neoadjuvant ICI therapy. In the 4 previously described studies radiographic response by traditional RECIST criteria was not an effective marker of response. Furthermore, pathologic response rates in the studies ranged from 18% to 42% and it is unclear whether this correlated with long-term survival outcomes. Since the diagnosis and subsequent treatment decisions involving HCC historically have not included tumor biopsy, the identification of prognostic and predictive biomarkers guiding treatment have lagged behind other tumor types. Undoubtedly, this is an unmet need and investigators leveraging the preliminary results from the aforementioned studies will be able to identify and validate biomarkers in the future.

FUTURE DIRECTION-ONGOING NEOADJUVANT CLINICAL TRIALS

Numerous clinical trials are currently investigating the role of different immune modulators either as monotherapy or as combination therapy in the neoadjuvant setting. Key questions being addressed include efficacy, safety, predictive biomarkers, and length of treatment. **Table 1** provides an overview of the neoadjuvant studies currently open for accrual.

SUMMARY

Immunotherapy has rapidly changed the standard of care in multiple areas of oncology. Given success in the setting of unresectable HCC and the advantages of neoadjuvant therapy, many trials are demonstrating the safety and feasibility of combination of ICI/TKIs in patients with resectable or locally advanced HCC. We look forward to the ongoing and future trials with neoadjuvant therapy to possibly guide treatment decisions and increase survival in early-stage HCC.

CLINICS CARE POINTS

- Advances in systemic therapy, especially ICIs, have increased survival outcomes in advanced HCC and are now starting to be used in the neoadjuvant setting.
- Neoadjuvant ICI therapy in HCC has demonstrated promising preliminary results with limited toxicity and no evidence of delaying surgery in patients with early-stage, resectable disease.
- Despite the encouraging preliminary results, further investigations are needed to determine the optimal duration of therapy, validate endpoints, and identify biomarkers to guide treatment decisions.

REFERENCES

1. Sung H, Ferlay J, Siegel RL, et al. Global Cancer Statistics 2020: GLOBOCAN Estimates of Incidence and Mortality Worldwide for 36 Cancers in 185 Countries. CA Cancer J Clin 2021;71(3):209–49.

2. Han J, Wang B, Liu W, et al. Declining disease burden of HCC in the United States, 1992-2017: A population-based analysis. Hepatology 2022;76(3):576–88.

3. Konyn P, Ahmed A, Kim D. Current epidemiology in hepatocellular carcinoma. Expert Rev Gastroenterol Hepatol 2021;15(11):1295–307.

4. Akateh C, Black SM, Conteh L, et al. Neoadjuvant and adjuvant treatment strategies for hepatocellular carcinoma. World J Gastroenterol 2019;25(28):3704–21.

5. Marubashi S, Gotoh K, Akita H, et al. Anatomical versus non-anatomical resection for hepatocellular carcinoma. Br J Surg 2015;102(7):776–84.

6. Tabrizian P, Jibara G, Shrager B, et al. Recurrence of hepatocellular cancer after resection: patterns, treatments, and prognosis. Ann Surg 2015;261(5):947–55.

7. Portolani N, Coniglio A, Ghidoni S, et al. Early and late recurrence after liver resection for hepatocellular carcinoma: prognostic and therapeutic implications. Ann Surg 2006;243(2):229–35.

8. Laschtowitz A, Roderburg C, Tacke F, et al. Preoperative Immunotherapy in Hepatocellular Carcinoma: Current State of the Art. J Hepatocell Carcinoma 2023; 10:181–91.

9. Pellicoro A, Ramachandran P, Iredale JP, et al. Liver fibrosis and repair: immune regulation of wound healing in a solid organ. Nat Rev Immunol 2014;14(3): 181–94.

10. Marron TU, Schwartz M, Corbett V, et al. Neoadjuvant Immunotherapy for Hepatocellular Carcinoma. J Hepatocell Carcinoma 2022;9:571–81.

11. Ho WJ, Zhu Q, Durham J, et al. Neoadjuvant Cabozantinib and Nivolumab Converts Locally Advanced HCC into Resectable Disease with Enhanced Antitumor Immunity. Nat Cancer 2021;2(9):891–903.

12. Zhang T, Zhang L, Xu Y, et al. Neoadjuvant therapy and immunotherapy strategies for hepatocellular carcinoma. Am J Cancer Res 2020;10(6):1658–67.

13. Finn OJ. Cancer immunology. N Engl J Med 2008;358(25):2704–15.

14. Calderaro J, Rousseau B, Amaddeo G, et al. Programmed death ligand 1 expression in hepatocellular carcinoma: Relationship With clinical and pathological features. Hepatology 2016;64(6):2038–46.

15. Garris CS, Arlauckas SP, Kohler RH, et al. Successful Anti-PD-1 Cancer Immunotherapy Requires T Cell-Dendritic Cell Crosstalk Involving the Cytokines IFN-γ and IL-12. Immunity 2018;49(6):1148–61.e7.

16. Huang AC, Orlowski RJ, Xu X, et al. A single dose of neoadjuvant PD-1 blockade predicts clinical outcomes in resectable melanoma. Nat Med 2019;25(3):454–61.

17. Blank CU, Rozeman EA, Fanchi LF, et al. Neoadjuvant versus adjuvant ipilimumab plus nivolumab in macroscopic stage III melanoma. Nat Med 2018;24(11): 1655–61.

18. Forde PM, Chaft JE, Smith KN, et al. Neoadjuvant PD-1 Blockade in Resectable Lung Cancer. N Engl J Med 2018;378(21):1976–86.

19. Liu J, Blake SJ, Yong MC, et al. Improved Efficacy of Neoadjuvant Compared to Adjuvant Immunotherapy to Eradicate Metastatic Disease. Cancer Discov 2016; 6(12):1382–99.

20. Rizvi NA, Hellmann MD, Snyder A, et al. Cancer immunology. Mutational landscape determines sensitivity to PD-1 blockade in non-small cell lung cancer. Science 2015;348(6230):124–8.

21. Tsushima F, Yao S, Shin T, et al. Interaction between B7-H1 and PD-1 determines initiation and reversal of T-cell anergy. Blood 2007;110(1):180–5.

22. Topalian SL, Taube JM, Pardoll DM. Neoadjuvant checkpoint blockade for cancer immunotherapy. Science 2020;367(6477).

23. Patel SP, Othus M, Chen Y, et al. Neoadjuvant-Adjuvant or Adjuvant-Only Pembrolizumab in Advanced Melanoma. N Engl J Med 2023;388(9):813–23.
24. Kudo M, Finn RS, Qin S, et al. Lenvatinib versus sorafenib in first-line treatment of patients with unresectable hepatocellular carcinoma: a randomised phase 3 non-inferiority trial. Lancet 2018;391(10126):1163–73.
25. Bruix J, Qin S, Merle P, et al. Regorafenib for patients with hepatocellular carcinoma who progressed on sorafenib treatment (RESORCE): a randomised, double-blind, placebo-controlled, phase 3 trial. Lancet 2017;389(10064):56–66.
26. Abou-Alfa GK, Meyer T, Cheng AL, et al. Cabozantinib in Patients with Advanced and Progressing Hepatocellular Carcinoma. N Engl J Med 2018;379(1):54–63.
27. Finn RS, Qin S, Ikeda M, et al. Atezolizumab plus Bevacizumab in Unresectable Hepatocellular Carcinoma. N Engl J Med 2020;382(20):1894–905.
28. Kaseb AO, Hasanov E, Cao HST, et al. Perioperative nivolumab monotherapy versus nivolumab plus ipilimumab in resectable hepatocellular carcinoma: a randomised, open-label, phase 2 trial. Lancet Gastroenterol Hepatol 2022;7(3):208–18.
29. Marron TU, Fiel MI, Hamon P, et al. Neoadjuvant cemiplimab for resectable hepatocellular carcinoma: a single-arm, open-label, phase 2 trial. Lancet Gastroenterol Hepatol 2022;7(3):219–29.
30. Magen A, Hamon P, Fiaschi N, et al. Intratumoral dendritic cell-CD4(+) T helper cell niches enable CD8(+) T cell differentiation following PD-1 blockade in hepatocellular carcinoma. Nat Med 2023;29(6):1389–99.
31. Xia Y, Tang W, Qian X, et al. Efficacy and safety of camrelizumab plus apatinib during the perioperative period in resectable hepatocellular carcinoma: a single-arm, open label, phase II clinical trial. J Immunother Cancer 2022;10(4).
32. Llovet JM, Villanueva A, Marrero JA, et al. Trial Design and Endpoints in Hepatocellular Carcinoma: AASLD Consensus Conference. Hepatology 2021;73(Suppl 1):158–91.

Expanding Indications for Surgical Resection in Hepatocellular Carcinoma

What is the Evidence?

Gloria Y. Chang, MD[a], Adam C. Yopp, MD[b],*

KEYWORDS

- Hepatic resection • Hepatocellular carcinoma • Surgical resection
- Portal vein tumor thrombosis

KEY POINTS

- Hepatic resection is one of the mainstays of curative therapy for hepatocellular carcinoma (HCC).
- Hepatic functional reserve can be evaluated using tests measuring indocynanine green clearance.
- The ultimate goal of hepatic resection for HCC should remain obtaining an appropriate oncological margin while maintaining sufficient functional liver remnant.

INTRODUCTION

Hepatocellular carcinoma (HCC) is the third leading cause of cancer-related deaths worldwide and the fastest-rising cause of cancer related mortality in the United States.[1,2] Factors determining outcome following HCC diagnosis are complex and heterogenous in nature, dependent not only on tumor burden and biology, but on underlying liver function and patient performance status. These complexities require maintaining a tenuous balance between tumor- and patient-related factors with decisions regarding treatment strategies best made in the context of a multidisciplinary team approach.[3]

Surgical resection is the one of the mainstay curative treatment options in patients with localized, early-stage HCC associated with 5 year overall survival rates

[a] Department of Surgery, Division of Surgical Oncology, University of Texas Southwestern Medical Center, Dallas, TX 75390, USA; [b] Department of Surgery, Division of Surgical Oncology, University of Texas Southwestern Medical Center, 5323 Harry Hines Boulevard, Dallas, TX 75390, USA
* Corresponding author. Department of Surgery, Division of Surgical Oncology, University of Texas Southwestern Medical Center, 5323 Harry Hines Boulevard, Dallas, TX 75390.
E-mail address: adam.yopp@utsouthwestern.edu

Surg Oncol Clin N Am 33 (2024) 99–109
https://doi.org/10.1016/j.soc.2023.07.004

approaching 60%.[4,5] As such, clinical practice guidelines have recommended curative surgical resection in early stage HCC.[6] However, owing to heterogeneity of the patient population and low utilization of HCC screening, only 10% to 37% of patients presenting with HCC are candidates for surgical resection based on traditional indications.[7,8] With improvements in surgical approaches and perioperative care as well as the advent of direct-acting antivirals in hepatitis C treatment and more efficacious systemic therapy regimens in the neoadjuvant and adjuvant settings, more patients may be eligible for surgical resection outside traditional guideline recommendations.

Herein, we discuss the indications for surgical resection in HCC related to patient-related factors and review the evidence for expanding surgical indications focusing on patients presenting with macrovascular tumor invasion or multifocal tumors.

SURGICAL RESECTION FOR EARLY-STAGE HEPATOCELLULAR CARCINOMA

Hepatic resection is one of the mainstays of curative therapy for HCC. The appropriate selection of resectable candidates requires careful consideration of a multitude of factors including tumor burden (size and number of nodules, presence of vascular involvement, extrahepatic spread), patient factors (performance status, underlying liver function), and availability of other therapies (access to transplantation, interventional procedures, immunotherapies).

The existence of a multitude of HCC staging systems exemplifies the complexity of evaluating patients for curative surgical resection. According to the Barcelona Clinic Liver Cancer (BCLC) system endorsed by the American Association for the Study of Liver Diseases (AASLD) and the European Association for the Study of the Liver (EASL), early stage (0/A) disease with a solitary tumor is recommended for surgical resection. BCLC stage 0 constitutes patients with a single nodule $\leq$ 2 cm in size with preserved liver function and BCLC stage A represents a solitary lesion or up to 3 nodules $\leq$ 3 cm in size with preserved liver function and good patient performance status.[9] The ultimate goal of hepatic resection for HCC should remain obtaining an appropriate oncological margin while maintaining sufficient functional liver remnant.

Although perioperative mortality following hepatic resection for HCC has decreased over the past 3 decades,[10,11] as indications for resection continue to expand, careful preoperative assessment of the degree of functional impairment of the liver is crucial to ensuring that oncological benefits outweigh the risks of posthepatectomy liver failure (PHLF). PHLF, defined by the International Study Group of Liver Surgery as an increased prothrombin time and concomitant hyperbilirubinemia on or after postoperative day 5, is associated with perioperative mortality rates of more than 50%.[12]

Preoperative Assessment: Clinical and Blood Tests

Multiple validated tools are used to stratify patients based on preresection liver function to determine both feasibility of resection and the extent of resection tolerability to lessen the risks of PHLF. In the West, the two most utilized prognostic tools are Child–Pugh (CP) classification and Model for End-Stage Liver Disease (MELD) score. In 1964, Child and Turcotte developed a classification based on serum albumin, total bilirubin, and prothrombin time, as well as the presence and grade of hepatic encephalopathy and ascites, to predict short-term mortality following portacaval shunt surgery.[13] Although widely used to stratify patients for hepatic resection of HCC, neither the original Child Turcotte score nor the Pugh modification was designed specifically for this purpose.[14] Nevertheless, the Child Turcotte Pugh (CP) score continues to be widely used in surgical decision making for liver resection (LR). In most Western centers, LR is limited to CP A patients, with CP C status universally accepted as a contraindication to resection.

The MELD score, based on serum total bilirubin, international normalized ratio (INR), and creatinine, was first reported to predict early death following an elective transjugular intrahepatic portosystemic shunt placement but is now used primarily for allocation of organs for liver transplantation.[15] Multiple studies have suggested an elevated MELD score associated with PHLF following hepatectomy for HCC in cirrhotic patients. Teh and colleagues demonstrated that cirrhotic patients with cirrhosis and a MELD score of less than 9 have low risk of PHLF perioperative morbidity and patients with a MELD score $\geq$ 9 a greater risk of postoperative liver failure and perioperative mortality.[16–18]

The presence of portal hypertension, defined as a hepatic venous pressure gradient (HVPG) $\geq$ 10 mm Hg, has been defined by both AASLD and EASL guidelines as a contraindication to HCC-related hepatic resection.[19,20] On the basis of a study by Bruix and colleagues in 29 patients undergoing LR for HCC, elevated HVPG measures with concomitant thrombocytopenia was associated with decompensation following hepatic resection in CP A cirrhotic patients.[21] Twenty-three of the 29 study patients underwent at least a major hepatectomy (sectionectomy or greater), calling into question the applicability of their findings in operations involving the resection of minor LRs involving less than 3 segments. As HVPG is not normally measured in most centers due to its invasive nature, surrogates of absent clinically significant portal hypertension including platelet count greater than 100,000 per microliter, ascites, and grade III or higher portosystemic varices are more commonly used to determine candidates for resection[22]

In addition, hepatic functional reserve can be evaluated using tests measuring indocynanine green clearance (IGC). If hepatic IGC retention is greater than 20% at 15 minutes following injection, no more than one-sixth of the liver should be resected. If IGC retention is greater than 30%, then limited resection or ablative techniques are appropriate.[23] Currently the use of IGC is not performed outside of clinical trials in the United States.

EXPANDING INDICATIONS FOR RESECTION OF HEPATOCELLULAR CARCINOMA

In recent years, there has been an evolution in the indications for surgical resection for HCC, moving away from guideline recommended criterion limiting resection to patients with a solitary tumor and preserved liver function and performance status, to consideration of resection in tumors exhibiting multifocality (BCLC B) or macrovascular tumor invasion (BCLC C).[24–28]

Tsilimigras and colleagues in an international multi-institutional database study comprising Western institutions compared the oncological outcomes following curative intent hepatic resection between patients within (BCLC 0/A) and beyond (BCLC B/C) traditional criteria.[29] They reported a 5 year overall survival of 51.6% within the BCLC B/C group, a favorable comparison when taken in context with historical cohorts of patients treated with either locoregional and/or systemic therapy.[30,31]

A separate retrospective, single institution study performed in China by Guo and colleagues in a predominantly hepatitis B cohort demonstrated that surgical resection improved long-term survival among patients with BCLC-B and BCLC-C HCC compared with locoregional therapy or best supportive care when matched according to patient- and tumor-related factors.[32] These 2 studies highlight the heterogeneity of the intermediate and advanced HCC stages and the potential benefit of surgical resection in a carefully selected patient population. Hereafter, we will discuss separately the role for surgical resection in HCC taking into consideration multifocality and presence of macrovascular invasion with emphasis on contrasting outcome measures including overall survival from traditional guideline recommended treatment measures. As large tumor size in the absence of multifocality and macrovascular invasion is no longer considered outside of traditional guideline recommendations as a contraindication for surgical resection it will not be further discussed.[9]

Tumor Multifocality

AASLD and EASL guidelines using the BCLC staging and treatment algorithm, recommend patients presenting with multifocal HCC in the absence of vascular invasion (BCLC B or intermediate stage) to undergo either liver transplantation if within criteria and/or locoregional therapy consisting of transarterial chemoembolization (TACE) or radioembolization (TARE).[19,20] Multifocality encompasses a wide variation in tumor number ranging from 2 to innumerable masses and as such, careful selection of patients for hepatic resection is needed based on identifying preoperative factors predicting early tumor recurrences. This is especially paramount as resection of multifocal tumors oftentimes includes a larger parenchymal resection increasing the potential of PHLF.

Of note, the BCLC-B group is composed of a large, heterogeneous population, and current BCLC guidelines may potentially overlook a select subgroup that may still benefit from surgical resection especially in a cohort that lack liver transplant options due to organ shortage (especially in Eastern countries), socioeconomic factors, or tumors outside standard or expanded transplant criteria.[33] Recently, several studies have suggested broadening the indications for hepatic resection in conjunction with the identification of preoperative indices aimed at guiding decision making in this cohort of patients.[32–34]

The first step in determining the applicability of hepatic resection in patients presenting with multifocal HCC in the absence of vascular invasion is whether tumor-, patient-, or hospital-based criteria for transplant are met. Especially in the presence of underlying liver dysfunction, liver transplantion in the setting of multifocality offers the most efficacious outcome compared with either resection, systemic, or locoregional therapies.[35]

In patients presenting with multifocal HCC within Milan criteria ($\leq$ 3 tumors and $\leq$ 3 cm in size), 5 year overall survival rates range from 49% to 69%[19,22,28] following hepatic resection. These survival rates are favorable compared with those seen in Western guidelines recommending locoregional therapies including TACE and TARE with 3 year survival rates of 26% to 29%.[36,37] These favorable results have led to many centers in Eastern countries to preferentially offer surgical resection in patients with multifocal HCC within Milan criteria who are not transplant candidates.[33,38–40]

As most patients with multifocal HCC tumor presentation within Milan or expanded transplant criteria in Western countries preferential undergo liver transplantation due to access of suitable donor livers there is uncertainity on the role of hepatic resection for multifocal tumors outside transplant criteria. In the multifocal cohort outside of transplant criteria outcomes are not as favorable as 5 year overall survival rates range from 12% to 24%.[24,29] The major limitation of these surgical series is their retrospective nature with multifocality determined on pathology results from surgical resections rather than *a priori* based on preoperative imaging studies. Recent studies have demonstrated that surgical resection may provide a greater benefit compared with locoregional therapies alone in patients with multifocal tumors outside of the Milan criteria.[34,41]

However, owing to high rates of recurrence and increasing extent of parenchymal resection with associated perioperative morbidities predictors are needed to better stratify patients who will have the greatest benefit from resection. Rather than using clinicopathological factors associated with outcomes only available after surgery including tumor size, tumor differentiation, cirrhosis, and microvascular invasion, predictive models have been identified to better stratify patients.[42] These predictive models although promising need further validation before widespread acceptance.

Presence of Tumor Macrovascular Invasion

HCC has a known proclivity for macrovascular invasion and presents most frequently as portal vein tumor thrombosis (PVTT), observed in 30% to 50% of newly diagnosed tumors.[43] The presence of PVTT is associated with a poor overall prognosis secondary to associated intra- and extra-hepatic tumor dissemination via hematogenous spread and the potential sequalae of associated clinical manifestations of portal hypertension.

The BCLC classification system classifies patients with HCC and concomitant PVTT as BCLC-C (advanced stage) and historically systemic therapy consisting of tyrosine kinase inhibitors or more recently combination immunotherapies have been recommended.[9,44,45] Even with the evolution of more efficacious systemic therapies, the median overall survival in patients presenting with PVTT is generally less than 1 year.[46] However, the paradigm of not offering surgical resection in this cohort of patients has been recently challenged by experienced centers from both Western and Eastern centers resulting in favorable survival and perioperative outcomes.[33]

Patients presenting with PVTT secondary to HCC present a diverse population with varying prognosis depending on the location and extent of involvement of the PVTT, severity of liver dysfunction and portal hypertension, and patient functional status. To delineate subtypes within the larger group of patients with HCC and concomitant PVTT, two main PVTT classification systems have been proposed. The Liver Cancer Study Group of Japan, perhaps the most widely used PVTT classification system in the most recent iteration describes 5 grades of PVTT ranging from Vp0 to Vp4 based on invasion or presence of macrovascular tumor thrombus in the main trunk versus first- or second-order branches of the portal vein[47] (**Fig. 1**). The Cheng classification system first described by Shi and colleagues stratifies the tumor thrombus also into 5 separate categories but not only incorporates macroscopic PVTT but also microscopic vascular invasion[48] (**Fig. 2**). The use of these 2 widely used PVTT classification systems allows clinicians to better stratify patients for treatment, including hepatic resection.

The overall goal of hepatic resection for HCC with concomitant PVTT includes not only obtaining a margin negative parenchymal resection but also thrombus extirpation within the portal system to mitigate further clinical manifestation of portal hypertension and hematogenous tumor dissemination. Given that, surgical options in the presence of HCC-related PVTT include: (1) partial hepatectomy with en bloc resection of ipsilateral tumor thrombus, (2) partial hepatectomy with enbloc vascular resection and reconstruction, or (3) partial hepatectomy with thrombectomy. The extent of PVTT determines the operative approach and the perioperative outcomes.

In patients presenting with HCC and concomitant Vp1-2 or Cheng classification Group 1 PVTT (limited to second-order or segmental portal branches or more distally), partial hepatectomy with en bloc resection of ipsilateral tumor thrombus is appropriate and has a favorable prognosis among PVTT-associated HCC. In the 22nd report of the Nationwide Follow-Up Survey of Primary Liver Cancer in Japan, resected HCC tumors with Vp1 or Vp2 PVTT were found to have median overall survival (OS) of 73.4 months and 38.0 months and 5 year OS of 55.7% and 44.1%, respectively.[49] In contrast, Vp1

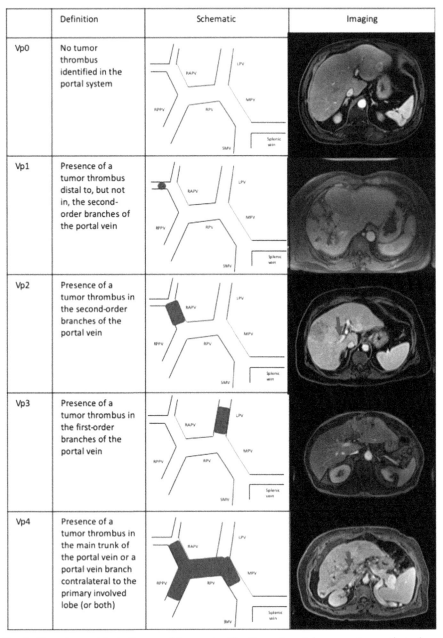

	Definition	Schematic	Imaging
Vp0	No tumor thrombus identified in the portal system		
Vp1	Presence of a tumor thrombus distal to, but not in, the second-order branches of the portal vein		
Vp2	Presence of a tumor thrombus in the second-order branches of the portal vein		
Vp3	Presence of a tumor thrombus in the first-order branches of the portal vein		
Vp4	Presence of a tumor thrombus in the main trunk of the portal vein or a portal vein branch contralateral to the primary involved lobe (or both)		

Fig. 1. Liver Cancer Study Group of Japan classification of portal venous tumor thrombus.

or Vp2-associated HCC treated with systemic therapy was reported to have median OS of 16.2 and 8.2 months, respectively. A number of retrospective studies include Vp3 (involving first-order branches of the portal vein) PVTT within the group of PVTT-associated HCC that may still benefit from LR, in the presence of preserved liver function.[50,51] Kokudo and colleagues reported that in patients with CP class A or B

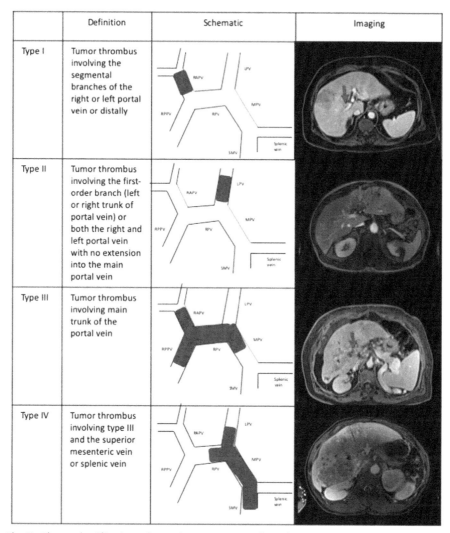

	Definition	Schematic	Imaging
Type I	Tumor thrombus involving the segmental branches of the right or left portal vein or distally		
Type II	Tumor thrombus involving the first-order branch (left or right trunk of portal vein) or both the right and left portal vein with no extension into the main portal vein		
Type III	Tumor thrombus involving main trunk of the portal vein		
Type IV	Tumor thrombus involving type III and the superior mesenteric vein or splenic vein		

Fig. 2. Cheng classification of portal venous tumor thrombus.

liver function with HCC involving PVTT, undergoing LR was associated with a signifi-cantly higher OS compared with other treatments ($P < .001$).[50] A subgroup analysis for propensity score-matched patient groups demonstrated a significant survival advan-tage in patients with Vp1–Vp3 but not in Vp4 PVTT (hazard ratio, 0.84; 95% confidence interval, 0.63–1.12).

A significant concern regarding LR for PVTT-associated HCC is the high rate of postoperative recurrence. Models to help with prognostication and the selection of patients who may benefit most from LR are paramount to expanding indications. Zhang and colleagues developed the Eastern Hepatobiliary Surgery Hospital (EHBH)/PVTT scoring system from a retrospective cohort including patients with PVTT-associated HCC limited to a first-order branch or above. The EHBH/PVTT score includes total bilirubin, alpha-fetoprotein, tumor diameter, and satellite lesions and distinguishes between two groups: ≤ 3 points and greater than 3 points, which have distinct median OS (17.0 vs 7.9 months, $P < .001$, respectively). The development of this model excluded Vp4 patients and thus it remains uncertain whether it can be applied to this group of patients.[52] A nomogram to predict postoperative early recurrence in patients with PVTT-associated HCC undergoing hepatic resection has been reported, using factors including hepatitis B surface antigen, PVTT, HBV DNA, satellite nodules, alpha-fetoprotein, and tumor diameter.[53]

Taking into account the high rate of recurrence seen in HCC tumors presenting with concomitant Vp4 PVTT coupled with the higher perioperative morbidity and mortality observed in this cohort of patients, hepatic resection should only be considered in select patients with Vp1–Vp3 PVTT based on prognostic indices.

Future Considerations

As surgical techniques and perioperative management of patients with HCC have continued to evolve, perhaps the most exciting development that will unlikely continue to expand the indications in surgical resection for HCC is the growing efficacy of systemic therapy in the neoadjuvant and adjuvant setting. Multiple clinical trials discussed elsewhere in this issue in further detail are undergoing and likely will change the surgical management of HCC.

SUMMARY

Available therapies for HCC have experienced tremendous growth in the last decade alongside parallel improvements in surgical technique and perioperative care for hepatic resection. Historically, hepatic resection for HCC has been reserved for patients with solitary tumors without vascular invasion. However, in well-selected patients HCC tumors multifocal in nature or with vascular invasion should be considered for hepatic resection.

CLINICS CARE POINTS

- Advances in surgical technique, perioperative care, and the availability of additional treatment agents and modalities have expanded the surgical indications for HCC.
- In well-selected patients, LR can be successfully performed with significant survival benefit for patients with multifocal HCC (particularly for those with 3 or fewer lesions) not otherwise eligible for transplantation and HCC associated with Vp1–Vp3 PVTT.
- With the evolution of systemic therapy options in the neoadjuvant and adjuvant setting, there may be an increasing role for surgical resection.

REFERENCES

1. Sung H, Ferlay J, Siegel RL, et al. Global Cancer Statistics 2020: GLOBOCAN Estimates of Incidence and Mortality Worldwide for 36 Cancers in 185 Countries. CA Cancer J Clin 2021;71(3):209–49.
2. Rahib L, Smith BD, Aizenberg R, et al. Projecting cancer incidence and deaths to 2030: the unexpected burden of thyroid, liver, and pancreas cancers in the United States. Cancer Res 2014;74(11):2913–21.
3. Yopp AC, Mansour JC, Beg MS, et al. Establishment of a multidisciplinary hepatocellular carcinoma clinic is associated with improved clinical outcome. Ann Surg Oncol 2014;21(4):1287–95.

4. Pang TC, Lam VW. Surgical management of hepatocellular carcinoma. World J Hepatol 2015;7(2):245–52.

5. Zhu H, Xing H, Yu B, et al. Long-term survival and recurrence after curative resection for hepatocellular carcinoma in patients with chronic hepatitis C virus infection: a multicenter observational study from China. HPB (Oxford) 2020;22(12): 1793–802.

6. Singal AG, Llovet JM, Yarchoan M, et al. AASLD practice guidance on prevention, diagnosis, and treatment of hepatocellular carcinoma. Hepatology 2023. https://doi.org/10.1097/HEP.0000000000000466.

7. Fong Y, Sun RL, Jarnagin W, et al. An analysis of 412 cases of hepatocellular carcinoma at a Western center. Ann Surg 1999;229(6):790–9 [discussion: 799-800].

8. Fan ST, Lo CM, Liu CL, et al. Hepatectomy for hepatocellular carcinoma: toward zero hospital deaths. Ann Surg 1999;229(3):322–30.

9. Reig M, Forner A, Rimola J, et al. BCLC strategy for prognosis prediction and treatment recommendation: The 2022 update. J Hepatol 2022;76(3):681–93.

10. Dokmak S, Fteriche FS, Borscheid R, et al. 2012 Liver resections in the 21st century: we are far from zero mortality. HPB (Oxford) 2013;15(11):908–15.

11. Kenjo A, Miyata H, Gotoh M, et al. Risk stratification of 7,732 hepatectomy cases in 2011 from the National Clinical Database for Japan. J Am Coll Surg 2014; 218(3):412–22.

12. Balzan S, Belghiti J, Farges O, et al. The "50-50 criteria" on postoperative day 5: an accurate predictor of liver failure and death after hepatectomy. Ann Surg 2005; 242(6):824–8 [discussion: 828-829].

13. Child CG, Turcotte JG. Surgery and portal hypertension. Major Probl Clin Surg 1964;1:1–85.

14. Pugh RN, Murray-Lyon IM, Dawson JL, et al. Transection of the oesophagus for bleeding oesophageal varices. Br J Surg 1973;60(8):646–9.

15. Malinchoc M, Kamath PS, Gordon FD, et al. A model to predict poor survival in patients undergoing transjugular intrahepatic portosystemic shunts. Hepatology 2000;31(4):864–71.

16. Teh SH, Christein J, Donohue J, et al. Hepatic resection of hepatocellular carcinoma in patients with cirrhosis: Model of End-Stage Liver Disease (MELD) score predicts perioperative mortality. J Gastrointest Surg 2005;9(9):1207–15 [discussion: 1215].

17. Cucchetti A, Ercolani G, Vivarelli M, et al. Impact of model for end-stage liver disease (MELD) score on prognosis after hepatectomy for hepatocellular carcinoma on cirrhosis. Liver Transpl 2006;12(6):966–71.

18. Delis SG, Bakoyiannis A, Dervenis C, et al. Perioperative risk assessment for hepatocellular carcinoma by using the MELD score. J Gastrointest Surg 2009; 13(12):2268–75.

19. Bruix J, Reig M, Rimola J, et al. Clinical decision making and research in hepatocellular carcinoma: pivotal role of imaging techniques. Hepatology 2011; 54(6):2238–44.

20. Bruix J. Liver cancer: still a long way to go. Hepatology 2011;54(1):1–2.

21. Bruix J, Castells A, Bosch J, et al. Surgical resection of hepatocellular carcinoma in cirrhotic patients: prognostic value of preoperative portal pressure. Gastroenterology 1996;111(4):1018–22.

22. Maithel SK, Kneuertz PJ, Kooby DA, et al. Importance of low preoperative platelet count in selecting patients for resection of hepatocellular carcinoma: a multi-institutional analysis. J Am Coll Surg 2011;212(4):638–48 [discussion: 648-650].

23. Makuuchi M, Imamura H, Sugawara Y, et al. Progress in surgical treatment of hepatocellular carcinoma. Oncology 2002;62(Suppl 1):74–81.

24. Tsilimigras DI, Bagante F, Moris D, et al. Defining the chance of cure after resection for hepatocellular carcinoma within and beyond the Barcelona Clinic Liver Cancer guidelines: A multi-institutional analysis of 1,010 patients. Surgery 2019;166(6):967–74.

25. Ng KK, Vauthey JN, Pawlik TM, et al. Is hepatic resection for large or multinodular hepatocellular carcinoma justified? Results from a multi-institutional database. Ann Surg Oncol 2005;12(5):364–73.

26. Pawlik TM, Poon RT, Abdalla EK, et al. Critical appraisal of the clinical and pathologic predictors of survival after resection of large hepatocellular carcinoma. Arch Surg 2005;140(5):450–7 [discussion: 457-458].

27. Pandey D, Lee KH, Wai CT, et al. Long term outcome and prognostic factors for large hepatocellular carcinoma (10 cm or more) after surgical resection. Ann Surg Oncol 2007;14(10):2817–23.

28. Tsilimigras DI, Bagante F, Sahara K, et al. Prognosis After Resection of Barcelona Clinic Liver Cancer (BCLC) Stage 0, A, and B Hepatocellular Carcinoma: A Comprehensive Assessment of the Current BCLC Classification. Ann Surg Oncol 2019;26(11):3693–700.

29. Tsilimigras DI, Bagante F, Moris D, et al. Recurrence Patterns and Outcomes after Resection of Hepatocellular Carcinoma within and beyond the Barcelona Clinic Liver Cancer Criteria. Ann Surg Oncol 2020;27(7):2321–31.

30. Labgaa I, Demartines N, Melloul E. Surgical Resection Versus Transarterial Chemoembolization for Intermediate Stage Hepatocellular Carcinoma (BCLC-B): An Unsolved Question. Hepatology 2019;69(2):923.

31. Guo H, Wu T, Lu Q, et al. Surgical resection improves long-term survival of patients with hepatocellular carcinoma across different Barcelona Clinic Liver Cancer stages. Cancer Manag Res 2018;10:361–9.

32. Kudo M, Arizumi T, Ueshima K, et al. Subclassification of BCLC B Stage Hepatocellular Carcinoma and Treatment Strategies: Proposal of Modified Bolondi's Subclassification (Kinki Criteria). Dig Dis 2015;33(6):751–8.

33. Torzilli G, Belghiti J, Kokudo N, et al. A snapshot of the effective indications and results of surgery for hepatocellular carcinoma in tertiary referral centers: is it adherent to the EASL/AASLD recommendations?: an observational study of the HCC East-West study group. Ann Surg 2013;257(5):929–37.

34. Wada H, Eguchi H, Noda T, et al. Selection criteria for hepatic resection in intermediate-stage (BCLC stage B) multiple hepatocellular carcinoma. Surgery 2016;160(5):1227–35.

35. Wong LL, Landsittel DP, Kwee SA. Liver Transplantation vs Partial Hepatectomy for Stage T2 Multifocal Hepatocellular Carcinoma <3 cm without Vascular Invasion: A Propensity-Score Matched Survival Analysis. J Am Coll Surg 2023.

36. Lo CM, Ngan H, Tso WK, et al. Randomized controlled trial of transarterial lipiodol chemoembolization for unresectable hepatocellular carcinoma. Hepatology 2002;35(5):1164–71.

37. Llovet JM, Real MI, Montana X, et al. Arterial embolisation or chemoembolisation versus symptomatic treatment in patients with unresectable hepatocellular carcinoma: a randomised controlled trial. Lancet 2002;359(9319):1734–9.

38. Choo SP, Tan WL, Goh BKP, et al. Comparison of hepatocellular carcinoma in Eastern versus Western populations. Cancer 2016;122(22):3430–46.

39. Omata M, Cheng AL, Kokudo N, et al. Asia-Pacific clinical practice guidelines on the management of hepatocellular carcinoma: a 2017 update. Hepatol Int 2017; 11(4):317–70.
40. Zhong JH, Xiang BD, Gong WF, et al. Comparison of long-term survival of patients with BCLC stage B hepatocellular carcinoma after liver resection or transarterial chemoembolization. PLoS One 2013;8(7):e68193.
41. Hyun MH, Lee YS, Kim JH, et al. Hepatic resection compared to chemoembolization in intermediate- to advanced-stage hepatocellular carcinoma: A meta-analysis of high-quality studies. Hepatology 2018;68(3):977–93.
42. Tsilimigras DI, Hyer JM, Paredes AZ, et al. Tumor Burden Dictates Prognosis Among Patients Undergoing Resection of Intrahepatic Cholangiocarcinoma: A Tool to Guide Post-Resection Adjuvant Chemotherapy? Ann Surg Oncol 2021; 28(4):1970–8.
43. Cerrito L, Annicchiarico BE, Iezzi R, et al. Treatment of hepatocellular carcinoma in patients with portal vein tumor thrombosis: Beyond the known frontiers. World J Gastroenterol 2019;25(31):4360–82.
44. Finn RS, Qin S, Ikeda M, et al. Atezolizumab plus Bevacizumab in Unresectable Hepatocellular Carcinoma. N Engl J Med 2020;382(20):1894–905.
45. Llovet JM, Ricci S, Mazzaferro V, et al. Sorafenib in advanced hepatocellular carcinoma. N Engl J Med 2008;359(4):378–90.
46. Mokdad AA, Singal AG, Marrero JA, et al. Vascular Invasion and Metastasis is Predictive of Outcome in Barcelona Clinic Liver Cancer Stage C Hepatocellular Carcinoma. J Natl Compr Canc Netw 2017;15(2):197–204.
47. Liver Cancer Study Group of Japan. The general rules for the clinical and pathological study of primary liver cancer. Liver Cancer Study Group of Japan. Jpn J Surg 1989;19(1):98–129.
48. Shi J, Lai EC, Li N, et al. A new classification for hepatocellular carcinoma with portal vein tumor thrombus. J Hepatobiliary Pancreat Sci 2011;18(1):74–80.
49. Kudo M, Izumi N, Kokudo N, et al. Report of the 22nd nationwide follow-up Survey of Primary Liver Cancer in Japan (2012-2013). Hepatol Res 2022;52(1):5–66.
50. Kokudo T, Hasegawa K, Matsuyama Y, et al. Survival benefit of liver resection for hepatocellular carcinoma associated with portal vein invasion. J Hepatol 2016; 65(5):938–43.
51. Kondo K, Chijiiwa K, Kai M, et al. Surgical strategy for hepatocellular carcinoma patients with portal vein tumor thrombus based on prognostic factors. J Gastrointest Surg 2009;13(6):1078–83.
52. Zhang XP, Gao YZ, Chen ZH, et al. An Eastern Hepatobiliary Surgery Hospital/ Portal Vein Tumor Thrombus Scoring System as an Aid to Decision Making on Hepatectomy for Hepatocellular Carcinoma Patients With Portal Vein Tumor Thrombus: A Multicenter Study. Hepatology 2019;69(5):2076–90.
53. Zhang XP, Chen ZH, Zhou TF, et al. A nomogram to predict early postoperative recurrence of hepatocellular carcinoma with portal vein tumour thrombus after R0 liver resection: A large-scale, multicenter study. Eur J Surg Oncol 2019; 45(9):1644–51.

Minimally Invasive Robotic Techniques for Hepatocellular Carcinoma Resection: How I Do It

Aradhya Nigam, MD[a], Jason S. Hawksworth, MD[b],*,
Emily R. Winslow, MD[c]

KEYWORDS

- Hepatocellular carcinoma • Minimally invasive • Hepatectomy • Robotic

KEY POINTS

- Despite an increase in the incidence of hepatocellular carcinoma, adoption of minimally invasive liver resection has remained slow in the United States.
- Advancements in laparoscopic and robotic technology have enabled surgeons to safely perform minimally invasive liver resection for hepatocellular carcinoma.
- Minimally invasive liver resection combined with ERAS protocol have vastly reduced hospital stays for patients and reduced hospital costs compared with open surgery.
- We demonstrate that the majority of major hepatectomies can be performed robotically with a standardized set up for port placement.
- Use of the laparoscopic cavitron ultrasonic surgical aspirator for parenchymal transection during robotic cases facilitates precise identification of intrahepatic structures in minimally invasive liver resection.

 Video content accompanies this article at http://www.surgonc.theclinics.com.

INTRODUCTION

Since the 1980s, the incidence of hepatocellular carcinoma has more than tripled.[1] Although advancements in minimally invasive techniques and recognition of technical

[a] Department of Surgery, Medstar Georgetown University Hospital, 3800 Reservoir Road, NW, 4PHC, Washington, DC 20007, USA; [b] Division of Abdominal Organ Transplantation, Columbia University Irving Medical Center, 622 West 168th Street, PH14-105, New York, NY 20032, USA; [c] Department of Transplant Surgery, Medstar Georgetown University Hospital, 3800 Reservoir Road, NW, 2PHC, Washington, DC 20007, USA
* Corresponding author. Division of Abdominal Organ Transplantation, Columbia University Irving Medical Center, 622 West 168th Street, PH14-105, New York, NY 20032.
E-mail address: jsnhawk@hotmail.com

Surg Oncol Clin N Am 33 (2024) 111–132
https://doi.org/10.1016/j.soc.2023.06.009

feasibility have led to a greater proportion of patients receiving minimally invasive liver resection, more than 90% of hepatocellular carcinoma resections are still performed open. This is despite increasing evidence that minimally invasive surgery provides patients with improved outcomes and decreased hospital stays, while allowing surgeons the ability to perform margin negative resections similar to open procedures. As a result, minimally invasive surgery has developed into an important option for patients with resectable hepatocellular carcinoma and should be incorporated into the practice of all surgeons performing liver surgery.

In this review, our approach and methodology behind performing minimally invasive liver resection for hepatocellular carcinoma is described. The historical and current trends in minimally invasive liver resection are reviewed and institutional criteria used for minimally invasive resection discussed. In the second portion of the review, the surgical considerations for performing various major liver resections including right and left hepatectomy, left lateral sectionectomy, and central hepatectomy are defined. It is important to note that our institutional practice has significantly transitioned to robotic resection for all minimally invasive liver resections owing to improved observed outcomes, technical versatility, and without increased costs.[2] As a result, use of a standardized robotic port placement and laparoscopic cavitron ultrasonic surgical aspirator (CUSA) in all major hepatectomies is described. Through this discussion, our aim is to conceptualize and demonstrate the feasibility of minimally invasive approaches for hepatocellular carcinoma resection.

HISTORY OF MINIMALLY INVASIVE TECHNIQUES IN HEPATOCELLULAR CARCINOMA RESECTION

The evolution of hepatocellular carcinoma resection from open to minimally invasive techniques has had a complex history (**Fig. 1**).[3–5] Liver resection was first reported in 1886 by Luis for the resection of a large hepatic adenoma in a 76-year-old woman who died postoperatively due to hemorrhage. Subsequently, the first successful resection for a left liver tumor was performed in 1888 by Carl von Langenbuch. In 1911, Wendel reported the first right liver resection for primary hepatocellular carcinoma; however, details on the extent of resection were left unreported.[6] With improved

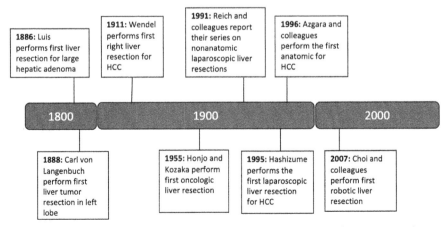

Fig. 1. Timeline of minimally invasive liver resection. Major events in liver resection history that contributed to the development of minimally invasive surgery for hepatocellular carcinoma resection.

understanding in liver anatomy and advancements in surgical management of patients, recognition that resection of hepatocellular carcinoma would require more formal resections became apparent. In 1955, Honjo and Araki[7] described their experience with a formal anatomic, staged resection of a patient with gastric cancer metastases to the liver with their description of the dissection of the hepatic hilum. These cases laid the groundwork for studying and guiding optimal resection principles for patients that eventually led to single-stage approaches and advanced techniques for the management of hepatocellular carcinoma.

Throughout the 1980s and 1990s the use of minimally invasive surgery was gaining increased traction for a variety of intraabdominal pathology.[8] With improvements in technique, minimally invasive liver resection for hepatocellular carcinoma was progressively introduced. In 1991, Reich and colleagues[9] reported their case series of 2 women who underwent nonanatomic liver resection of benign liver pathology reported at respective "liver edges." The first laparoscopic resection of a hepatocellular carcinoma was performed and reported by Hashizume in 1995 for a 2-cm cancer in Couinaud segment 5.[10] The following year, Azagra and colleagues[11] described the first formal laparoscopic anatomic resection with a left lateral hepatectomy for hepatocellular carcinoma. The first reported robotic liver resection was performed in 2007 by Choi and colleagues for a 2.4-cm left lateral segment mass.[12]

TRENDS IN THE USE OF MINIMALLY INVASIVE SURGERY FOR HEPATOCELLULAR CARCINOMA RESECTION

The adoption of minimally invasive surgery for hepatocellular carcinoma remains slow in the United States.[13,14] Initial development of minimally invasive techniques was hampered by technical difficulty and risk of complications including hemorrhage, air embolism, bile leakage, and tumor seeding.[15] Over time, a greater number of institutions began to report improved outcomes with laparoscopic liver resections compared with open surgery.[15-19] Recognition of minimally techniques for hepatocellular carcinoma, both domestically and internationally (**Table 1**), paved the way for its increased adoption.

Globally, hepatocellular carcinoma remains the most common indication for minimally invasive liver resection, representing about 50% of resections.[15] Although the prevalence of minimally invasive techniques for hepatocellular carcinoma in the United States still lags compared with East Asian countries, its use in malignant liver disease remains on the increase. In their evaluation of the National Inpatient Sample (NIS) and National Surgical Quality Improvement Project (NSQIP), He and colleagues observed a progressive increase in the utilization of minimally invasive techniques for hepatocellular carcinoma in the United States from approximately 1% of cases in 2000 to 6.1% in 2012.[20]

The first breakthrough for the international acceptance of minimally invasive techniques for liver resection came in 2008 during the First International Consensus Conference with subsequent publication of the Louisville Consensus Guidelines in 2009.[21] The guidelines set the stage for minimally invasive liver surgery by acknowledging laparoscopy as a "safe and effective approach to the management of surgical liver disease." In addition, the consortium set forth commonly used terminology for minimally invasive liver surgery including pure laparoscopy, hand-assisted laparoscopy, and hybrid technique (**Table 2**). After publication of the Louisville Consensus Guidelines, several groups reported their institutional experience with laparoscopic surgery.[22] The Second International Consensus Conference met in 2015 to reevaluate the use of minimally invasive techniques for liver surgery, expanding on their prior guidelines and

Table 1
International laparoscopic liver resection consensus conferences

Conference	Year	Statement	Position Established
First International Laparoscopic Liver Resection Consensus Conference[21]	2008	Louisville	• Reviewed the feasibility and safety of minimally invasive liver resection • Defined types of minimally invasive liver resection
Second International Laparoscopic Liver Resection Consensus Conference[23]	2015	Morioka	• Established minimally invasive surgery to be as safe as open resection • Discussed optimal perioperative management (preoperative evaluation, bleeding control, parenchymal transection) • Suggested patients have educational program for minimally invasive surgery
European Guidelines Meeting[24]	2018	Southampton	• Reviewed indications of minimally invasive liver resection • Reviewed techniques for minimally invasive liver resection • Discussed learning curves and implementation • Established robotic surgery as effective as laparoscopy
Third International Laparoscopic Liver Resection Consensus Conference[78]	2018	Seoul	• Established the feasibility and safety of laparoscopic living donor hepatectomy
Joint Initiative of the International Laparoscopic Liver Society and Asian-Pacific Hepato-Pancreato-Biliary Association[79]	2021	—	• International acceptance of minimally invasive living donor liver transplant • Demonstrated effectiveness of robotic living donor liver transplant

Table 2 Types of laparoscopic liver resections as defined by the first international laparoscopic liver resection consensus conferences	
Types of Laparoscopic Resection	Definition
Pure	Liver resection performed solely through laparoscopic ports
Hand-Assisted	Liver resection used with assistance of hand port
Hybrid	Procedure started as pure/hand-assisted but completed through a laparotomy incision

Buell JF, Cherqui D, Geller DA, et al. The international position on laparoscopic liver surgery: The Louisville Statement, 2008. Ann Surg. 2009 Nov;250(5):825-30. https://doi.org/10.1097/sla.0b013e 3181b3b2d8.

establishing the safety and efficacy of laparoscopic surgery for a variety of major and minor liver resections.[23] The guidelines further commented on the use of robotic surgery for liver resection, stating strong evidence for its use in experienced hands, as evidence remained limited to case series and cohort studies. Findings from the Second Consensus Conference were further reaffirmed in the 2018 European Consensus Guidelines, which described minimally invasive liver resection for a broad range of complex liver pathology.[24] Use of robotic surgery by this time had been encouraged and in fact touted for its reduced hospital costs compared with open surgery.

The consensus guidelines consistently reiterated the critical importance of clinical expertise in approaching complex liver resections. Although proficiency remains dependent on provider experience and technical abilities, Chua and colleagues[25] published their systematic review stating that the "learning curve" for minimally invasive liver resection as approximately 50 cases for laparoscopy and 25 cases for robotic approaches and was replicated by Fukumori and colleagues in Denmark.[26] However, use of these numbers as cutoffs has remained controversial, as other reports demonstrate case numbers for proficiency to be much higher.[27]

INDICATIONS AND ELIGIBILITY FOR RESECTION

The Louisiana Consensus Statement outlined that minimally invasive liver resection should optimally be reserved for patients with small (<5 cm), solitary lesions located at the periphery.[21] However, the utility and safety of minimally invasive surgery has progressively evolved. Takahara and colleagues reported their observations of a large cohort of patients in a multiinstitutional study of patients who underwent liver resection in Japan.[28] Using propensity score matching, the group observed that minimally invasive techniques were associated with decreased morbidity, as minimally invasive patients demonstrated decreased blood loss, shorter hospital stay, and less complications, while having no significant difference in survival or recurrence outcomes; this was further demonstrated in cirrhotic patients in whom minimally invasive liver resection for hepatocellular carcinoma was associated with less morbidity and demonstrated decreased postoperative ascites and liver failure.

The indications for robotic intervention remain similar to laparoscopy but remain subject to the expertise of the provider.[29] Di Benedetto and colleagues recently conducted a multinational retrospective study to investigate the outcomes experienced in robotic liver resection compared with open surgery for hepatocellular carcinoma.[30] Their findings highlight that robotic resection was associated with increased operative time and perioperative blood loss; however, patients had shorter hospital/intensive care unit stays and experienced less postoperative complications and liver failure. Our group has transitioned to the use of robotic liver resection for hepatocellular carcinoma owing to its improved ability to perform and visualize complex resections along with its improved outcomes and complete oncologic resection.[2]

PRINCIPLES OF HEPATOCELLULAR CARCINOMA RESECTION

Surgical resection for hepatocellular carcinoma includes both anatomic and nonanatomic resections.[31–33] Anatomic resections for hepatocellular carcinoma ensure adequate margins while ensuring complete removal of portal system inflow and venous outflow to the respective lesion. Classically, the Brisbane 2000 Terminology was used to describe 6 major hepatic resections: left lateral sectionectomy, right hepatectomy, left hepatectomy, right trisectionectomy, and left trisectionectomy, and finally right posterior sectionectomy.[34] More recently, the adoption of minimally invasive surgery and preoperative diagnostics have allowed for better definition of lesions and have called to question whether parenchymal preserving procedures could be performed. As a result, the Brisbane terminology was recently discussed and updated in the Tokyo 2020 Terminology[35] consensus statement. The Tokyo terminology looked to better define anatomic resections for hepatic resection based on "cone unit"[36] resections and allowing for parenchymal sparing using intraoperative color dye or indocyanine green (ICG) imaging to define resection margins. Although our group has acknowledged the Tokyo terminology, our institutional practice has primarily been to perform formal anatomic resection using the Brisbane terminology. However, we have incorporated ICG staining to facilitate and aid intraoperative ultrasound in delineating our margins of resection. Further adjustments to resection parameters remain, pending future trials and societal recommendations.

Nonanatomic resection remains an alternative approach to resection defined as carcinoma resection with tumor-free margins irrespective of liver segment anatomy. Anatomic resections have classically been advocated for due to the potential to remove micrometastatic disease along portal vein tributaries and reduced recurrence rates in retrospective studies.[37,38] Only one report has compared nonanatomic and anatomic resection in a randomized trial, demonstrating that anatomic resection compared with nonanatomic significantly reduced time to recurrence and had decreased recurrence at 2 years; however, interestingly no differences in recurrence-free survival and overall survival were observed.[39] As previously stated, anatomic resection remains standard of care for patients able to tolerate formal resection, but nonanatomic resections have still been considered for patients who require liver parenchymal preservation and cirrhotic patients unable to undergo transplantation.

SURGICAL CONSIDERATIONS IN MINIMALLY INVASIVE HEPATOCELLULAR CARCINOMA RESECTION
Preoperative Assessment of Patients

Similar to open surgery, preoperative assessment of a minimally invasive surgery candidate requires accurate staging along with selecting medically appropriate patients. Several staging systems exist for predicting advanced disease (**Table 3**).[40–45] Our group uses the Barcelona Clinic Liver Cancer (BCLC) classification system to assess objective resectability.[46,47] The staging system evaluates several factors including Child-Pugh status, ECOG status, and stage to stratify patients into 5 stages: very early (BCLC 0), early (BCLC A), intermediate (BCLC B), advanced (BCLC C), and terminal (BCLC D) stage disease. In addition, we use MRI and triphasic liver–specific protocol computed tomography scan to evaluate patients with contraindications to

Table 3
Staging systems for predicting prognosis in hepatocellular carcinoma

Staging System	Year	Variables	Advantages	Disadvantages
AJCC TNM Staging System (8th Edition)	2017	Tumor size (T) Nodal status (N) Distant metastasis (M)	• Validated for resection and transplantation	• Excludes cirrhosis • Excludes AFP • Excludes MELD
Okuda System	1985	Tumor size Ascites Albumin Bilirubin	• Included cirrhosis as part of prognostication	• Purely clinical system • Not applicable to early stage HCC • Excluded vascular invasion and AFP • Does not distinguish multifocal tumors
The Cancer of the Liver Italian Program (CLIP) Staging System	1998	Child-Pugh score Tumor size Number of lesions Serum AFP Presence of PVT[a]	• Prognostic for overall survival	• Excludes performance status • Overemphasizes potential impact of PVT
Barcelona Cancer Liver Cancer (BCLC) Staging System	1999	ECOG status Tumor extent Vascular invasion Extrahepatic disease	• Accounts for performance status • Accounts for vascular invasion • Prognostic for survival	• Excludes cirrhotic variables • Questions over generalizability
Albumin-Bilirubin (ALBI) score	2015	Albumin Bilirubin	• Objective measure of liver function in HCC • Validated in multiple centers • Risk stratification for TACE[c]	• Variable outcomes based on population studied • Inability to guide resectability
Risk Estimation of Tumor Recurrence After Transplantation (RETREAT)	2017	Microvascular invasion Baseline AFP Tumor sum[b]	• Predict recurrence after intervention	• Not widely validated • Unclear if applicable to HCC resection

[a] PVT: portal vein thrombosis.
[b] Tumor sum: largest tumor diameter + Number of viable tumors.
[c] TACE: transarterial chemoembolization.

resection including extrahepatic disease, multilobar disease, involvement of the main bile duct, or invasion into the main portal vein or inferior vena cava.[48] For large tumors (>5 cm), liver biopsy is considered to discern the extent of liver fibrosis/cirrhosis.

In addition to evaluating criteria for resectability, we assess the future liver remnant (FLR) in all patients undergoing resection.[49] Cutoffs for proceeding with surgery are subjected to discussion but have been defined as greater than 20% for otherwise normal livers, greater than 30% for patients who had prior chemotherapy or hepatic steatosis, and greater than 40% for cirrhotics.[50,51] For patients with borderline FLRs, portal vein embolization of the diseased side is considered in an attempt to hypertrophy the remnant liver.[47,52] Recently, liver venous deprivation or "dual embolization" of the both portal and hepatic veins has been introduced to further optimize hypertrophy and is used at our institution in borderline cases.[53,54] If embolization is pursued, our institution typically reevaluates FLR approximately 3 to 4 weeks postembolization. All patients planning resection for hepatocellular carcinoma are further discussed in our multidisciplinary team conference encompassing medical oncology, hepatobiliary surgery, hepatology, diagnostic radiology, and interventional radiology to ensure appropriate management of patients.

After the decision to proceed with surgery is made, patients are reevaluated in the office to discuss surgical approach. For patients undergoing minimally invasive resection, cardiopulmonary status is assessed to ensure patients can tolerate pneumoperitoneum/insufflation. For patients with an extensive cardiac history, they are risk stratified by their cardiologist, and electrocardiogram/stress tests are advocated for high-risk patients. In addition, baseline laboratory work is collected to include preoperative complete blood count, type and cross, coagulation laboratories, basic metabolic panel, and liver function panel. Platelets and prothrombin time/international normalized ratio are carefully assessed to ensure adequate underlying function of the liver. Finally, baseline AFP is obtained to aid in postoperative surveillance.

Use of Enhanced Recovery After Surgery for Liver Resection

ERAS protocols have demonstrated efficacy in the perioperative care of patients.[55–57] The initial development of ERAS protocols in liver resection drew concerns over surgical complexity and associated coagulopathy, potential for massive fluid shifts, and gravity of complications. On the contrary, utilization of ERAS protocols in open liver surgery demonstrated decreased complications, reduced hospital stay, and improvements in perioperative quality of life.[58] For minimally invasive liver surgery, similar improvements in patient outcomes have been observed with utilization of ERAS protocols without an impact on conversion to open or readmission rates.

Several ERAS protocols have been proposed for use in liver surgery. For our patients undergoing minimally invasive hepatectomy, a standard institutionalized protocol has been developed. In the preoperative holding unit, patients are provided multimodal pain control, including celecoxib, acetaminophen, and gabapentin. A tap block is performed whenever feasible. Postoperatively, patients are given ketorolac, acetaminophen, and gabapentin with PRN narcotics and nausea control. Patients are given a clear liquid diet and bowel regimen and encouraged to be out of bed. On postoperative day 1, patients are advanced to a regular diet with protein shakes, and foley is discontinued in the morning. Patients are typically discharged on postoperative day 1 or 2 if they meet the following criteria for discharge: (1) patients are out-of-bed ambulating, (2) pain controlled, (3) tolerating diet without nausea/vomiting, (4) and ensuring adequate liver function. Patients are discharged home with gabapentin, acetaminophen, tramadol, and oxycodone as needed and bowel regimen.

Anesthesia Considerations for Minimally Invasive Liver Resection

Minimally invasive liver resection is performed under general anesthesia with controlled ventilation.[59] For patients with concern for liver disease, cis-atracurium is used as a muscle relaxant. Maintenance induction is given with either sevoflurane or isoflurane, given the need for liver resection and hemodynamic changes. For hemodynamic monitoring, an arterial line is placed for continuous blood pressure monitoring. A central line is placed selectively for access and to monitor central venous pressures (CVP). A low-target CVP less than 5 mm Hg has been associated with decreased blood loss, decreased variation in hemodynamics, and shorter hospital stay.[60] In discussion with the anesthesia team, intravenous fluid administration is limited preoperatively and perioperatively. Refractory elevated CVPs are managed with diuresis and, if needed, vasoactive agents.

Perioperative Antibiotics

The efficacy of perioperative antibiotics in liver surgery remains controversial with consensus over optimal antibiotic strategy unestablished.[61] We use preoperative antibiotics to cover for skin flora and prophylaxis against surgical site infections using cefazolin or vancomycin (in cases of penicillin allergy) for skin coverage. Redosing of cefazolin is done every 4 hours for the length of the surgery. Postoperative antibiotics are not given.

Robotic Port Types and Placement

Port placement in our cases remain standardized for all hepatectomies and have been used on the Da Vinci Si and Xi systems (**Fig. 2**).[62] We begin by making an infraumbilical or Pfannenstiel incision and place a 12-mm assist port. The site is used for multiple

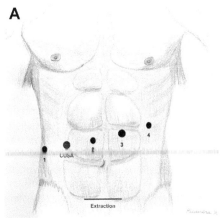
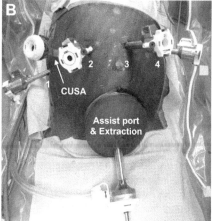

Fig. 2. Port placement for major hepatectomy. (*A*) Robotic liver resection port placement in the upper abdomen. Port #1 and #3 serve as working ports, with #1 being a 8 mm and #3 a 12 mm port. Port #2 is an 8 mm camera port that is placed in line with the portal vein. Port #4 is an 8 mm used for retraction during the case. Between ports #1 and #2 a 12 mm assistant port is placed that accommodates the laparoscopic CUSA. An additional Pfannenstiel or infraumbilical incision is made to place an assist port. (*B*) Port placement before robot docking. (Hawksworth, J., Radkani, P., Nguyen, B. et al. Improving safety of robotic major hepatectomy with extrahepatic inflow control and laparoscopic CUSA parenchymal transection: technical description and initial experience. Surg Endosc 36, 3270-3276 (2022). https://doi.org/10.1007/s00464-021-08639-z.)

reasons including insufflation during the case, suction during parenchymal transection, and for specimen extraction at the conclusion of the case. Four robotic ports are then placed along the upper abdomen. Port #1 (8 mm) is placed in the anterior medial axillary line as a working port. Port #2 (8 mm) is our camera port that is placed along the right midclavicular line in line with the portal vein. Port #3 (12 mm) is an additional working port placed to the left of midline and can be used to accommodate the robotic stapler. Port #4 (8 mm) is used for retraction. We place an additional 12-mm assist port between port #1 and port #2 about 8 to 12 cm below the costal margin that allows accommodation of the laparoscopic CUSA without interfering with the additional robotic instruments (see *Parenchymal Transection* section). Port placement is visualized in **Fig. 5**.

Parenchymal Transection

Several techniques are available to the surgeon for parenchymal transection during minimally invasive cases.[63,64] Broadly, devices can be categorized into transection devices (ultrasonic dissector, Water Jet) and Energy devices (Bipolar, Sealing devices, Ultrasonic shears). Studies comparing transection devices have been limited but ultimately are subject to surgeon preferences and type of surgery. At our institution, we have previously described the use of the CUSA for use in robotic parenchymal transection. As briefly described in the prior section, introduction of an additional assist port in line with the liver allows for optimally parenchymal transection in any major hepatectomy. Our institutional experience has found use of the laparoscopic CUSA during robotic hepatectomy to be more efficient than use of energy devices, which we still use for vessel/bile duct transection. Furthermore, after introduction of the CUSA for parenchymal transection, we report low rates of blood transfusion requirements and need for conversion to open.[62]

Use of Indocyanine Green in Minimally Invasive Liver Resection

The use of ICG in liver resection has developed into an effective tool for guiding parenchymal transection, particularly in minimally invasive liver resection.[65–67] Although ICG is metabolized by the liver, it is also excreted into the biliary system, thus allowing it to be used in multiple phases of liver resection.[68] As a result, the use of ICG in parenchymal transection has greatly increased. In our practice, ICG imaging is used for 3 major reasons in minimally invasive liver resection: (1) guide parenchymal transection after inflow control with "negative staining" to delineate precise liver demarcation, (2) perform an ICG cholangiogram to delineate intrahepatic biliary anatomy during various hepatectomies (**Fig. 3**), and (3) inject tumor as a "positive staining"[69,70] to ensure adequate resection, particularly in nonanatomic resections. The multimodal use during liver transection demonstrates its utility during hepatic transection; however, its use remains limited by variable sensitivity, particularly in cirrhotic patients, and low penetration depth up to 10 mm.[67] Thus, our practice is to use ICG to complement ultrasound imaging when identifying major structures and determining transection planes.

Drain Placement

The use of drains after liver resection remains controversial.[71–75] The recent publication of the ND-trial by Arita and colleagues[76] randomized 400 patients undergoing hepatic resection without biliary reconstruction and found that a significantly greater proportion of patients who had drains placed experienced severe primary complications compared with those who had no drains placed. Our indications for drain placement in minimally invasive liver resection generally include patients undergoing central

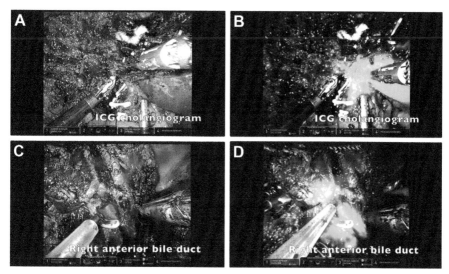

Fig. 3. ICG cholangiogram. Right hilar plate dissection during robotic right hepatectomy. (*A*) ICG cholangiogram demonstrating hepatic duct confluence and confirming division of right hepatic duct. (*B*) Right anterior bile duct intrahepatic dissection during robotic right anterior sectionectomy. (*C*) Identification of right anterior sector bile duct with ICG cholangiogram confirming biliary anatomy (*D*).

resection and nonanatomic resections or having intraoperative concern for developing a postoperative bile leak.

TYPES OF HEPATOCELLULAR CARCINOMA RESECTION PROCEDURE

Advancement of minimally invasive techniques for liver resection has led to improved patient outcomes and hospital stays. Although traditionally our group has used both laparoscopic and robotic approaches to hepatocellular resection, we have progressively transitioned to a robotic-only approach, although the steps and surgical principles for liver resection remain similar. Our decision to transition to robotic hepatectomy is multifactorial. For one, the improved optics allows a more detailed, 3-dimensional view of the operation. Second, the use of articulating instruments vastly improves the surgeon's ability to perform complex maneuvers, particularly in complex liver surgery. Finally, the used algorithms reduce the fatigue and tremor associated with laparoscopic surgery. The procedures described later describe our methodology for robotic hepatectomies.

ROBOTIC RIGHT HEPATECTOMY/ROBOTIC RIGHT POSTERIOR HEPATECTOMY

After intubation, the patient is placed in 12° reverse Trendelenburg and 5 to 10° right side up. A bump is placed under the right hemiabdomen. A Pfannenstiel incision is made and a hand port placed. A 12-mm assist port is introduced through the hand port for insufflation to 12 to 15 mm Hg. The camera is introduced to inspect the liver and rule out extrahepatic disease/distant metastasis. The additional robotic ports are then placed across the upper abdomen as previously described (see *Robotic Port Types and Placement*).

The falciform ligament is taken down, and the extrahepatic right hepatic vein is exposed. Intraoperative ultrasound is used to identify the target lesion. In addition, the ultrasound is used to identify the hepatic veins, portal vein, and additional lesions in the liver. The middle hepatic vein location is marked on the liver surface (**Fig. 4**A). We then proceed with inflow control. The right liver hilum is exposed by using the cystic duct to retract the common bile duct medially (**Fig. 4**B). The right hepatic artery is dissected and exposed. The right hepatic artery is occluded with a bulldog, and left hepatic artery flow is confirmed with doppler ultrasound. The right hepatic artery is then clipped and divided (**Fig. 4**C). The portal vein bifurcation is then identified and dissected. Once the right portal vein is adequately dissected and distinct from the left portal vein, it is ligated with a combination of suture ligation and clips (**Fig. 4**D). At this point, we inject 2.5 ug of ICG systemically to confirm liver demarcation (**Fig. 4**E). Umbilical tape is passed around the hepatoduodenal ligament and Rummel tourniquet used around a short (5 cm) 18-Fr red rubber catheter in the event a full pringle is needed during parenchymal transection.

After inflow control, we proceed with mobilization of the right liver. The hepatoduodenal ligament and right triangular ligaments are divided, and the liver is mobilized from the infrahepatic inferior vena cava to the right hepatic vein. All short hepatic veins are carefully dissected and subsequently either clipped and divided using vessel sealer until the base of the right hepatic vein is visualized (**Fig. 4**F). Once mobilization of the liver is complete, we proceed with parenchymal transection using the laparoscopic CUSA (**Fig. 4**G). Using the demarcated right liver edge after ICG injection, the liver is carefully transected. All bile ducts and vessel tributaries are clipped and divided. The parenchymal transection is carried down to the right hilar plate (**Fig. 4**H). Before dividing the right hilar plate, an ICG cholangiogram is performed to identify the hepatic confluence and avoid injury to the left hepatic duct. The right hilar plate is typically divided with a robotic stapler (**Fig. 4**I). The parenchymal transection is carried up to the right hepatic vein. The right hepatic vein is dissected and transected with a robotic stapler, completing the parenchymal transection. The cut surface of the liver is visualized for hemostasis and biliary leakage. Ultrasound with Doppler is used to confirm liver remnant inflow patency (**Fig. 4**J). The liver specimen is then retrieved through the Pfannenstiel incision. See Video 1 for a robotic right hepatectomy.

For right posterior hepatectomy, the steps are similar to right hepatectomy. For inflow control, the right posterior sector hepatic artery is identified, dissected (**Fig. 5**A), and ligated followed by the right posterior sector portal vein (**Fig. 5**B). Ultrasound with Doppler is used to confirm the inflow anatomy before dividing the vessels. Umbilical tape is placed around the hepatoduodenal ligament in the event a Pringle maneuver is required. The right liver is fully mobilized. The table is now rotated to 15 to 20° right side up to accommodate the posterior parenchymal transection. Ultrasound is used to identify the right hepatic vein and mark a parenchymal transection plane to ensure a negative margin (**Fig. 5**C). ICG is administered to confirm demarcation of the right posterior sector and guide the parenchymal transection (**Fig. 5**D). Parenchymal transection is performed with the laparoscopic CUSA between segments 6/7 from 5/8. Any larger branches of the right hepatic vein are identified and transected using the robotic stapler. See Video 2 for a robotic right posterior hepatectomy.

ROBOTIC LEFT HEPATECTOMY/LEFT LATERAL SECTIONECTOMY

Positioning and port placement for left hepatectomy are similar to right hepatectomy. The falciform is taken down and extrahepatic hepatic veins dissected and exposed. The left triangular ligament is divided to mobilize the left liver. Intraoperative ultrasound is used to visualize the lesion, portal vein, and hepatic veins and rule out additional lesions in the liver. The middle hepatic vein is marked and the parenchymal transection plane planned. We then proceed with inflow control by exposing the left liver hilum

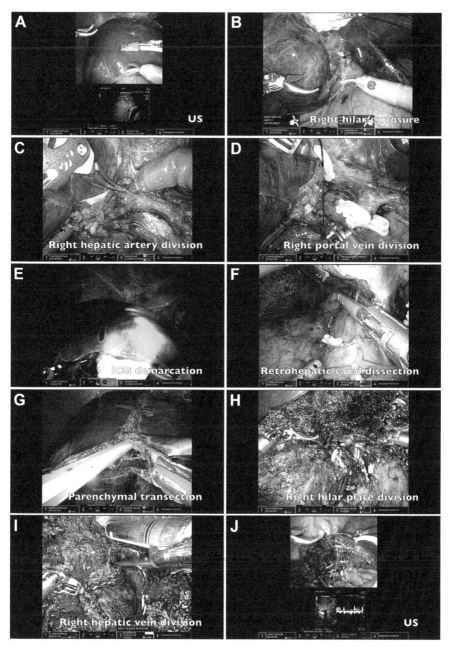

Fig. 4. Robotic right hepatectomy. Ultrasound is introduced to identify the biliary and vascular anatomy of the liver and the location of the tumor (*A*). The right liver hilum is exposed by retracting the common bile duct medial (*B*). Inflow control includes identifying and ligating the right hepatic artery (*C*) and portal vein (*D*). ICG is administered to demarcate the transection plane (*E*). After mobilization of the liver the retrohepatic caval dissection is performed by dividing short hepatic veins up to the level of the right hepatic vein (*F*). The liver parenchyma is transected using a CUSA (*G*). The parenchymal transection is carried down to the right hilar plate (*H*), which is divided with a robotic stapler. The parenchymal

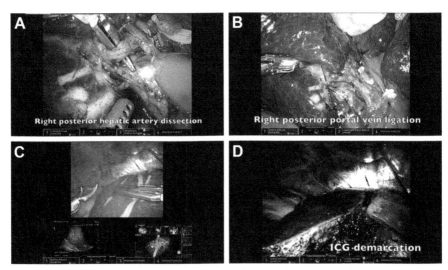

Fig. 5. Robotic right posterior hepatectomy. Robotic right posterior hepatectomy is performed with a similar approach as right hepatectomy. The right liver hilum is exposed, and the right posterior sector hepatic artery is identified and ligated (*A*) followed by the right posterior sector portal vein branch (*B*). An ultrasound is used to identify the pertinent vascular and biliary structures and mark the planned parenchymal transection plane (*C*), which is also guided following ICG administration (*D*). Parenchymal transection is performed with the laparoscopic CUSA. See Video 2 for a robotic right posterior hepatectomy.

below the umbilical fissure. The left hepatic artery is dissected and isolated as it enters the umbilical fissure and clipped and ligated at this location (**Fig. 6**A). The portal vein bifurcation is then identified and left portal vein isolated. It is important to note that adequate dissection may require division of the caudate lobe branches. The left portal vein is then divided using suture ligation and clips (**Fig. 6**B). ICG is injected systemically to demarcate the left lobe of the liver (**Fig. 6**C). Umbilical tape is placed around the hepatoduodenal ligament in the event a Pringle maneuver is required.

Parenchymal transection is performed along the demarcated dissection line using the laparoscopic CUSA as described (**Fig. 6**D). The parenchymal transection is carried down to the left hilar plate (**Fig. 6**E). ICG cholangiogram is used to confirm the anatomy and identify the biliary confluence. The left bile duct is divided using either clips or the robotic stapler. The parenchymal transection is carried up to the left hepatic vein. Finally, the left hepatic vein is divided with a stapler (**Fig. 6**F). The specimen is then removed through the Pfannenstiel incision and liver surface evaluated for hemostasis and bile leaks. See Video 3 for a robotic left hepatectomy.

Our approach to a left lateral sectionectomy is similar to left hepatectomy, although hilar dissection is typically not required (**Fig. 7**). After positioning the patient and docking the robot the left liver is mobilized. Ultrasound introduced to confirm the lesion is present in the left lateral liver. The left hepatic vein and respective pedicles to segment

---

transection proceeds up to the right hepatic vein, which is also divided with the robotic stapler (*I*). Hepatic inflow to the left liver remnant is confirmed with ultrasound (*J*). See Video 1 for a robotic right hepatectomy.

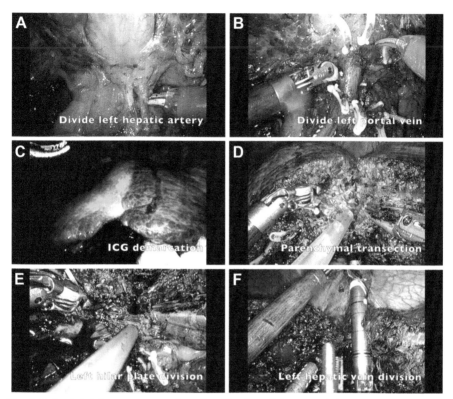

Fig. 6. Robotic left hepatectomy. After identification of the major biliary vascular structures with ultrasound (US), the left liver hilum is identified below the umbilical fissure. The left hepatic artery (A) and left portal vein (B) are identified and divided. ICG is injected to demarcate the liver plane (C). After mobilization of the liver, parenchymal transection is performed using the CUSA (D) down to the hilar plate (E), which is then divided with a robotic stapler. The parenchymal transection is carried up to the left hepatic vein, which is dissected and divided with the robotic stapler (F). See Video 3 for a robotic left hepatectomy.

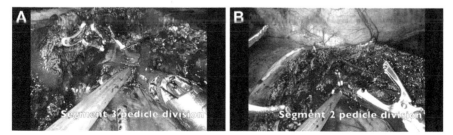

Fig. 7. Robotic left lateral sectionectomy. Left lateral sectionectomy is performed without extensive dissection of the hilum. After using the ultrasound to identify the left lateral structures and mobilization of the left lateral liver, the CUSA is used to divide the liver just medial to the falciform ligament. The pedicles to segment 3 (A) and 2 (B) are identified and ligated with clips and divided. The parenchymal transection is carried to the left hepatic vein, which is divided with the robotic stapler. See Video 4 for a robotic left lateral hepatectomy.

2 and segment 3 are visualized with the ultrasound and marked on the liver surface. The left triangular ligament is then divided to mobilize the left lateral liver. The laparoscopic CUSA is used to transect segments 2/3 medial to the falciform ligament. The segment 2 and 3 pedicles are identified intraparenchymally and divided with clips or staples. Finally, the left hepatic vein is divided with a stapler and specimen removed via the Pfannenstiel incision. See Video 4 for a robotic left lateral hepatectomy.

ROBOTIC RIGHT ANTERIOR SECTIONECTOMY AND CENTRAL HEPATECTOMY

Central resections of the liver, although not previously described in the Brisbane 2000 Terminology, have proved to be oncologic sound operations that allow for parenchymal preservation. Right anterior sectionectomy (segments 5 and 8) and central hepatectomy (segments 4, 5, and 8) have previously been described but less well reported in minimally invasive surgery, perhaps owing to its technical difficulty. However, the robotic approach enables precise resection of the central liver while allowing for the technical versatility to access difficult areas of the procedure.[77]

Our approach, patient positioning, and port placement are similar to previously described major hepatectomies. For right anterior sectionectomy (segments 5 and 8), we obtain inflow control by isolating and dissecting the right anterior sector right hepatic artery, which is subsequently clipped and divided (**Fig. 8**A). The right anterior sector portal vein is then identified, dissected, and divided using a combination of suture ligation and clips (**Fig. 8**B). Ultrasound with Doppler is used to confirm the inflow anatomy before dividing the right anterior sector hepatic artery and portal vein branches. ICG is administered to demonstrate demarcation of the right anterior sector (**Fig. 8**C). Umbilical tape is placed around the hepatoduodenal ligament in the event a Pringle maneuver is required.

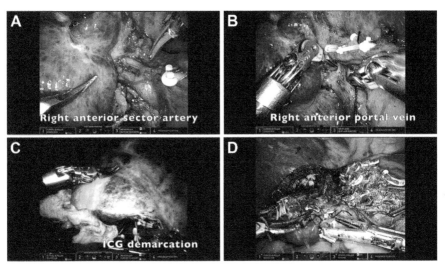

Fig. 8. Robotic right anterior sectionectomy. After right hilar exposure, the right anterior sector hepatic artery (A) and portal vein (B) are identified and divided. Ultrasound is used to identify the vascular and biliary structures in the liver and ICG used to demarcate the medial and lateral edges of the transection plane (C). Parenchymal transection is performed with the CUSA along both the segment 5/8–segment 6/7 and segment 5/8–segment 4 planes. The resection bed is inspected for bleeding or bile leakage (D). See Video 5 for a robotic right anterior sectionectomy.

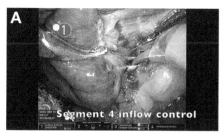
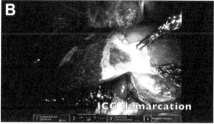

Fig. 9. Central hepatectomy. After hilar exposure, the inflow control is obtained by identifying and ligating the right anterior sector and segment 4 branches hepatic artery and portal vein branches (*A*). ICG is used to confirm inflow control and facilitate demarcation of the transection planes (*B*). Parenchymal transection is performed as previously described. See Video 6 for a robotic central hepatectomy.

The right liver is mobilized, and the parenchyma transection planes are marked with ultrasound. The laparoscopic CUSA is used for parenchymal transection and all bile and vessel tributaries and controlled and divided using energy vessel devices and/ or clips. Parenchymal transection occurs medially between segment 5/8 and segment 4a/4b and laterally between segment 5/8 and segment 6/7. Major hepatic vein branches are divided with the robotic stapler. Hemostasis is confirmed, and signs of bile leaks are evaluated (**Fig. 8**D). See Video 5 for a robotic right anterior sectionectomy.

Central hepatectomy (segment 4, 5, and 8) is similarly performed. The right anterior sector branches of the right hepatic artery and portal veins are divided. In addition, the vascular arterial and portal branches to segment 4 are identified, dissected, and divided along the umbilical fissure (**Fig. 9**A). ICG is administered to demonstrate central liver demarcation (**Fig. 9**B). Parenchymal division is accomplished using the CUSA medially between segment 4a/4b and segment 2/3 and laterally between segment 5/8 and segment 6/7. The middle hepatic vein is then divided and ligated using the robotic stapler. Hemostasis is confirmed, and signs of bile leaks are evaluated. See Video 6 for a robotic central hepatectomy.

SUMMARY

Minimally invasive liver resection has proved to be an important advancement for patients with resectable hepatocellular carcinoma by improving outcomes while preserving oncologic resection principles. The combination of minimally invasive techniques and ERAS protocols has allowed most of the uncomplicated patients undergoing major hepatectomy to be discharged on postoperative day 1 or 2 without readmission or long-term complications. As a result, particularly in high-volume centers, minimally invasive liver resection has developed into an effective approach to hepatocellular carcinoma resection. In this review, our approach to performing robotic hepatectomies was described in detail, including use of a standardized port placement and integration of the laparoscopic CUSA. Better understanding of the procedure and improved outcomes associated with minimally invasive techniques can hopefully lead to increased adoption for hepatocellular carcinoma resection.

DISCLOSURE

The authors have no disclosures or conflicts of interest.

SUPPLEMENTARY DATA

Supplementary data related to this article can be found online at https://doi.org/10.1016/j.soc.2023.06.009.

REFERENCES

1. American Cancer Society. Cancer facts & figures 2022. Atlanta: American Cancer Society; 2022. Available at: https://www.cancer.org/content/dam/cancer-org/research/cancer-facts-and-statistics/annual-cancer-facts-and-figures/2022/2022-cancer-facts-and-figures.pdf. Access: March 22, 2023.
2. Hawksworth J, Llore N, Holzner ML, et al. Robotic Hepatectomy Is a Safe and Cost-Effective Alternative to Conventional Open Hepatectomy: a Single-Center Preliminary Experience. J Gastrointest Surg 2021;25(3):825–8.
3. Kokudo N, Takemura N, Ito K, et al. The history of liver surgery: Achievements over the past 50 years. Ann Gastroenterol Surg 2020;4(2):109–17.
4. Tanabe KK. The past 60 years in liver surgery. Cancer 2008;113(7 Suppl):1888–96.
5. Mittler J, McGillicuddy JW, Chavin KD. Laparoscopic liver resection in the treatment of hepatocellular carcinoma. Clin Liver Dis 2011;15(2):371–84, vii-x.
6. Foster JH. History of liver surgery. Arch Surg 1991;126(3):381–7.
7. Honjo I, Araki C. Total resection of the right lobe of the liver; report of a successful case. J Int Coll Surg 1955;23(1 Pt 1):23–8.
8. Alkatout I, Mechler U, Mettler L, et al. The Development of Laparoscopy-A Historical Overview. Front Surg 2021;8:799442.
9. Reich H, McGlynn F, DeCaprio J, et al. Laparoscopic excision of benign liver lesions. Obstet Gynecol 1991;78(5 Pt 2):956–8.
10. Hashizume M, Takenaka K, Yanaga K, et al. Laparoscopic hepatic resection for hepatocellular carcinoma. Surg Endosc 1995;9(12):1289–91.
11. Azagra JS, Goergen M, Gilbart E, et al. Laparoscopic anatomical (hepatic) left lateral segmentectomy-technical aspects. Surg Endosc 1996;10(7):758–61.
12. Choi SB, Park JS, Kim JK, et al. Early experiences of robotic-assisted laparoscopic liver resection. Yonsei Med J 2008;49(4):632–8.
13. Caruso S, Patriti A, Ceccarelli G, et al. Minimally invasive liver resection: has the time come to consider robotics a valid assistance? Hepatobiliary Surg Nutr 2018;7(3):195–8.
14. Vanounou T, Steel JL, Nguyen KT, et al. Comparing the clinical and economic impact of laparoscopic versus open liver resection. Ann Surg Oncol 2010;17(4):998–1009.
15. Ciria R, Cherqui D, Geller DA, et al. Comparative Short-term Benefits of Laparoscopic Liver Resection: 9000 Cases and Climbing. Ann Surg 2016;263(4):761–77.
16. Cherqui D, Laurent A, Mocellin N, et al. Liver resection for transplantable hepatocellular carcinoma: long-term survival and role of secondary liver transplantation. Ann Surg 2009;250(5):738–46.
17. Dagher I, Belli G, Fantini C, et al. Laparoscopic hepatectomy for hepatocellular carcinoma: a European experience. J Am Coll Surg 2010;211(1):16–23.
18. Vigano L, Tayar C, Laurent A, et al. Laparoscopic liver resection: a systematic review. J Hepatobiliary Pancreat Surg 2009;16(4):410–21.
19. Aldrighetti L, Guzzetti E, Pulitano C, et al. Case-matched analysis of totally laparoscopic versus open liver resection for HCC: short and middle term results. J Surg Oncol 2010;102(1):82–6.

20. He J, Amini N, Spolverato G, et al. National trends with a laparoscopic liver resection: results from a population-based analysis. HPB (Oxford) 2015;17(10):919–26.
21. Buell JF, Cherqui D, Geller DA, et al. The international position on laparoscopic liver surgery: The Louisville Statement, 2008. Ann Surg 2009;250(5):825–30.
22. Fancellu A, Rosman AS, Sanna V, et al. Meta-analysis of trials comparing minimally-invasive and open liver resections for hepatocellular carcinoma. J Surg Res 2011;171(1):e33–45.
23. Wakabayashi G, Cherqui D, Geller DA, et al. Recommendations for laparoscopic liver resection: a report from the second international consensus conference held in Morioka. Ann Surg 2015;261(4):619–29.
24. Abu Hilal M, Aldrighetti L, Dagher I, et al. The Southampton Consensus Guidelines for Laparoscopic Liver Surgery: From Indication to Implementation. Ann Surg 2018;268(1):11–8.
25. Chua D, Syn N, Koh YX, et al. Learning curves in minimally invasive hepatectomy: systematic review and meta-regression analysis. Br J Surg 2021;108(4):351–8.
26. Fukumori D, Tschuor C, Penninga L, et al. Learning curves in robot-assisted minimally invasive liver surgery at a high-volume center in Denmark: Report of the first 100 patients and review of literature. Scand J Surg 2023;31. https://doi.org/10.1177/14574969221146003. 14574969221146003.
27. Krenzien F, Benzing C, Feldbrügge L, et al. Complexity-adjusted learning curves for robotic and laparoscopic liver resection: a word of caution. Annals of Surgery Open 2022;3(1):e131.
28. Takahara T, Wakabayashi G, Beppu T, et al. Long-term and perioperative outcomes of laparoscopic versus open liver resection for hepatocellular carcinoma with propensity score matching: a multi-institutional Japanese study. J Hepatobiliary Pancreat Sci 2015;22(10):721–7.
29. Giulianotti PC, Bianco FM, Daskalaki D, et al. Robotic liver surgery: technical aspects and review of the literature. Hepatobiliary Surg Nutr 2016;5(4):311–21.
30. Di Benedetto F, Magistri P, Di Sandro S, et al. Safety and Efficacy of Robotic vs Open Liver Resection for Hepatocellular Carcinoma. JAMA Surg 2023;158(1):46–54.
31. Nevarez NM, Yopp AC. Anatomic *vs*. non-anatomic liver resection for hepatocellular carcinoma: standard of care or unfilled promises? Hepatoma Research 2021;7:66.
32. Liu H, Hu FJ, Li H, et al. Anatomical vs nonanatomical liver resection for solitary hepatocellular carcinoma: A systematic review and meta-analysis. World J Gastrointest Oncol 2021;13(11):1833–46.
33. Xu H, Liu F, Hao X, et al. Laparoscopically anatomical versus non-anatomical liver resection for large hepatocellular carcinoma. HPB (Oxford) 2020;22(1):136–43.
34. Strasberg JB SM, Clavien P-A, Gadzijev E, et al. The Brisbane 2000 Terminology of Liver Anatomy and Resections. HPB (Oxford) 2000;2(3):333–9.
35. Wakabayashi G, Cherqui D, Geller DA, et al. The Tokyo 2020 terminology of liver anatomy and resections: Updates of the Brisbane 2000 system. J Hepatobiliary Pancreat Sci 2022;29(1):6–15.
36. Takasaki K, Kobayashi S, Tanaka S, et al. Highly anatomically systematized hepatic resection with Glissonean sheath code transection at the hepatic hilus. Int Surg 1990;75(2):73–7.
37. Cucchetti A, Cescon M, Ercolani G, et al. A comprehensive meta-regression analysis on outcome of anatomic resection versus nonanatomic resection for hepatocellular carcinoma. Ann Surg Oncol 2012;19(12):3697–705.

38. Zhou Y, Xu D, Wu L, et al. Meta-analysis of anatomic resection versus nonanatomic resection for hepatocellular carcinoma. Langenbeck's Arch Surg 2011; 396(7):1109–17.
39. Feng X, Su Y, Zheng S, et al. A double blinded prospective randomized trial comparing the effect of anatomic versus non-anatomic resection on hepatocellular carcinoma recurrence. HPB (Oxford) 2017;19(8):667–74.
40. Amin MB, Greene FL, Edge SB, et al. The Eighth Edition AJCC Cancer Staging Manual: Continuing to build a bridge from a population-based to a more "personalized" approach to cancer staging. CA Cancer J Clin 2017;67(2):93–9.
41. Okuda K, Ohtsuki T, Obata H, et al. Natural history of hepatocellular carcinoma and prognosis in relation to treatment. Study of 850 patients. Cancer 1985; 56(4):918–28.
42. A new prognostic system for hepatocellular carcinoma: a retrospective study of 435 patients: the Cancer of the Liver Italian Program (CLIP) investigators. Hepatology 1998;28(3):751–5.
43. Llovet JM, Bru C, Bruix J. Prognosis of hepatocellular carcinoma: the BCLC staging classification. Semin Liver Dis 1999;19(3):329–38.
44. Johnson PJ, Berhane S, Kagebayashi C, et al. Assessment of liver function in patients with hepatocellular carcinoma: a new evidence-based approach-the ALBI grade. J Clin Oncol 2015;33(6):550–8.
45. Mehta N, Heimbach J, Harnois DM, et al. Validation of a Risk Estimation of Tumor Recurrence After Transplant (RETREAT) Score for Hepatocellular Carcinoma Recurrence After Liver Transplant. JAMA Oncol 2017;3(4):493–500.
46. Reig M, Forner A, Rimola J, et al. BCLC strategy for prognosis prediction and treatment recommendation: The 2022 update. J Hepatol 2022;76(3):681–93.
47. Vauthey JN, Dixon E, Abdalla EK, et al. Pretreatment assessment of hepatocellular carcinoma: expert consensus statement. HPB (Oxford) 2010;12(5):289–99.
48. Belghiti J, Kianmanesh R. Surgical treatment of hepatocellular carcinoma. HPB (Oxford) 2005;7(1):42–9.
49. Chapelle T, Op de Beeck B, Roeyen G, et al. Measuring future liver remnant function prior to hepatectomy may guide the indication for portal vein occlusion and avoid posthepatectomy liver failure: a prospective interventional study. HPB (Oxford) 2017;19(2):108–17.
50. Guglielmi A, Ruzzenente A, Conci S, et al. How much remnant is enough in liver resection? Dig Surg 2012;29(1):6–17.
51. Dixon E, Abdalla E, Schwarz RE, et al. AHPBA/SSO/SSAT sponsored Consensus Conference on Multidisciplinary Treatment of Hepatocellular Carcinoma. HPB (Oxford) 2010;12(5):287–8.
52. Ribero D, Chun YS, Vauthey JN. Standardized liver volumetry for portal vein embolization. Semin Intervent Radiol 2008;25(2):104–9.
53. Gavriilidis P, Marangoni G, Ahmad J, et al. Simultaneous portal and hepatic vein embolization is better than portal embolization or ALPPS for hypertrophy of future liver remnant before major hepatectomy: A systematic review and network meta-analysis. Hepatobiliary Pancreat Dis Int 2022. https://doi.org/10.1016/j.hbpd.2022.08.013.
54. Gruttadauria S, Di Francesco F, Miraglia R. Liver venous deprivation: an interesting approach for regenerative liver surgery. Updates Surg 2022;74(1):385–6.
55. van Dam RM, Hendry PO, Coolsen MM, et al. Initial experience with a multimodal enhanced recovery programme in patients undergoing liver resection. Br J Surg 2008;95(8):969–75.

56. Noba L, Rodgers S, Chandler C, et al. Enhanced Recovery After Surgery (ERAS) Reduces Hospital Costs and Improve Clinical Outcomes in Liver Surgery: a Systematic Review and Meta-Analysis. J Gastrointest Surg 2020;24(4):918–32.

57. Joliat GR, Kobayashi K, Hasegawa K, et al. Guidelines for Perioperative Care for Liver Surgery: Enhanced Recovery After Surgery (ERAS) Society Recommendations 2022. World J Surg 2023;47(1):11–34.

58. Agarwal V, Divatia JV. Enhanced recovery after surgery in liver resection: current concepts and controversies. Korean J Anesthesiol 2019;72(2):119–29.

59. Tympa A, Theodoraki K, Tsaroucha A, et al. Anesthetic Considerations in Hepatectomies under Hepatic Vascular Control. HPB Surg 2012;2012:720754.

60. Hughes MJ, Ventham NT, Harrison EM, et al. Central venous pressure and liver resection: a systematic review and meta-analysis. HPB (Oxford) 2015;17(10): 863–71.

61. Guo T, Ding R, Yang J, et al. Evaluation of different antibiotic prophylaxis strategies for hepatectomy: A network meta-analysis. Medicine (Baltim) 2019;98(26): e16241.

62. Hawksworth J, Radkani P, Nguyen B, et al. Improving safety of robotic major hepatectomy with extrahepatic inflow control and laparoscopic CUSA parenchymal transection: technical description and initial experience. Surg Endosc 2022; 36(5):3270–6.

63. Pamecha V, Gurusamy KS, Sharma D, et al. Techniques for liver parenchymal transection: a meta-analysis of randomized controlled trials. HPB (Oxford) 2009;11(4):275–81.

64. Scatton O, Brustia R, Belli G, et al. What kind of energy devices should be used for laparoscopic liver resection? Recommendations from a systematic review. J Hepatobiliary Pancreat Sci 2015;22(5):327–34.

65. Marino MV, Podda M, Fernandez CC, et al. The application of indocyanine green-fluorescence imaging during robotic-assisted liver resection for malignant tumors: a single-arm feasibility cohort study. HPB (Oxford) 2020;22(3):422–31.

66. Ishizawa T, Fukushima N, Shibahara J, et al. Real-time identification of liver cancers by using indocyanine green fluorescent imaging. Cancer 2009;115(11): 2491–504.

67. Wakabayashi T, Cacciaguerra AB, Abe Y, et al. Indocyanine Green Fluorescence Navigation in Liver Surgery: A Systematic Review on Dose and Timing of Administration. Ann Surg 2022;275(6):1025–34.

68. Boni L, David G, Mangano A, et al. Clinical applications of indocyanine green (ICG) enhanced fluorescence in laparoscopic surgery. Surg Endosc 2015; 29(7):2046–55.

69. Lim C, Vibert E, Azoulay D, et al. Indocyanine green fluorescence imaging in the surgical management of liver cancers: current facts and future implications. J Visc Surg 2014;151(2):117–24.

70. Rossi G, Tarasconi A, Baiocchi G, et al. Fluorescence guided surgery in liver tumors: applications and advantages. Acta Biomed 2018;89(9-S):135–40.

71. Belghiti J, Kabbej M, Sauvanet A, et al. Drainage after elective hepatic resection. A randomized trial. Ann Surg 1993;218(6):748–53.

72. Fong Y, Brennan MF, Brown K, et al. Drainage is unnecessary after elective liver resection. Am J Surg 1996;171(1):158–62.

73. Liu CL, Fan ST, Lo CM, et al. Abdominal drainage after hepatic resection is contraindicated in patients with chronic liver diseases. Ann Surg 2004;239(2):194–201.

74. Fuster J, Llovet JM, Garcia-Valdecasas JC, et al. Abdominal drainage after liver resection for hepatocellular carcinoma in cirrhotic patients: a randomized controlled study. Hepatogastroenterology 2004;51(56):536–40.
75. Sun HC, Qin LX, Lu L, et al. Randomized clinical trial of the effects of abdominal drainage after elective hepatectomy using the crushing clamp method. Br J Surg 2006;93(4):422–6.
76. Arita J, Sakamaki K, Saiura A, et al. Drain Placement After Uncomplicated Hepatic Resection Increases Severe Postoperative Complication Rate: A Japanese Multi-institutional Randomized Controlled Trial (ND-trial). Ann Surg 2021;273(2):224–31.
77. Hawksworth J, Radkani P, Filice R, et al. Robotic Central Hepatectomy and Right Anterior Sectionectomy: Minimally Invasive Parenchyma Sparing Surgery for Central Liver Tumors. J Gastrointest Surg 2023;27(2):407–10.
78. Han HS, Cho JY, Kaneko H, et al. Expert Panel Statement on Laparoscopic Living Donor Hepatectomy. Dig Surg 2018;35(4):284–8.
79. Cherqui D, Ciria R, Kwon CHD, et al. Expert Consensus Guidelines on Minimally Invasive Donor Hepatectomy for Living Donor Liver Transplantation From Innovation to Implementation: A Joint Initiative From the International Laparoscopic Liver Society (ILLS) and the Asian-Pacific Hepato-Pancreato-Biliary Association (A-PHPBA). Ann Surg 2021;273(1):96–108.

Optimal Liver Transplantation Criteria for Hepatocellular Carcinoma

Mignote Yilma, MD[a,b], Neil Mehta, MD[c],*

KEYWORDS

- Hepatocellular carcinoma • Liver transplantation • AFP • Locoregional therapy
- Downstaging • Milan criteria

KEY POINTS

- Liver transplant is the treatment of choice for patients with early-stage hepatocellular carcinoma (HCC) in the setting of portal hypertension and/or decompensated liver disease.
- In the United States, alpha-fetoprotein (AFP) greater than 1000 ng/mL is considered a contraindication for liver transplant. Although a decrease in AFP to less than 500 ng/mL with locoregional therapy has been associated with comparable posttransplant survival, AFP cutoffs as low as 20 ng/mL can be used to identify patients who might benefit from liver transplantation.
- Liver transplant patient selection might prioritize response to locoregional therapy for deceased donor liver transplant, while prioritizing both biomarker and radiographic response for living donor liver transplant.
- Complete locoregional response for a single small tumor (with low AFP and compensated liver disease) can be used to identify patients with low transplant urgency who might not derive much benefit from transplant.
- Optimal liver transplant selection for patients with HCC should consider tumor burden, biological and radiographic response to locoregional therapy, and organ availability.

INTRODUCTION

Patients with hepatocellular carcinoma (HCC) derive optimal benefit from liver transplantation (LT), but this requires balancing their risk of waitlist dropout from tumor progression with their risk of tumor recurrence post-LT. In 1996, the Milan criteria (1 lesion

[a] Department of Surgery, University of California San Francisco, 513 Parnassus Avenue, S-321, San Francisco, CA 94143, USA; [b] National Clinician Scholars Program, University of California San Francisco, 513 Parnassus Avenue, S-321, San Francisco, CA 94143, USA; [c] Department of Medicine, University of California San Francisco, Connie Frank Transplant Center, 400 Parnassus Avenue 7th Floor, San Francisco, CA 94143, USA
* Corresponding author.
E-mail address: Neil.mehta@ucsf.edu
Twitter: @mignoteyilmaMD (M.Y.)

Surg Oncol Clin N Am 33 (2024) 133–142
https://doi.org/10.1016/j.soc.2023.06.011
1055-3207/24/© 2023 Elsevier Inc. All rights reserved.

≤5 cm, 2–3 lesions ≤3 cm)[1] was introduced as selection criteria for patients with HCC for LT. In early 2002, the Model for End-Stage Liver Disease (MELD) exception points were introduced in the United States, giving priority to patients with HCC,[2] which inadvertently led to increased waitlist dropout for non-HCC patients.[3] In response, a 6-month wait period requirement before awarding MELD exception points and an MELD exception cap were enacted.[4,5] Although Markov models suggest a minimum acceptable 5-year post-LT survival threshold of 61% for those beyond Milan criteria,[6] careful patient selection criteria based on tumor burden and biomarkers has shown 5-year post-LT survival of 80%.[7] Although this is the current landscape in which LT for HCC exists, the story starts with the greater debate of what the optimal LT cutoff for HCC is, which requires balancing the risk of tumor progression with risk of tumor recurrence.

TRANSPLANT SURVIVAL AND WAITLIST URGENCY

For non-HCC patients, MELD-Na > 15 has been a proposed cutoff for LT, with decreased survival benefit in those with MELD-Na below this threshold. Nevertheless, this "transplant benefit," the number of years gained by LT minus the number of years gained by alternative treatments,[8] has not been clearly established for patients with HCC. Based solely on tumor burden, the University of California San Francisco (UCSF) criteria (single tumor ≤6.5 cm or ≤3 lesions with largest one ≤4.5 cm, and total tumor diameter ≤8 cm)[7] predicts 81% 5-year post-LT survival. As the upper limit of tumor burden increases, the post-LT survival drops slightly below this threshold. For instance, patients beyond Milan but within "up-to-7" (sum of largest tumor and number of tumors <7)[9] have 5-year post-LT survival of 71%.

With advances in local-regional therapy (LRT), we have started to identify patients with long waitlist survival who might derive no benefit from LT compared with alternative treatments. In a study of more than 2100 patients with HCC,[10] MELD score less than 13, within Milan criteria, alpha-fetoprotein (AFP), and radiologic response to LRT were used to identify a subset of patients who derived no benefit from LT compared with alternative treatments. Similarly, Mehta and colleagues[11] identified a subset of patients with HCC within Milan criteria who had a low risk of waitlist dropout as those with low tumor burden (1 tumor 2–3 cm), complete response to LRT, and posttreatment AFP level ≤20 ng/mL. A United Network of Organ Sharing (UNOS) study similarly found that patients with 1 tumor of 2 to 3 cm, AFP < 20 ng/mL, Child-Pugh A disease, and MELD-Na < 15 have low risk of waitlist dropout.[12] Because patients with HCC appear to have lower 5-year survival benefit from LT when compared with non-HCC patients,[13] identifying patients with long waitlist survival allows us to judiciously select patients for LT. In addition, LRT can be used to bridge patients within Milan criteria who are on the waitlist, thus reducing their risk of waitlist dropout from tumor progression.[14] Patients with waitlist time greater than 6 months are recommended to undergo bridging therapy, with complete pathologic response predicting reduced post-LT recurrence as well as improved recurrence-free survival.[15,16]

HEPATOCELLULAR CARCINOMA DOWNSTAGING

Patients beyond Milan criteria can be downstaged to within Milan criteria, which has emerged as a reliable tool to select patients for LT.[17] For patients downstaged to within Milan criteria, their 5-year post-LT survival after successful downstaging appears to be similar to those within Milan criteria.[18] Given the limited supply of organs, response to down-staging can be used as a prognostic marker to select patients with favorable tumor biology,[19] thus maximizing transplant survival benefit. The Region 5

Down-staging protocol,[20] which has been accepted as the national policy in the US (UNOS Down-Staging [UNOS-DS]), has led to 80% and 87% post-LT 5-year survival and recurrence-free estimates, respectively. A more recent analysis of beyond Milan criteria patients found 52% and 21% 10-year post-LT survival and recurrence rate, respectively, in those downstaged compared with 62% and 13% in those always within Milan criteria.[21] Despite the organ shortage, LT continues to be the best available therapy for patients beyond Milan criteria who undergo downstaging, with a recent randomized trial finding 5-year overall survival of 78% in those who undergo LT versus 31% in those who did not.[17]

Down-staging to within Milan criteria should be paired with period of waiting to decrease risk of recurrence.[22] A UNOS study of more than 6000 patients with HCC found short waitlist time was an independent predictor of poor patient survival.[23] On the other hand, long waitlist time could lead to waitlist dropout owing to aggressive tumor biology. In the United States, there is a 6-month delay before granting MELD exception point, a time that allows us to assess tumor behavior as well as an opportunity to improve patient selection.[24] A multicenter study of more than 1000 patients with HCC within Milan criteria found the optimal time from HCC diagnosis to deceased donor LT (DDLT) was 6 to 18 months, with similar 5-year post-LT survival estimates for those within the optimal timeframe and increased risk of recurrence within 5 years of LT for those outside of the optimal timeframe.[25]

RADIOGRAPHIC AND BIOCHEMICAL RESPONSE TO LOCOREGIONAL THERAPY

Down-staging protocols are only as good as the means through which they are assessed, with 20% to 30% of tumor stage being underestimated by preoperative imaging.[26,27] Treatment response assessment using the Liver Imaging Reporting and Data System[28] or modified Response Evaluation Criteria in Solid Tumors (mRECIST)[29] in those receiving LRT can help classify tumor progression using objective response that have been shown to predict improved patient survival.[30,31] A recent multicenter prospective study from the MERITS-LT consortium[32] of 209 patients who met UNOS-DS criteria and had successfully been downstaged to within Milan criteria found no difference in mRECIST between transarterial chemoembolization and yttrium-90 radioembolization. Although greater than 80% of patients were successfully down-staged, 43% were under-staged (exceeded T2 criteria) based on explant histology. This suggests that pre-LT imaging might underestimate tumor burden, and additional efforts should be made to better estimate post-LRT response, including utilization of additional LRT treatments, for example, when viable tumor or tumors or increasing AFP is noted.

Tumor size and biochemical markers continue to be used in patient selection for LT, with responses to LRT allowing us to expand on previously accepted cutoffs. In patients within Milan criteria, AFP level beyond 1000 ng/mL is widely accepted as a contraindication for LT.[33,34] Several other cutoff levels have been suggested with patient selection models advocating for AFP cutoff levels as low as 200 ng/mL[33] and 400 ng/mL,[35] with outcomes beginning to worsen at AFP levels as low as 16 ng/mL.[36] In patients with AFP > 1000 ng/mL, a decrease in AFP to less than 500 ng/mL and 100 ng/mL in those who undergo LRT was associated with 67.0% and 88.4% post-LT survival,[37] with AFP responders to LRT having better post-LT outcomes compared with AFP nonresponders.[38]

MOVING TOWARD OPTIMAL SELECTION CRITERIA

Although patients with HCC have similar post-LT survival estimates to non-HCC patients,[39] their post-LT mortality risk is driven by the rate of HCC recurrence.[40] As such, LT selection criteria for patients with HCC centers on identifying not only those who will have similar post-LT survival as non-HCC patients but also those who will have a low risk of recurrence. The current patient selection criteria in the United States require HCC to be within or downstaged to within Milan criteria and AFP beyond 1000 ng/mL to be reduced to less than 500 ng/mL after LRT.[41] Even after being down-staged, patients initially beyond UNOS-DS need to be carefully selected for LT. For instance, "all-comers" (defined as exceeding UNOS-DS with any number of tumors with total diameter >8 cm but without extrahepatic disease or macrovascular invasion) have lower probability of being successfully downstaged to within Milan criteria and have higher probability of dropout within 2 years of listing owing to tumor progression.[42] In addition, patients with high tumor burden and that require down-staging have a high risk of being understaged.[32,43] As such, the recommendation is to perform additional LRT to reduce tumor burden, with downstaging to within Milan being the minimal requirement for LT.[44]

There are several other selection models (**Fig. 1**, **Table 1**) based on donor type (DDLT or living donor LT [LDLT]), tumor burden, biological marker, and additional factors. Using tumor differentiation and cancer-related symptoms, the extended Toronto criteria (ETC)[45] predicts 68% 5-year post-LT survival for those beyond Milan but within ETC. Although these extended criteria have 5-year estimated post-LT survival estimates that fall slightly below that of within Milan criteria, they do not consider the effects of LRT.[20] Beyond tumor burden, the next set of LT selection criteria incorporate AFP, acknowledging the importance of this biomarker in HCC. The AFP French model[34] identified a low-risk group (largest tumor ≤3 cm and ≤3 tumors and AFP ≤100 ng/mL) with 5-year post-LT survival of 68%. Continuing with the theme of tumor size and biomarkers, the total tumor volume (TTV)-AFP model found 75.0% 4-year post-LT survival for those beyond Milan but within TTV-AFP (defined as TTV ≤115 cm and AFP ≤400 ng/).[46] The Metroticket 2.0[33] model stratified patients based on the sum of tumor number and size, and AFP to predict 5-year post-LT survival, outperforming Milan, UCSF, and Up-to-7 criteria. Although these selection criteria had incorporated AFP, none had looked at the change in AFP. New York/California score,

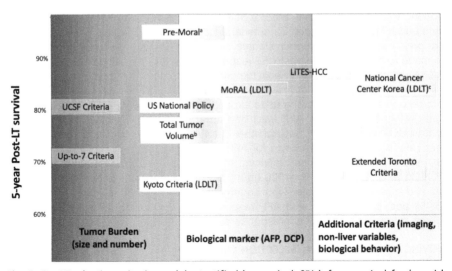

Fig. 1. Pre-LT selection criteria models stratified by survival. [a]Risk-free survival for low-risk group. [b]Four years. [c]Includes tumor size.

Table 1
Pre–liver transplantation selection criteria

Selection Criteria	Tumor Burden	Biological Marker	Additional Criteria	AUROC
UCSF Criteria[7]	Single tumor ≤6.5 cm or ≤3 lesions with largest one ≤4.5 cm, and total tumor diameter ≤8 cm			
Up-to-7 Criteria[9]	Sum of largest tumor and number of tumors <7			
US National Policy[20]	Milan or DS to within Milan	AFP >1000 ng/mL → <500 ng/mL		0.8
Total Tumor Volume (TTV)-AFP[46]	TTV ≤115 cm^3	AFP ≤400 ng/mL		0.57[a]
French AFP[34]	Largest tumor ≤3 cm and ≤3 tumors in lowest risk	AFP		0.78[a]
Metroticket 2.0[33]	Sum of tumor number and size	AFP		
Pre-MORAL[49]	Largest tumor size ≤3 cm for lowest risk	AFP <200 ng/mL for lowest risk	NLR <5 for lowest risk	0.82
HALT-HCC[50]	Tumor number and largest tumor size	Natural log of AFP	MELD-Na	0.61
LiTES-HCC[51]	Total tumor diameter	AFP, AFP-response	Bilirubin, international normalized ratio, estimated glomerular filtration rate, chronic kidney disease, age, diabetes, cause	0.65[b]
Kyoto (LDLT)[54]	Tumor number ≤10, maximal diameter ≤5 cm	DCP ≤400 mAU/mL		
Moral (LDLT)[52]		$\sqrt{AFP}, \sqrt{DCP}$		0.84
National Cancer Center Korea (LDLT)[53]	Tumor diameter <10 cm		Negative ^{18}F-FDG PET	0.80

Abbreviations: AUROC, area under the receiver operating characteristic; DS, downstaged.
[a] c-statistic.
[b] Ten-year area under the curve in validation cohort.

which incorporates AFP response (defined as the difference between maximum and final pre-LT AFP) to stratify patients into risk groups,[38] had a higher performance compared with Milan, French-AFP, and Metroticket 2.0.[47]

Although AFP was the first biomarker to be used in these selection criteria, additional biomarkers have been identified and used in pre-LT selection criteria. In addition to AFP, AFP-L3 greater than 35%, des-γ carboxyprothrombin (DCP) greater than 7.5 ng/mL,[48] and neutrophil-to-lymphocyte ratio (NLR) greater than 5[49] have been associated with worse post-LT outcome. Using NLR (lower risk <5), AFP (lowest risk <200 ng/mL), and tumor size, the pre-MORAL model[49] found 5-year recurrence-free survival of 56% in high-risk versus 99% in low-risk group. The Hazard Associated with Liver Transplantation for HCC (HALT-HCC)[50] scoring model added MELD-Na to tumor burden and AFP and found worsening 5-year overall survival (79% in those with low vs 62% in those with high HALT-HCC score). A new criterion, Liver Transplant Expected Survival-HCC (LiTES-HCC),[51] uses 11 HCC- and non-HCC–specific variables to predict 86.3% post-LT overall survival at 5 years of follow-up. Each of these criteria have further fine-tuned LT selection criteria by using various biomarkers, with each one trying to identify the optimal LT cutoff for DDLT.

In recognition of the different organ donor types, selection criteria have been developed specifically for LDLT patients with HCC. The MoRAL[52] score found 83% 5-year post-LT survival for those with low score (protein induced by vitamin K absence-II and AFP) undergoing LDLT. The National Cancer Center Korea[53] uses tumor diameter less than 10 cm and negative ^{18}F-fluorodeoxyglucose (^{18}F-FDG) PET to predict 84% post-LT survival for patients who meet this criteria and undergo LDLT. The Kyoto criteria[54] found an 82% post-LT survival for those who underwent LDLT using tumor number ≤10, maximal diameter ≤5 cm, and serum DCP ≤400 mAU/mL. Last, Bhangui and colleagues[55] was able to risk-stratify 405 LDLT patients into low-, medium-, and high-risk groups based on pre-LT AFP ≥100 ng/mL, tumor beyond UCSF criteria, and ^{18}F-FDG PET avidity, with 9.3%, 25.0%, and 46.0% risk of recurrence, respectively.

SUMMARY

LT continues to be the optimal treatment for HCC. Considerations for LT among this patient population must take into consideration organ demand and supply, as well as tumor progression with risk of recurrence post-LT. In the United States, Milan (and UNOS-DS for those beyond Milan) criteria have been used to maximize the number of years gained by LT versus by alternative treatments. Advances in LRT have allowed us to downstage patients to within Milan criteria with newer pre-LT selection criteria incorporating dynamic and additional biomarkers as well as imaging modality to risk-stratify patients as we continue to look for the optimal LT cutoff for patients with HCC. Although it is impossible to compare all the LT selection models, the optimal LT criteria should be transplant-center specific, accounting for organ availability (DDLT versus LLDT) and dynamic response to LRT.

CLINICS CARE POINTS

- In non-resection candidates, liver transplantation (LT) is the preferred treatment for early-stage HCC.
- For patients beyond Milan criteria but who otherwise appear to be acceptable candidates for LT, local-regional therapy should be considered for downstaging though patients beyond UNOS-DS criteria have worse intention-to-treat outcomes.

- Response to locoregional therapy should not only be monitored with cross-sectional imaging but also with AFP to assess tumor biology

DISCLOSURE

The authors have nothing to disclose.

REFERENCES

1. Mazzaferro V, Regalia E, Doci R, et al. Liver transplantation for the treatment of small hepatocellular carcinomas in patients with cirrhosis. N Engl J Med 1996; 334(11):693–700.
2. Pomfret EA, Washburn K, Wald C, et al. Report of a national conference on liver allocation in patients with hepatocellular carcinoma in the United States. Liver Transplant 2010;16(3):262–78.
3. Goldberg D, French B, Abt P, et al. Increasing disparity in waitlist mortality rates with increased model for end-stage liver disease scores for candidates with hepatocellular carcinoma versus candidates without hepatocellular carcinoma. Liver Transplant 2012;18(4):434–43.
4. Ishaque T, Massie AB, Bowring MG, et al. Liver transplantation and waitlist mortality for HCC and non-HCC candidates following the 2015 HCC exception policy change. Am J Transplant 2019;19(2):564–72.
5. Nagai S, Kitajima T, Yeddula S, et al. Effect of mandatory 6-month waiting period on waitlist and transplant outcomes in patients with hepatocellular carcinoma. Hepatology 2020;72(6):2051–62.
6. Singal AG, Lampertico P, Nahon P. Epidemiology and surveillance for hepatocellular carcinoma: new trends. J Hepatol 2020;72(2):250–61.
7. Yao FY, Ferrell L, Bass NM, et al. Liver transplantation for hepatocellular carcinoma: expansion of the tumor size limits does not adversely impact survival. Hepatology 2001;33(6):1394–403.
8. Merion RM, Schaubel DE, Dykstra DM, et al. The survival benefit of liver transplantation. Am J Transplant 2005;5(2):307–13.
9. Mazzaferro V, Llovet JM, Miceli R, et al. Predicting survival after liver transplantation in patients with hepatocellular carcinoma beyond the Milan criteria: a retrospective, exploratory analysis. Lancet Oncol 2009;10(1):35–43.
10. Lai Q, Vitale A, Iesari S, et al. Intention-to-treat survival benefit of liver transplantation in patients with hepatocellular cancer. Hepatology 2017;00(0).1910–9.
11. Mehta N, Dodge JL, Goel A, et al. Identification of liver transplant candidates with hepatocellular carcinoma and a very low dropout risk: implications for the current organ allocation policy. Liver Transplant 2013;19(12):1343–53.
12. Mehta N, Dodge JL, Hirose R, et al. Predictors of low risk for dropout from the liver transplant waiting list for hepatocellular carcinoma in long wait time regions: implications for organ allocation. Am J Transplant 2019;19(8):2210–8.
13. Berry K, Ioannou GN. Comparison of liver transplant-related survival benefit in patients with versus without hepatocellular carcinoma in the United States. Gastroenterology 2015;149(3):669–80 [quiz: e15-6].
14. Crocetti L, Bozzi E, Scalise P, et al. Locoregional treatments for bridging and downstaging HCC to liver transplantation. Cancers 2021;13(21).
15. Agopian VG, Morshedi MM, McWilliams J, et al. Complete pathologic response to pretransplant locoregional therapy for hepatocellular carcinoma defines cancer

cure after liver transplantation: analysis of 501 consecutively treated patients. Ann Surg 2015;262(3):536–45 [discussion: 43-5].

16. Otto G, Herber S, Heise M, et al. Response to transarterial chemoembolization as a biological selection criterion for liver transplantation in hepatocellular carcinoma. Liver Transplant 2006;12(8):1260–7.

17. Mazzaferro V, Citterio D, Bhoori S, et al. Liver transplantation in hepatocellular carcinoma after tumour downstaging (XXL): a randomised, controlled, phase 2b/3 trial. Lancet Oncol 2020;21(7):947–56.

18. Yao FY, Mehta N, Flemming J, et al. Downstaging of hepatocellular cancer before liver transplant: long-term outcome compared to tumors within Milan criteria. Hepatology 2015;61(6):1968–77.

19. Yao FY, Fidelman N. Reassessing the boundaries of liver transplantation for hepatocellular carcinoma: where do we stand with tumor down-staging? Hepatology 2016;63(3):1014–25.

20. Mehta N, Guy J, Frenette CT, et al. Excellent outcomes of liver transplantation following down-staging of hepatocellular carcinoma to within milan criteria: a multicenter study. Clin Gastroenterol Hepatol 2018;16(6):955–64.

21. Tabrizian P, Holzner ML, Mehta N, et al. Ten-year outcomes of liver transplant and downstaging for hepatocellular carcinoma. JAMA Surg 2022;157(9):779–88.

22. Roberts JP, Venook A, Kerlan R, et al. Hepatocellular carcinoma: ablate and wait versus rapid transplantation. Liver Transplant 2010;16(8):925–9.

23. Halazun KJ, Patzer RE, Rana AA, et al. Standing the test of time: outcomes of a decade of prioritizing patients with hepatocellular carcinoma, results of the UNOS natural geographic experiment. Hepatology 2014;60(6):1957–62.

24. Mehta N, Yao FY. What are the optimal liver transplantation criteria for hepatocellular carcinoma? Clin Liver Dis 2019;13(1):20–5.

25. Mehta N, Heimbach J, Lee D. et al. Wait time of less than 6 and greater than 18 months predicts hepatocellular carcinoma recurrence after liver transplantation: proposing a wait time "sweet spot", Transplantation, 101 (9): 2071-2078, 2017.

26. Yao FY, Xiao L, Bass NM, et al. Liver transplantation for hepatocellular carcinoma: validation of the UCSF-expanded criteria based on preoperative imaging. Am J Transplant 2007;7(11):2587–96.

27. Duffy JP, Vardanian A, Benjamin E, et al. Liver transplantation criteria for hepatocellular carcinoma should be expanded: a 22-year experience with 467 patients at UCLA. Ann Surg 2007;246(3):502–9 [discussion: 9-11].

28. Chernyak V, Fowler KJ, Kamaya A, et al. Liver imaging reporting and data system (LI-RADS) version 2018: imaging of hepatocellular carcinoma in at-risk patients. Radiology 2018;289(3):816–30.

29. Lencioni R. and Llovet JM. Modified RECIST (mRECIST) assessment for hepatocellular carcinoma, Semin Liver Dis, 2010, 30 (1): 052–060.

30. Ormiston WEL, Yarmohammadi H, Lobaugh S, et al. Post-treatment CT LI-RADS categories: predictors of overall survival in hepatocellular carcinoma post bland transarterial embolization. Abdom Radiol (NY) 2021;46(8):3738–47.

31. Vincenzi B, Di Maio M, Silletta M, et al. Prognostic relevance of objective response according to EASL Criteria and mRECIST criteria in hepatocellular carcinoma patients treated with loco-regional therapies: a literature-based meta-analysis. PLoS One 2015;10(7):e0133488.

32. Mehta N, Frenette C, Tabrizian P, et al. Downstaging outcomes for hepatocellular carcinoma: results from the multicenter evaluation of reduction in tumor size before liver transplantation (MERITS-LT) consortium. Gastroenterology 2021; 161(5):1502–12.

33. Mazzaferro V, Sposito C, Zhou J, et al. Metroticket 2.0 model for analysis of competing risks of death after liver transplantation for hepatocellular carcinoma. Gastroenterology 2018;154(1):128–39.
34. Duvoux C, Roudot-Thoraval F, Decaens T, et al. Liver transplantation for hepatocellular carcinoma: a model including α-fetoprotein improves the performance of Milan criteria. Gastroenterology 2012;143(4):986–94.e3 [quiz: e14-5].
35. Toso C, Meeberg G, Hernandez-Alejandro R, et al. Total tumor volume and alpha-fetoprotein for selection of transplant candidates with hepatocellular carcinoma: a prospective validation, *Hepatology*, 62 (1):158-65, 2015.
36. Berry K, Ioannou GN. Serum alpha-fetoprotein level independently predicts post-transplant survival in patients with hepatocellular carcinoma. Liver Transplant 2013;19(6):634–45.
37. Mehta N, Dodge JL, Roberts JP, et al. Alpha-fetoprotein decrease from > 1,000 to < 500 ng/mL in patients with hepatocellular carcinoma leads to improved post-transplant outcomes, *Hepatology*, 69 (3): 1193-1205, 2019.
38. Halazun KJ, Tabrizian P, Najjar M, et al. Is it time to abandon the Milan criteria?: results of a bicoastal US collaboration to redefine hepatocellular carcinoma liver transplantation selection policies. Ann Surg 2018;268(4):690–9.
39. Kwong A, Kim W, Lake J, et al. OPTN/SRTR 2018 annual data report: liver. Am J Transplant 2020;20:193–299.
40. Mehta N, Heimbach J, Harnois DM, et al. Validation of a risk estimation of tumor recurrence after transplant (RETREAT) score for hepatocellular carcinoma recurrence after liver transplant. JAMA Oncol 2017;3(4):493–500.
41. Hameed B, Mehta N, Sapisochin G, et al. Alpha-fetoprotein level > 1000 ng/mL as an exclusion criterion for liver transplantation in patients with hepatocellular carcinoma meeting the Milan criteria. Liver Transplant 2014;20(8):945–51.
42. Sinha J, Mehta N, Dodge JL, et al. Are there upper limits in tumor burden for down-staging of hepatocellular carcinoma to liver transplant? Analysis of the all-comers protocol. Hepatology 2019;70(4):1185–96.
43. Mehta N, Dodge JL, Grab JD, et al. National experience on down-staging of hepatocellular carcinoma before liver transplant: influence of tumor burden, alpha-fetoprotein, and wait time. Hepatology 2020;71(3):943–54.
44. Yao FY, Fidelman N, Mehta N. The key role of staging definitions for assessment of downstaging for hepatocellular carcinoma. Semin Liver Dis 2021;41(2):117–27.
45. Sapisochin G, Goldaracena N, Laurence JM, et al. The extended Toronto criteria for liver transplantation in patients with hepatocellular carcinoma: A prospective validation study. Hepatology 2016;64(6):2077–88.
46. Toso C, Meeberg G, Hernandez-Alejandro R, et al. Total tumor volume and alpha-fetoprotein for selection of transplant candidates with hepatocellular carcinoma: a prospective validation. Hepatology 2015;62(1):158–65.
47. Halazun KJ, Rosenblatt RE, Mehta N, et al. Dynamic α-fetoprotein response and outcomes after liver transplant for hepatocellular carcinoma. JAMA Surgery 2021; 156(6):559–67.
48. Chaiteerakij R, Zhang X, Addissie BD, et al. Combinations of biomarkers and M ilan criteria for predicting hepatocellular carcinoma recurrence after liver transplantation. Liver Transplant 2015;21(5):599–606.
49. Halazun KJ, Najjar M, Abdelmessih RM, et al. Recurrence after liver transplantation for hepatocellular carcinoma: a new MORAL to the story. Ann Surg 2017; 265(3):557–64.
50. Sasaki K, Firl DJ, Hashimoto K, et al. Development and validation of the HALT-HCC score to predict mortality in liver transplant recipients with hepatocellular

carcinoma: a retrospective cohort analysis. Lancet Gastroenterol Hepatol 2017; 2(8):595–603.

51. Goldberg D, Mantero A, Newcomb C, et al. Predicting survival after liver transplantation in patients with hepatocellular carcinoma using the LiTES-HCC score. J Hepatol 2021;74(6):1398–406.

52. Lee JH, Cho Y, Kim HY, et al. Serum tumor markers provide refined prognostication in selecting liver transplantation candidate for hepatocellular carcinoma patients beyond the milan criteria. Ann Surg 2016;263(5):842–50.

53. Lee SD, Lee B, Kim SH, et al. Proposal of new expanded selection criteria using total tumor size and (18)F-fluorodeoxyglucose - positron emission tomography/ computed tomography for living donor liver transplantation in patients with hepatocellular carcinoma: The National Cancer Center Korea criteria. World J Transplant 2016;6(2):411–22.

54. Kaido T, Ogawa K, Mori A, et al. Usefulness of the Kyoto criteria as expanded selection criteria for liver transplantation for hepatocellular carcinoma. Surgery 2013;154(5):1053–60.

55. Bhangui P, Saigal S, Gautam D, et al. Incorporating tumor biology to predict hepatocellular carcinoma recurrence in patients undergoing living donor liver transplantation using expanded selection criteria. Liver Transplant 2021;27(2):209–21.

Downstaging Hepatocellular Carcinoma before Transplantation

Role of Immunotherapy Versus Locoregional Approaches

Jessica Lindemann, MD, PhD, Jennifer Yu, MD, MPHS,
Maria Bernadette Majella Doyle, MD, MBA*

KEYWORDS

- Hepatocellular carcinoma • Liver transplantation • Downstage
- Locoregional therapy • Immunotherapy

KEY POINTS

- Hepatocellular carcinoma (HCC) continues to be a leading cause of cancer-related death in the United States.
- Transarterial chemoembolization is the current preferred modality for liver-directed therapy as a bridge to transplant in patients with HCC; recent evidence suggests that radioembolization may prolong time to progression when compared with chemoembolization.
- Combination therapies have already begun to show promise in maintaining disease control and may ultimately prove to be lifesaving in patients who are able to undergo liver transplant.

INTRODUCTION

Primary liver cancer was the third most common cause of death due to cancer worldwide in 2020, and it is estimated that more than 1 million people will develop liver cancer annually by the year 2025.[1] Hepatocellular carcinoma (HCC) is the most common type, accounting for 80% to 90% of all liver cancers.[1,2] Surgical resection and liver transplantation remain the mainstay of curative treatment of HCC. However, the risks associated with surgical resection are significantly greater in patients with liver

Department of Surgery, Division of Abdominal Organ Transplantation, Washington University School of Medicine, 660 South Euclid Avenue, Campus Box 8109, St Louis, MO 63110, USA
* Corresponding author. Department of Surgery, Section of Abdominal Transplantation, Washington University School of Medicine, 660 South Euclid Avenue, Campus Box 8109, St Louis, MO 63110.
E-mail address: doylem@wustl.edu

Surg Oncol Clin N Am 33 (2024) 143–158
https://doi.org/10.1016/j.soc.2023.07.001
1055-3207/24/© 2023 Elsevier Inc. All rights reserved.

cirrhosis, which is present in most patients with HCC. Additionally, a limited resection for HCC leaves behind diseased liver parenchyma at risk of developing new HCCs in the future. There is an estimated 35% risk of recurrence at 1 year,[3] 40% to 50% recurrence at 3 years,[4–6] and up to 70% risk of recurrence at 5 years after resection.[7–10] Therefore, liver transplantation remains the treatment of choice for cure in patients who fall within transplant criteria.

LIVER TRANSPLANTATION IN THE MANAGEMENT OF HEPATOCELLULAR CARCINOMA

The Barcelona Clinic Liver Cancer (BCLC) criteria are the most widely used criteria to guide management for HCC.[11] The criteria were first proposed more than 20 years ago and are updated regularly, representing the most up-to-date, evidence-based classification system for delineating treatment of HCC.[2,12] The most recently updated version from 2022 demonstrates the ever-increasing complexity in medical decision-making as well as the major advances that have been made in the field during the last 2 decades.[12] Many of these advancements, including locoregional interventions and immunotherapies, can be used to downstage patients with HCC and have led to the expansion of eligibility criteria for liver transplantation in the treatment of HCC. As in all surgical interventions, appropriate patient selection is critical to the success of the operation. In liver transplantation, where a limited resource is being used to treat a malignant condition, it is particularly important that patients are selected appropriately to ensure comparable survival after liver transplant for other nonmalignant conditions. The Milan criteria for liver transplantation, first proposed 25 years ago, remain the benchmark for the selection of patients with HCC in the United States.[13] However, it has become clear that tumor number and size alone do not fully predict overall survival. There have been multiple observational studies that have demonstrated a survival benefit for select patients transplanted outside of the Milan criteria.[14–19] Importantly, in a study comparing outcomes after patients with HCC underwent living liver transplantation, a higher posttransplant recurrence rate was demonstrated in patients who underwent expedited transplant through living liver donation. This suggests that some time spent on the waitlist may help determine individual tumor biology and identify those patients who are perhaps more likely to recur after transplantation.[20,21] This supports the current Organ Procurement and Transplantation Network/United Network for Organ Sharing (OPTN/UNOS) policy in the United States, which requires a 6-month waiting period on the liver transplant list before exception points are granted to patients listed for transplantation as treatment of HCC.[2]

Role of Locoregional Therapy in Downstaging

The current US national guidelines for liver transplantation in HCC include disease within the Milan criteria, or sustained response to local-regional therapy if downstaged to within Milan criteria.[22] Additionally, alpha fetoprotein (AFP) levels need to be less than 500 ng/mL after local-regional therapy if they were greater than 1000 ng/mL at time of diagnosis.[22] These criteria result in an overall survival of 80% at 5-years after liver transplantation, comparable to an overall survival after liver transplantation for nonmalignant indications.[13] The University of San Francisco (UCSF) downstaging protocol for granting priority listing for liver transplant for HCC is currently the nationally adopted protocol used in the United States, referred to as the United Network for Organ Sharing Downstaging criteria (UNOS-DS).[23,24] The initial selection criteria are listed in **Box 1** and include 3 distinct groups of patients.[25] The first group consists

---

Box 1
United Network for organ sharing downstaging criteria

UNOS-DS Criteria

Inclusion:
HCC exceeding Milan criteria but meeting one of the following:
1. Single lesion 5.1–8 cm
2. Two to three lesions each less than 5 cm with the sum of the maximal tumor diameters less than 8 cm
3. Four to five lesions each less than 3 cm with the sum of the maximal tumor diameters less than 8 cm
Absence of vascular invasion or extrahepatic disease based on cross-sectional imaging

Criteria for successful downstaging:
Residual tumor size and diameter within Milan criteria (1 lesion <5 cm, 2–3 lesions <3 cm)
1. Only viable tumor(s) are considered; tumor diameter measurements should not include the area of necrosis from tumor-directed therapy
2. If there is more than one area of residual tumor enhancement, then the diameter of the entire lesion should be counted toward the overall tumor burden

Additional guidelines:
1. A minimal observation period of 3 months between successful downstaging and liver transplantation is required.

From Tan DJH, Lim WH, Yong JN, et al. UNOS Down-Staging Criteria for Liver Transplantation of Hepatocellular Carcinoma: Systematic Review and Meta-Analysis of 25 Studies. Clin Gastroenterol Hepatol 2023;21(6):1475-84; with permission.

---

of patients with 1 lesion greater than 5 cm but not larger than 8 cm; the second group consists of patients having 2 or 3 lesions with at least one greater than 3 cm but not more than 5 cm with a total tumor diameter less than or equal to 8 cm; and the third group consists of patients with 4 to 5 lesions each less than 3 cm with a total tumor diameter up to 8 cm.[25]

For patients in the United States who present outside of Milan criteria and who are expected to have a transplant wait time of greater than 6 months, local-regional therapy for downstaging tumors to within Milan criteria is often used. This strategy helps control tumor growth while on the waiting list, reducing the risk of dropout before transplantation. It also provides a method for assessing tumor biology because patients who progress despite locoregional therapy have been shown to have a worse outcome after liver transplantation.[26] This is sometimes referred to as the "ablate and wait" strategy, where a waiting period of at least 3 months but often 6 months is used to assess for an early progression of disease before transplantation.[27] Options for locoregional therapy include transarterial chemoembolization (TACE), transarterial radioembolization (TARE) most often with Yttrium-90 (Y-90), radiofrequency ablation (RFA), and microwave ablation (MWA) techniques, as well as percutaneous ethanol injection (PEI).

Transarterial embolization

There are multiple forms of transarterial embolization (TAE) including bland embolization, chemoembolization (TACE), and embolization using drug-eluting beads (DEB-TACE). The TAE or bland embolization technique involves using small particles to selectively occlude the arterial supply to the tumor, which results in hypoxia, cell death, and subsequently, tumor necrosis.[28] Similarly, in TACE, the arterial supply to the tumor is selectively occluded; however, in this technique, an emulsion of chemotherapy drug and an oil-based contrast agent is given at high concentrations directly into the tumor, which is usually followed by injection of a gel foam. This serves to both reduce the bioavailability of the chemotherapeutic agent and decrease blood flow to the tumor.[29,30] In the DEB-TACE technique, microspheres coated with doxorubicin are selectively delivered into the arterial blood supply of the tumor. This results in a sustained release of chemotherapy directly into the tumor while also occluding the tumor blood supply.[28]

Of all the available locoregional therapy options, including TARE, RFA, and MWA, TACE was the first treatment to be supported with level one evidence.[31,32] As such, it is the recommended first-line modality for downstaging HCC and serves as the reference standard for comparison of other treatment modalities.[12,33,34] In randomized controlled trials comparing TACE versus DEB-TACE, there was no statistically significant difference in response rates or survival between the 2 techniques; therefore, use is generally guided by local practice preference.[35,36]

Transarterial radioembolization
Recently, TARE has had promising results in liver-directed therapy for downstaging before transplantation, including the potential benefit of immunomodulatory effects resulting in tumor suppression.[37–39] However, this intervention has not yet been widely adapted in downstaging algorithms. The technique, also referred to as selective internal radiation therapy (SIRT), most often uses the Y-90 radionuclide bound to either glass or resin microspheres that are delivered directly to the tumor.[32] This approach limits the dose of radiation to the liver parenchyma beyond the tumor and results in a relatively low incidence of postradioembolization complications.[40]

There are several published studies investigating the role of TARE versus TACE in downstaging of HCC before liver transplantation, some of which favor TARE for its limited side effect profile, longer time to progression, and improved tumor necrosis at transplant hepatectomy.[37,38,41,42] In a randomized controlled trial of TACE versus TARE investigating time to progression following treatment, patients who underwent Y-90 radioembolization had a significantly longer median time to progression compared with the TACE group (26 vs 6.8 months, $P < .012$).[41] Longer time to progression may have significant implications for patients on waiting lists for liver transplantation, potentially reducing dropout rates. Sarwar and colleagues evaluated complete pathologic necrosis on explanted livers following TACE, TARE and thermal ablation using data from the UNOS database spanning a period of 8 years.[42] Significantly more patients underwent TACE compared with TARE (70% vs 11%); however, those patients who underwent TARE or thermal ablation were more likely to have complete pathologic necrosis of the tumor in the explanted liver (OR 1.92; 95% CI 1.57–2.36; $P < .001$ and OR 2.19; 95% CI 1.86–2.57; $P < .001$), a factor known to be associated with an improved survival in patients undergoing liver transplantation after locoregional therapy.[42]

Radiofrequency ablation and microwave ablation
Both the RFA and MWA techniques can be performed via laparotomy, laparoscopy, and percutaneous approaches. RFA results in cell death from frictional heating, which occurs after image-guided (usually ultrasound or computed tomography) insertion of the needle-like applicator into the targeted tissue followed by application of a high frequency (375–480 kHz) alternating current.[43] Similarly, MWA probes are also placed under image guidance and result in tissue heating and cell death through excitation of water molecules within the tissue after application of a frequency of 900 to 2450 MHz.[43] Although MWA has the propensity to more reliably provide slightly larger

treatment zones (3–5 cm), both modalities are limited by the risk of thermal injury to critical structures. RFA in particular is susceptible to the heat-sink effect, where the flow of blood results in a cooling effect in tumors located near large blood vessels, although the MWA technique is also susceptible to this phenomenon.[43] It is important to note that thermal ablation is relatively contraindicated not only for tumors near major blood vessels but also near biliary structures, bowel, and the diaphragm due to the risk of thermal injury or incomplete treatment.[44]

Kolarich and colleagues compared waitlist mortality and dropout among liver transplant candidates with HCC who underwent RFA versus TACE as a bridge to transplant using 10 years of data from the Scientific Registry of Transplant Recipients.[45] The authors found no difference in waitlist mortality or dropout for those patients outside Milan criteria who underwent TACE versus RFA (HR 0.91, 95% CI 0.79–1.03).[45] Wu and colleagues performed a cost-effectiveness analysis comparing ablation, TACE, and TARE approaches to liver-directed therapy and found that ablation is the most cost-effective strategy for bridge to liver transplant in patients with single, small HCC less than or equal to 3 cm.[46] Ablation was most effective if the waitlist dropout rate was less than 2% and the rate of transplantation was more than 15% quarterly. If the rate of transplantation increased to a rate of 24% quarterly, then TARE was most effective. TACE only became cost effective when the risk of dropout was less than 1% and the rate of transplantation was more than 45% quarterly. However, in a prospective study comparing RFA to observation alone in patients with HCC awaiting transplant, no survival benefit was identified over the observation-alone group.[47] In the absence of data to support improved outcomes in patients with HCC awaiting transplant who undergo thermal ablation, TACE remains the preferred liver-directed therapy.

Percutaneous ethanol injection

This technique, which consists of injecting 95% ethanol into liver tumors to induce coagulative necrosis, microvascular thrombosis, and ischemia, is one of the first percutaneous ablative techniques performed in clinical practice.[43] However, several publications suggest higher recurrence rates and lower overall survival with the use of PEI compared with other treatment modalities, which has led to limited use of PEI.[43,48,49] In a recent study, Lazzarotto-da-Silva and colleagues examined the dropout rates and posttransplant recurrence free survival with the use of PEI versus TACE as a bridge to transplant in patients with HCC.[50] The authors found similar dropout rates due to tumor progression as well as complete/near-complete pathologic response rates in the explanted liver among all groups. Five-year recurrence-free survival rates of 55.6% for PEI alone, 55.1% for TACE alone, and 71.4% for PEI + TACE with no statistically significant difference in recurrence free survival ($P = .42$), supporting the use of PEI or PEI + TACE as an acceptable alternative bridging therapy to transplantation for the treatment of HCC in those patients where chemo/radioembolization or thermal ablation may be technically challenging.

Role of Immunotherapy in Advanced Hepatocellular Carcinoma

Unlike other solid organ tumors, traditional cytotoxic chemotherapy has not shown great efficacy in the treatment of HCC, and the advent of molecularly targeted therapy and immunotherapy during the past decade has triggered a torrent of interest in new systemic options. In the most recent guidelines by the National Comprehensive Cancer Network and the European Society for Medical Oncology, several Food and Drug Administration (FDA)-approved immunomodulatory agents currently form the backbone of systemic treatment of advanced staged HCC.[51–53]

Tyrosine kinase inhibitors

As the first targeted systemic therapy to be approved by the FDA in treatment of advanced HCC, sorafenib is an oral multikinase inhibitor, which blocks tumor cell proliferation and prevents tumor angiogenesis through inhibition of vascular endothelial growth factor receptors (VEGFRs).[54] In 2008, the SHARP Investigators Study Group established the effectiveness of sorafenib as a single-agent treatment in a multicenter, phase 3, double-blind, placebo-controlled trial, demonstrating an improvement in median overall survival from 7.9 months to 10.7 months (HR 0.69, 95% CI 0.55–0.87, $P < .001$). Furthermore, although time to symptomatic progression did not differ significantly between the 2 groups, the median time to radiologic progression was significantly longer in the sorafenib group (5.5 vs 2.8 months, HR 0.58, 95% CI 0.45–0.74, $P < .001$).[55] Overall, sorafenib was reasonably well tolerated, with the most common side effects being hand-foot skin syndromes and diarrhea. Subgroup analysis later revealed that sorafenib therapy following earlier curative treatment, including resection or LRT, showed a trend toward longer median overall survival and time to progression as well as a higher disease control rate compared with placebo.[56] Despite being the only effective treatment option in advanced HCC for the subsequent decade both in the United States and worldwide, sorafenib monotherapy has shown varying success in downstaging advanced HCC, given relatively low objective response rates less than 5%.[55,57] Limited data have shown conversion to surgical candidacy,[58] and its use as neoadjuvant therapy before transplantation has had conflicting results in small retrospective studies. Truesdale and colleagues found that pretransplantation sorafenib utilization in 10 patients was associated with increased biliary complications and possibly a higher incidence of acute cellular rejection[59]; however, Frenette and colleagues noted no difference in the rate of surgical complications or rejection in their group of 15 patients.[60] Small sample sizes and the retrospective nature of these studies make it challenging to draw widely applicable conclusions, and more studies are needed to delineate safety and efficacy of sorafenib in the neoadjuvant setting.

Since 2018, additional agents have joined the armamentarium, including lenvatinib, which is another oral multikinase inhibitor targeting VEGFRs, fibroblast growth factor receptors, platelet-derived growth factor receptors, as well as the proto-oncogene receptors RET and KIT. Kudo and colleagues demonstrated noninferiority of lenvatinib to sorafenib for patients with unresectable HCC, revealing a similar median survival time (13.6 vs 12.3 months, HR 0.92, 95% CI 0.79–1.06),[52] and more recent study has continued to support the benefit of lenvatinib in prolonging progression-free survival.[61,62] Regorafenib, initially used for patients with metastatic colorectal cancer and gastrointestinal stromal tumors, has also since been approved as second-line therapy after progression on sorafenib and has shown increased potency compared with its predecessor. In the RESORCE trial, researchers randomized patients previously treated with sorafenib to regorafenib or placebo, finding that regorafenib increased median survival (10.6 vs 7.8 months, HR 0.63, CI 0.50–0.79, $P < .001$),[63] which was further supported by a meta-analysis by Facciorusso and colleagues who noted a median overall survival of 11.08 months (95% CI 9.46–12.71) with a similar side effect profile and tolerability to sorafenib.[64] However, limited data currently exist regarding the use of these agents in the neoadjuvant setting although multiple clinical trials are underway, and their utility before liver transplantation is yet to be proven.

Immune checkpoint inhibitors

As understanding of the tumor microenvironment continues to grow exponentially, the landscape of immunotherapy in the treatment of advanced HCC is changing constantly. Immune checkpoint inhibitors (ICIs) have gained increasing traction because their efficacy surpasses that of multikinase inhibitor agents alone, and the combination of the programmed death-ligand 1 inhibitor atezolizumab with bevacizumab, a monoclonal antibody targeting VEGF, is now considered first-line therapy in advanced HCC over sorafenib.[53]

Beginning with the landmark Checkmate 040 trial, researchers demonstrated the safety and efficacy of nivolumab, a programmed cell death protein 1 (PD-1) inhibitor, combined with ipilimumab, a cytotoxic T-lymphocyte-associated protein 4 inhibitor, in patients who had previously failed sorafenib therapy.[65] Patients were randomized to 3 different regimens of the combination therapy, and a strong clinical benefit was seen across all arms, with high objective response rates and higher or comparable median overall survival compared with nivolumab monotherapy.[66] A subsequent CheckMate 459 trial also assessed nivolumab monotherapy versus sorafenib as first-line treatment in advanced HCC, and although no difference was found in median overall survival (16.4 vs 14.7 months, HR 0.85, 95% CI 0.72–1.02) or median time to progression (3.8 vs 3.9 months, HR 0.98, 95% CI 0.82 vs 1.18), its treatment durability and tolerable side effect profile support the use of nivolumab in patients who may be ineligible for tyrosine kinase inhibitors or who have progressed on other first-line agents.[67] Similarly, in the KEYNOTE-224 trial, Zhu and colleagues established the utility of pembrolizumab, another anti-PD-1 monoclonal antibody, with an objective response noted in 17% of patients and comparable time to progression (4.9 months) and median overall survival (12.9 months) to other monotherapy agents. The safety and toxicity profile of pembrolizumab was also deemed manageable given that the most common treatment-related events were grade 1 to 2 severity fatigue, diarrhea, pruritus, and rash.[68]

As noted earlier, the IMbrave150 trial has most recently revised the standard of care in advanced HCC, assessing the combination of atezolizumab and bevacizumab. An international trial comparing the dual ICI therapy against sorafenib in patients with unresectable HCC, IMbrave150 demonstrated that atezolizumab-bevacizumab results in significantly improved overall survival at 12 months (67.2% vs 54.6%) and progression-free survival (6.8 vs 4.3 months, HR 0.59, 95% CI 0.47–0.76, $P < .01$). Perhaps just as exciting, the authors found an overall response rate of 27%,[53] similar to other combination studies, at 36% with lenvatinib + pembrolizumab[69] and 50% with apatinib + camrelizumab.[70] The excellent response rate seen with ICIs has prompted renewed interest in the potential for downstaging unresectable HCC, and an increasing number of studies are evaluating combination multikinase inhibitors with ICIs. In a study by Zhu and colleagues, 63 Child-Pugh A/B patients with unresectable HCC received first-line treatment with combined therapy (lenvatinib or apatinib in conjunction with nivolumab, camrelizumab, pembrolizumab, or sintilimab), and 10 were subsequently downstaged adequately to undergo resection. All 10 had successful R0 resections, and 6 patients achieved a pathologic complete response in the resected liver specimen. Although 5 of the patients experienced posthepatectomy liver failure, the 12-month survival rate was 90%, and the 12-month recurrence-free survival rate was 80%.[71]

Combined locoregional and immunomodulatory treatment

Since the advent of sorafenib, significant interest has surrounded exploring the potential for combination therapy and exploiting the characteristics of each modality in complementary fashion. Much of the rationale stems from using sorafenib to inhibit the angiogenic effect of VEGF secondary to the hypoxic tissue environment triggered by TACE. Several studies with sorafenib and TACE have been able to demonstrate improved disease control, overall survival, and time to progression when both therapies are implemented concurrently in comparison to either therapy alone.[72–75] However, the SPACE trial, an international study in which 307 patients were randomized to sorafenib with DEB-TACE or placebo with DEB-TACE, no significant differences were noted in time to progression (169 days sorafenib vs 166 days placebo, HR 0.797, 95% CI 0.58–1.08, $P = .07$), although regional differences in the amount of combined treatment may have contributed to this outcome.[76] Similar results were also borne out in the TACE 2 trial, which did not find any difference in progression-free or overall survival in a group of 399 European patients. The authors found a median progression-free survival duration of 238 days in the sorafenib + DEB-TACE group versus 235 days in the placebo + DEB-TACE group (HR 0.99, 95% CI 0.77–1.27, $P = .94$) and a median overall survival of 631 versus 598 days (HR 0.91, 95% CI 0.67–1.24, $P = .57$).[77]

As one of the first head-to-head comparisons of systemic to locoregional radioembolization therapy, the SARAH trial randomized a group of European patients to sorafenib or to SIRT with Y90-loaded resin microspheres. Investigators found no significant difference in median overall survival between the 2 groups (sorafenib 9.9 vs SIRT 8.0 months, HR 1.15, 95% CI 0.94–1.41), although patients tolerated SIRT significantly better in quality of life analyses, with fewer treatment-related adverse events.[78] Similarly, in the SIRveNIB phase III trial, patients in an Asian-Pacific population were randomized to receive sorafenib or SIRT, and results concurred with those in the SARAH trial, with no significant difference in overall survival between the 2 groups. Notably, SIRT was much better tolerated in comparison to sorafenib, with significantly fewer adverse events.[79]

In the pretransplant domain, an ongoing trial (NCT05171335) by the Methodist group seeks to assess the efficacy of lenvatinib with TACE in eliciting tumor necrosis on liver explant at the time of transplantation.[80] This investigation was launched following promising preliminary data from their institution in a retrospective review of patients who had undergone TACE alone versus TACE with sorafenib before transplantation in patients with unresectable HCC. The researchers found that patients who had undergone neoadjuvant sorafenib in addition to TACE had trend toward improved 5-year disease-free survival (100% TACE + sorafenib vs 67.2% TACE alone, $P = .07$) although no difference in overall 5-year survival (77.8% vs 61.5%, $P = .51$).[81]

Role of immunotherapy in downstaging

Currently, there are limited but optimistic data to support the use of neoadjuvant systemic therapies in the treatment of HCC before liver transplantation.[82,83] Tyrosine kinase inhibitors and more recently ICIs have garnered increasing interest in the pretransplant setting, although the use of immunomodulatory therapies in transplant candidates has generally been avoided due to reports of severe rejection and graft loss.[84–86] The Mount Sinai group recently published a series of 9 patients who underwent liver transplantation for HCC following treatment with the PD-1 inhibitor nivolumab.[82] The authors reported no severe allograft rejection, losses, tumor recurrences, or deaths at a median follow-up of 16 months with near-complete tumor necrosis observed in one-third of explanted livers. However, in another retrospective analysis, the University of California San Diego team noted that in 5 patients who had received treatment with nivolumab, the 2 patients with their most recent dose less than 3 months before transplantation developed severe hepatic necrosis and biopsy-proven acute cellular rejection.[87] The potential importance of timing between checkpoint inhibitor therapy cessation and liver transplant was also suggested by a recent Chinese cohort study, in which 16 patients who received PD-1 inhibitor therapy underwent transplantation, 3 of whom were successfully downstaged from outside UCSF

A

B

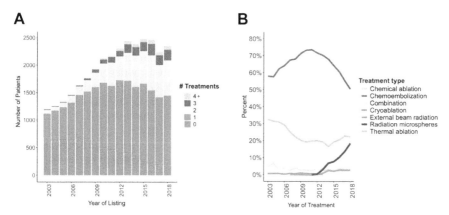

Fig. 1. (*A*) Number of treatments by year of listing. (*B*) Proportion of locoregional therapy (LRT) types by year of treatment. (*From* Kwong AJ, Ghaziani TT, Yao F, et al. National trends and waitlist outcomes of locoregional therapy among liver transplant candidates with hepatocellular carcinoma in the United States. Hepatol 2022;20(5):1142-50; with permission.)

criteria to within criteria. A variety of PD-1 inhibitors was noted, including nivolumab, pembrolizumab, sintilimab, and camrelizumab. Nine patients were diagnosed with rejection in the early postoperative period (mean 7 days after transplantation), with a significantly shorter time interval found in the rejection group between neoadjuvant ICI treatment and LT (21.0 vs 60 days, $P < .01$). All 9 patients were managed with immunosuppression modification, and no graft losses were noted. Of note, 14 of the 16 patients had also received combination targeted molecular therapy with lenvatinib or sorafenib.[88] As the experience with multimodal therapy in the pretransplant setting grows, it will be critical to further delineate protocols regarding dosing and timing of immunomodulatory therapy and to identify which patients would be most appropriate, considering individual tolerance of treatment and the risk of posttransplantation rejection. Most critically, appropriate timing of ICI therapy withdrawal while balancing the vagaries of the liver waitlist will be a necessary component of any treatment plan.

The remainder of evidence around PD-1 inhibitor use in this patient population is limited to case reports, and further investigations are required to determine whether this will be a viable treatment option in the future.[89]

Two ongoing trials, PLENTY202001 (NCT04125226) and Dulect2020-1 (NCT0443322), aim to assess combination systemic therapy in the neoadjuvant setting before liver transplantation. PLENTY202001 compares upfront pembrolizumab and lenvatinib for patients outside of Milan criteria against standard of care waitlist practice. Dulect2020-1 will evaluate the safety and efficacy of durvalumab with lenvatinib in participants with locally advanced HCC before liver transplantation as well as in participants with metastatic unresectable HCC.[90]

SUMMARY

HCC continues to be a leading cause of cancer-related death in the United States. With advances in locoregional therapy for unresectable HCC during the last 2 decades and the recent expansion of transplant criteria for HCC, as well as ongoing organ shortages, patients are spending more time on the waitlist, which has resulted in increased usage of locoregional therapies. This changing landscape is well displayed in **Fig. 1**, which demonstrates the number of treatments per patient by year of listing (A) and the proportion of locoregional therapy type by year of treatment (B).[91] Less than half of liver transplant candidates on the waiting list underwent locoregional therapy before listing in 2003, whereas 92.4% underwent some form of locoregional therapy in 2018.[91] Although TACE is the current preferred modality for liver-directed therapy as a bridge to transplant in patients with HCC, recent evidence suggests that radioembolization may prolong time to progression when compared with chemoembolization. In just the last 5 years, the proportion of radioembolization performed for HCC has increased significantly, from less than 5% in 2013 to 19% in 2018.[91]

Expanding on the proven value of locoregional therapies, the plethora of molecularly targeted therapies and ICIs under investigation represent the new horizon of treatment of HCC not only in advanced stages but also potentially at every stage of diagnosis and management. Although data remain sparse in the pretransplantation population, the possibility of downstaging patients previously considered unresectable or initially outside of transplant criteria is an extremely alluring strategy, which may prove vital in establishing transplant candidacy for an expanded host of patients. Combination therapies have already begun to show promise in maintaining disease control and may ultimately prove lifesaving in patients who are able to undergo liver transplant. Although it will be critical in the coming years to determine timing of therapy and appropriate postoperative immunosuppression strategies, both locoregional techniques and immunomodulation will change the history of liver transplant for HCC as we currently know it.

CLINICS CARE POINTS

- Hepatocellular carcinoma (HCC) continues to be a leading cause of cancer-related deaths in the United States.
- The current modality of choice for managing HCC beyond transplant criteria is transarterial chemoembolization; this can result in downstaging the disease burden, making patients eligible for liver transplantation.
- Recent evidence suggests that radioembolization may prolong time to progression for patients with HCC.
- There are early optimistic data suggesting that combination systemic and locoregional therapies, particularly using tyrosine kinase and check point inhibitors, may result in improved survival among liver transplant recipients with HCC.

DISCLOSURE

The authors have nothing to disclose.

REFERENCES

1. International Agency for Research on Cancer. Estimated age-standardized incidence rates (World) in 2020, liver, both sexes, all ages. 2020. Available at: https://gco.iarc.fr/today/online-analysismap?v=2020&mode=population&mode_population=continents&population=900&populations=900&key=asr&sex=0&cancer=11&type=0&statistic=5&prevalence=0&population_group=0&ages_group%5B%5D=0&ages_group%5B%5D=17&nb_items=10&group_cancer=1&include_nmsc=0&include_nmsc_other=0&projection=natural-earth&color_palette=default&map_scale=quantile&map_nb_colors=5&continent=0&show_ranking=0&rotate=%255B10%252C0%255D. Accessed April 2, 2023.

2. Llovet JM, Kelley RK, Villaneuva A, et al. Hepatocellular carcinoma. Nat Rev Dis Primers 2021;7(6):1–28.
3. Lu X, Zhao H, Yang H, et al. A prospective clinical study on early recurrence of hepatocellular carcinoma after hepatectomy. J Surg Oncol 2009;100:488–93.
4. Koike Y, Shiratori Y, Sato S, et al. Risk factors for recurring hepatocellular carcinoma differ according to infected hepatitis virus - an analysis of 236 consecutive patients with a single lesion. Hepatology 2000;32:1216–23.
5. Jaeck D, Bachellier P, Oussoultzoglou E, Weber JC, Wolf P. Surgical resection of hepatocellular carcinoma. Post-operative outcome and long-term results in Europe: an overview. Liver Transplant 2004;10:S58–63.
6. Sakon M, Umeshita K, Nagano H, et al. Clinical significance of hepatic resection in hepatocellular carcinoma: analysis by disease-free survival curves. Arch Surg 2000;135:1456–9.
7. Minagawa M, Makuuchi M, Takayama T, Kokudo N. Selection criteria for repeat hepatectomy in patients with recurrent hepatocellular carcinoma. Ann Surg 2003;238:703–10.
8. Bismuth H, Majno PE, Adam R. Liver transplantation for hepatocellular carcinoma. Semin Liver Dis 1999;19:311–22.
9. Llovet JM, Fuster J, Bruix J. Intention-to-treat analysis of surgical treatment for early hepatocellular carcinoma: resection versus transplantation. Hepatology 1999;30:1434–40.
10. Singal AG, Pillai A, Tiro J. Early detection, curative treatment, and survival rates for hepatocellular carcinoma surveillance in patients with cirrhosis: a meta-analysis. PLoS Med 2014;11(14):e1001624.
11. Llovet JM, Bru C, Bruix J. Prognosis of hepatocellular carcinoma: the BCLC staging classification. Semin Liver Dis 1999;19(3):329–38.
12. Reig M, Forner A, Rimola J, et al. BCLC strategy for prognosis prediction and treatment recommendation: the 2022 update. J Hepatol 2022;76(3):681–93.
13. Mehta N. Liver transplantation criteria for hepatocellular carcinoma, including posttransplant management. Clin Liver Dis 2021;17(5):332–6.
14. Yao FY, Ferrell L, Bass NM, et al. Liver transplantation for hepatocellular carcinoma: expansion of tumor size limits does not adversely impact survival. Hepatology 2001;33(6):1347–61.
15. Mazzaferro V, Llovet JM, Miceli R, et al. Predicting survival after liver transplantation in patients with hepatocellular carcinoma beyond the Milan criteria: a retrospective, exploratory analysis. Lancet Oncol 2009;10(1):35–43.
16. Shimamura T, Akamatsu N, Fujiyoshi M, et al. Expanded living-donor liver transplantation criteria for patients with hepatocellular carcinoma based on the Japanese nationwide survey: the 5-5-500 rule - a retrospective study. Transpl Int 2019; 32(4):356–68.
17. DuBay D, Sandroussi C, Sandhu L, et al. Liver transplantation for advanced hepatocellular carcinoma using poor tumor differentiation on biopsy as an exclusion criterion. Ann Surg 2011;253(1):166–72.
18. Duvoux C, Roudot-Thoraval F, Decaens T, et al. Liver transplantation for hepatocellular carcinoma: a model including α-fetoprotein improves the performance of Milan criteria. Gastroenterology 2012;143(4):986–94.
19. Toso C, Asthana S, Bigam DL, Shapiro AMJ, Kneteman NM. Reassessing selection criteria prior to liver transplantation for hepatocellular carcinoma utilizing the Scientific Registry of Transplant Recipients database. Hepatology 2009;832–8.
20. Kulik L, Abecassis M. Living donor liver transplantation for hepatocellular carcinoma. Gastroenterology 2004;127:S277–82.

21. Hayashi PH, Ludkowski M, Forman LM, et al. Hepatic artery chemoembolization for hepatocellular carcinoma in patients listed for liver transplantation. Am J Transplant 2004;4:782–7.

22. Marrero JA, Kulik LM, Sirlin C, et al. Diagnosis, staging, and management of hepatocellular carcinoma: 2018 practice guidance by the American Association for the Study of Liver Diseases. Hepatology 2018;68(2):723–50.

23. Roll GR, Roberts JP. Liver transplantation for hepatocellular carcinoma. In: Jarnagin WR, Allen PJ, Chapman WC, et al, editors. Blumgart's surgery of the liver, biliary tract and pancreas. 7th edition. Philadelphia: Elsevier; 2023. p. 1580–90.

24. Tan DJH, Lim WH, Yong JN, et al. UNOS Down-Staging Criteria for Liver Transplantation of Hepatocellular Carcinoma: Systematic Review and Meta-Analysis of 25 Studies. Clin Gastroenterol Hepatol 2023;21(6):1475–84.

25. Yao FY, Mehta N, Flemming J, et al. Downstaging of hepatocellular cancer before liver transplant: long-term outcome compared to tumors within Milan Criteria. Hepatology 2015;61(6):1968–77.

26. Lai Q, Vitale A, Lesari S, et al. Intention-to-treat survival benefit of liver transplantation in patients with hepatocellular cancer. Hepatology 2017;66(6):1910–9.

27. Roberts JP, Venook A, Kerlan R, Yao F. Hepatocellular carcinoma: Ablate and wait versus rapid transplantation. Liver Transplant 2010;16(8):925–9.

28. Mondaca S, Yarmohammadi H, Kemeny NE. Regional chemotherapy for biliary tract tumors and hepatocellular carcinoma. Surg Oncol Clin 2019;28(4):717–29.

29. Tsochatzis EA, Fatourou E, O'Beirne J, et al. Transarterial chemoembolization and bland embolization for hepatocellular carcinoma. World J Gastroenterol 2014; 20(12):3069–77.

30. Shah RP, Brown KT, Sofocleous CT. Arterially directed therapies for hepatocellular carcinoma. Am J Roentgenol 2011;197(4):W590–602.

31. Llovet JM, Real MI, Montana X, et al. Arterial embolisation or chemoembolisation versus symptomatic treatment in patients with unresectable hepatocellular carcinoma: a randomized controlled trial. Lancet 2002;359(9319):1734–9.

32. Taylor AC, Maddirela D, White SB. Role of Radioembolization for Biliary Tract and Primary Liver Cancer. Surg Oncol Clin 2019;28:731–43.

33. Yao FY, Fidelman N. Reassessing the boundaries of liver transplantation for hepatocellular carcinoma: where do we stand with tumor down-staging? Hepatology 2016;63:1014–25.

34. Parikh ND, Waljee AK, Singal AG. Downstaging hepatocellular carcinoma: a systematic review and pooled analysis. Liver Transplant 2015;21:1142–52.

35. Golfieri R, Giampalma E, Renzulli M, et al. Randomised controlled trial of doxorubicin-eluting beads vs conventional chemoembolisation for hepatocellular carcinoma. Br J Cancer 2014;111:255–64.

36. Lammer J, Malagari K, Vogl T, et al. Prospective randomized study of doxorubicin-eluting-bead embolization in the treatment of hepatocellular carcinoma: results of the PRECISION V study. Cardiovasc Intervent Radiol 2010;33: 41–52.

37. Lewandowski RJ, Kulik LM, Riaz A, et al. A comparative analysis of transarterial downstaging for hepatocellular carcinoma: chemoembolization versus radioembolization. Am J Transplant 2009;9:1920–8.

38. Salem R, Johnson GE, Kim E, et al. Yttrium-90 radioembolization for the treatment of solitary, unresectable HCC: the LEGACY study. Hepatology 2021;74:2242–52.

39. Chew V, Lee YH, Pan I, et al. Immune activation underlies a sustained clinical response to Yttrium-90 radioembolization in hepatocellular carcinoma. Gut 2019;68:335–46.
40. Riaz A, Lewandowski RJ, Kulik L, et al. Complications following radioembolization with yttrium-90 microspheres: a comprehensive literature review. J Vasc Intervent Radiol 2009;20(9):1121–30.
41. Salem R, Gordon AC, Mouli S, et al. Y90 radioembolization significantly prolongs time to progression compared with chemoembolization in patients with hepatocellular carcinoma. Gastroenterology 2016;151(6):1155–63.
42. Sarwar A, Bonder A, Hassan L, et al. Factors Associated With Complete Pathologic Necrosis of Hepatocellular Carcinoma on Explant Evaluation After Locoregional Therapy: A National Analysis Using the UNOS Database. Am J Roentgenol 2023;220(5):727–35.
43. Lorimer PD, Bilchik AJ. Radiofrequency ablation of liver tumors. In: Jarnagin WR, Allen PJ, Chapman WC, et al, editors. Blumgart's surgery of the liver, biliary tract and pancreas. 7th edition. Philadelphia: Elsevier; 2023. p. 1321–33.
44. Pompili M, Saviano A, de Matthaeis N, et al. Long-term effectiveness of resection and radiofrequency ablation for single hepatocellular carcinoma 3 cm. Results of a multicenter Italian survey. J Hepatol 2013;59:89–97.
45. Kolarich AR, Ishaque T, Ruck J, et al. Radiofrequency Ablation versus Transarterial Chemoembolization in Patients with Hepatocellular Carcinoma Awaiting Liver Transplant: An Analysis of the Scientific Registry of Transplant Recipients. J Vasc Intervent Radiol 2022;33(10):1222–9.
46. Wu X, Heller M, Kwong A, Fidelman N, Mehta N. Cost-Effectiveness Analysis of Interventional Liver-Directed Therapies for a Single, Small Hepatocellular Carcinoma in Liver Transplant Candidates. J Vasc Intervent Radiol 2023;16. S1051-S0443.
47. Porrett PM, Peterman H, Rosen M, et al. Lack of benefit of pre-transplant locoregional hepatic therapy for hepatocellular cancer in the current MELD era. Liver Transplant 2006;12:665–73.
48. Weis S, Franke A, Mössner J, Jakobsen JC, Schoppmeyer K. Radiofrequency (thermal) ablation versus no intervention or other interventions for hepatocellular carcinoma. Cochrane Database Syst Rev 2013;43:CD003046.
49. Pompili M, De Matthaeis N, Saviano A, et al. Single hepatocellular carcinoma smaller than 2 cm: are ethanol injection and radiofrequency ablation equally effective? Anticancer Res 2015;35:325–32.
50. Lazzarotto-da-Silva G, Grezzana-Filho TJM, Scaffaro LA, et al. Percutaneous ethanol injection is an acceptable bridging therapy to hepatocellular carcinoma prior to liver transplantation. Langenbeck's Arch Surg 2023;408(1):26.
51. Kudo M, Finn RS, Qin S, et al. Lenvatinib versus sorafenib in first-line treatment of patients with unresectable hepatocellular carcinoma: a randomised phase 3 non-inferiority trial. Lancet 2018;391:1163–73.
52. Finn RS, Qin S, Ikeda M, et al. Atezolizumab plus bevacizumab in unresectable hepatocellular carcinoma. N Engl J Med 2020;382:1894–905.
53. AstraZeneca. Imfinzi plus tremelimumab significantly improved overall survival in HIMALAYA Phase III trial in 1st-line unresectable liver cancer. 2021. Available from: https://www.astrazeneca-us.com/media/press-releases/2021/imfinzi-plus-tremelimumab-significantly-improved-overall-survival-in-himalaya-phase-iii-trial-in-1st-line-unresectable-liver-cancer-10152021.html. Accessed 4 April 2023.
54. Wilhelm SM, Carter C, Tang L, et al. BAY 43-9006 Exhibits Broad Spectrum Oral Antitumor Activity and Targets the RAF/MEK/ERK Pathway and Receptor Tyrosine

Kinases Involved in Tumor Progression and Angiogenesis. Cancer Res 2004;64: 7099–109.

55. Llovet JM, Ricci S, Mazzaferro V, et al. Sorafenib in Advanced Hepatocellular Carcinoma. N Engl J Med 2008;359:378–90.

56. Bruix J, Raoul J-L, Sherman M, et al. Efficacy and safety of sorafenib in patients with advanced hepatocellular carcinoma: Subanalyses of a phase III trial. J Hepatol 2012;57:821–9.

57. Cheng AL, Kang YK, Chen Z, et al. Efficacy and safety of sorafenib in patients in the Asia-Pacific region with advanced hepatocellular carcinoma: a phase III randomised, double-blind, placebo-controlled trial. Lancet Oncol 2009;10:25–34.

58. Bertacco A, Vitale A, Mescoli C, Cillo U. Sorafenib treatment has the potential to downstage advanced hepatocellular carcinoma before liver resection. Per Med 2020;17:83–7.

59. Truesdale AE, Caldwell SH, Shah NL, et al. Sorafenib therapy for hepatocellular carcinoma prior to liver transplant is associated with increased complications after transplant. Transpl Int 2011;24:991–8.

60. Frenette CT, Boktour M, Burroughs SG, et al. Pre-transplant utilization of sorafenib is not associated with increased complications after liver transplantation. Transpl Int 2013;26:734–9.

61. Facciorusso A, Tartaglia N, Villani R, et al. Lenvatinib versus sorafenib as first-line therapy of advanced hepatocellular carcinoma: a systematic review and meta-analysis. Am J Transl Res 2021;13:2379–87.

62. Wang S, Wang Y, Yu J, Wu H, Zhou Y. Lenvatinib as First-Line Treatment for Unresectable Hepatocellular Carcinoma: A Systematic Review and Meta-Analysis. Cancers 2022;14.

63. Bruix J, Qin S, Merle P, et al. Regorafenib for patients with hepatocellular carcinoma who progressed on sorafenib treatment (RESORCE): a randomised, double-blind, placebo-controlled, phase 3 trial. Lancet 2017;389:56–66.

64. Facciorusso A, Abd El Aziz MA, Sacco R. Efficacy of Regorafenib in Hepatocellular Carcinoma Patients: A Systematic Review and Meta-Analysis. Cancers 2020;12:36.

65. El-Khoueiry AB, Sangro B, Yau T, et al. Nivolumab in patients with advanced hepatocellular carcinoma (CheckMate 040): an open-label, non-comparative, phase 1/2 dose escalation and expansion trial. Lancet 2017;389:2492–502.

66. Yau T, Kang Y-K, Kim T-Y, et al. Efficacy and Safety of Nivolumab Plus Ipilimumab in Patients With Advanced Hepatocellular Carcinoma Previously Treated With Sorafenib: The CheckMate 040 Randomized Clinical Trial. JAMA Oncol 2020;6: e204564.

67. Yau T, Park J-W, Finn RS, et al. Nivolumab versus sorafenib in advanced hepatocellular carcinoma (CheckMate 459): a randomised, multicentre, open-label, phase 3 trial. Lancet Oncol 2022;23:77–90.

68. Zhu AX, Finn RS, Edeline J, et al. Pembrolizumab in patients with advanced hepatocellular carcinoma previously treated with sorafenib (KEYNOTE-224): a non-randomised, open-label phase 2 trial. Lancet Oncol 2018;19:940–52.

69. Finn RS, Ikeda M, Zhu AX, et al. Phase Ib Study of Lenvatinib Plus Pembrolizumab in Patients With Unresectable Hepatocellular Carcinoma. J Clin Oncol 2020;38:2960–70.

70. Xu J, Zhang Y, Jia R, et al. Anti-PD-1 Antibody SHR-1210 Combined with Apatinib for Advanced Hepatocellular Carcinoma, Gastric, or Esophagogastric Junction Cancer: An Open-label, Dose Escalation and Expansion Study. Clin Cancer Res 2019;25:515–23.

71. Zhu XD, Huang C, Shen YH, et al. Downstaging and Resection of Initially Unresectable Hepatocellular Carcinoma with Tyrosine Kinase Inhibitor and Anti-PD-1 Antibody Combinations. Liver Cancer 2021;10:320–9.

72. Zhao Y, Wang WJ, Guan S, et al. Sorafenib combined with transarterial chemoembolization for the treatment of advanced hepatocellular carcinoma: a large-scale multicenter study of 222 patients. Ann Oncol 2013;24:1786–92.

73. Koch C, Göller M, Schott E, et al. Combination of Sorafenib and Transarterial Chemoembolization in Selected Patients with Advanced-Stage Hepatocellular Carcinoma: A Retrospective Cohort Study at Three German Liver Centers. Cancers 2021;13.

74. Ren B, Wang W, Shen J, Li W, Ni C, Zhu X. Transarterial Chemoembolization (TACE) Combined with Sorafenib *versus* TACE Alone for Unresectable Hepatocellular Carcinoma: A Propensity Score Matching Study. J Cancer 2019;10: 1189–96.

75. Patidar Y, Chandel K, Condati NK, Srinivasan SV, Mukund A, Sarin SK. Transarterial Chemoembolization (TACE) Combined With Sorafenib versus TACE in Patients With BCLC Stage C Hepatocellular Carcinoma – A Retrospective Study. J Clin Exp Hepatol 2022;12:745–54.

76. Lencioni R, Llovet JM, Han G, et al. Sorafenib or placebo plus TACE with doxorubicin-eluting beads for intermediate stage HCC: The SPACE trial. J Hepatol 2016;64:1090–8.

77. Meyer T, Fox R, Ma YT, et al. Sorafenib in combination with transarterial chemoembolisation in patients with unresectable hepatocellular carcinoma (TACE 2): a randomised placebo-controlled, double-blind, phase 3 trial. Lancet Gastroenterol Hepatol 2017;2:565–75.

78. Vilgrain V, Pereira H, Assenat E, et al. Efficacy and safety of selective internal radiotherapy with yttrium-90 resin microspheres compared with sorafenib in locally advanced and inoperable hepatocellular carcinoma (SARAH): an open-label randomised controlled phase 3 trial. Lancet Oncol 2017;18:1624–36.

79. Chow PKH, Gandhi M, Tan S-B, et al. SIRveNIB: Selective Internal Radiation Therapy Versus Sorafenib in Asia-Pacific Patients With Hepatocellular Carcinoma. J Clin Oncol 2018;36:1913–21.

80. Abdelrahim M, Esmail A, Saharia A, et al. P-161 Trial in progress: Neoadjuvant combination therapy of lenvatinib plus transcatheter arterial chemoembolization (TACE) for transplant-eligible patients with large hepatocellular carcinoma. Ann Oncol 2022;33:S307.

81. Esmail A, Kodali S, Graviss E, et al. P-163 Tyrosine kinase inhibitors (TKIs) plus transarterial chemoembolization (TACE) compared to TACE alone as downstaging therapy in transplant recipients with hepatocellular carcinoma. Ann Oncol 2022;33:S308.

82. Tabrizian P, Florman SS, Schwartz ME. PD-1 inhibitor as bridge therapy to liver transplantation? Am J Transplant 2021;21:1979–80.

83. Kang E, Martinez M, Moisander-Joyce H, et al. Stable liver graft post anti-PD1 therapy as a bridge to transplantation in an adolescent with hepatocellular carcinoma. Pediatr Transplant 2022;26:e14209.

84. Nordness MF, Hamel S, Godfrey CM, et al. Fatal hepatic necrosis after nivolumab as a bridge to liver transplant for HCC: Are checkpoint inhibitors safe for the pre-transplant patient? Am J Transplant 2020;20:879–83.

85. Abdel-Wahab N, Shah M, Suarez-Almazor ME. Adverse Events Associated with Immune Checkpoint Blockade in Patients with Cancer: A Systematic Review of Case Reports. PLoS One 2016;11:e0160221.

86. Wang DY, Johnson DB, Davis EJ. Toxicities Associated With PD-1/PD-L1 Blockade. Cancer J 2018;24:36–40.
87. Schnickel GT, Fabbri K, Hosseini M, et al. Liver transplantation for hepatocellular carcinoma following checkpoint inhibitor therapy with nivolumab. Am J Transplant 2022;22:1699–704.
88. Wang T, Chen Z, Liu Y, et al. Neoadjuvant programmed cell death 1 inhibitor before liver transplantation for HCC is not associated with increased graft loss. Liver Transplant 2023;29:598–606.
89. Lominadze Z, Hill K, Shaik MR, et al. Immunotherapy for Hepatocellular Carcinoma in the Setting of Liver Transplantation: A Review. Int J Mol Sci 2023;24:2358.
90. Katariya NN, Lizaola-Mayo BC, Chascsa DM, et al. Immune Checkpoint Inhibitors as Therapy to Down-Stage Hepatocellular Carcinoma Prior to Liver Transplantation. Cancers 2022;14:2056.
91. Kwong AJ, Ghaziani TT, Yao F, et al. National trends and waitlist outcomes of locoregional therapy among liver transplant candidates with hepatocellular carcinoma in the United States. Clin Gastroenterol Hepatol 2022;20:1142–50.

Management of Intermediate-Stage Hepatocellular Carcinoma
Systemic Versus Locoregional Therapy

Mikin Patel, MD[a], Anjana Pillai, MD[b],*

KEYWORDS

- Hepatocellular carcinoma • Locoregional therapy • Systemic therapy

KEY POINTS

- Management of intermediate-stage hepatocellular carcinoma (HCC) requires an individualized patient profile to determine an optimal treatment strategy.
- Locoregional treatments such as transarterial chemoembolization and transarterial radioembolization can be applied in intermediate-stage HCC to downstage to curative options or as destination therapy.
- Systemic therapy is often only applied in intermediate-stage HCC in the presence of infiltrative or bilobar disease.

Hepatocellular carcinoma (HCC) accounts for over 90% of primary liver cancers, is the sixth most common malignancy globally, and is the third most common cause of cancer-related mortality worldwide.[1–3] Unfortunately, only one-third of patients present with early stage disease, leading to dismal long-term survival.[4] However, significant advances in locoregional and systemic therapies have improved outcomes.[5] Prognosis depends on disease stage, and HCC is most commonly classified according to the Barcelona Clinic Liver Cancer (BCLC) staging system, which takes into account patient performance status, liver function, and tumor burden.[6]

By BCLC criteria, approximately 30% of patients with HCC present with intermediate-stage (BCLC B) disease.[7] Historically, transarterial chemoembolization (TACE) was the recommended treatment for BCLC B HCC. However, there have been major advances in the treatment of HCC since the original BCLC guidelines

[a] Department of Radiology, University of Chicago Medicine, Chicago, IL, USA; [b] Department of Medicine, University of Chicago Medicine, Chicago, IL, USA
* Corresponding author. Center for Liver Diseases, The University of Chicago Medicine, 5841 South Maryland Avenue, MC 7120, Chicago, IL 60637.
E-mail address: apillai1@medicine.bsd.uchicago.edu

Surg Oncol Clin N Am 33 (2024) 159–172
https://doi.org/10.1016/j.soc.2023.06.008
1055-3207/24/© 2023 Elsevier Inc. All rights reserved.

were published. The 2022 BCLC staging update now stratifies intermediate-stage HCC into subgroups, offering a more complex, nuanced recommendation of treatment strategies.[8]

DEFINING INTERMEDIATE-STAGE HEPATOCELLULAR CARCINOMA

Intermediate-stage (or BCLC B) HCC is defined as multifocal disease without vascular invasion or extrahepatic spread in a patient with preserved liver function and no cancer-related symptoms (performance status 0).[8] In terms of tumor burden, intermediate-stage HCC is traditionally classified as unresectable disease or beyond Milan Criteria (1 tumor over 5 cm or >3 tumors, each smaller than 3 cm) but without vascular invasion or metastasis (which would classify as advanced or terminal stage HCC). In practice, this encompasses a heterogeneous group of patients including those with

Well-defined HCC tumors too large to classify as early stage (BCLC A) disease
Well-defined tumors in both lobes of the liver (bilobar disease)
Diffuse, infiltrative tumor (**Fig. 1**)

Median survival for all patients with intermediate-stage HCC is 10 months, but because of heterogeneity within the category, median survival times range from 5 to 25 months for the subgroups described.[7,9,10] Alternative classification systems (including Hong Kong Liver Cancer [HKLC] staging, which has been well-validated in Asian patients with HCC, many of whom have chronic hepatitis B virus infection) have been proposed to better prognosticate and direct treatment, but none have earned widespread adoption.[11–14] Ultimately, management of intermediate-stage HCC requires developing an individualized patient profile to determine prognosis and treatment strategy.

SURGICAL MANAGEMENT OF INTERMEDIATE-STAGE HEPATOCELLULAR CARCINOMA
Liver Resection

Surgical resection is an option for carefully selected patients with intermediate-stage HCC and preserved liver function. HKLC guidelines recommend liver resection as the first-line treatment for stage 2b patients (preserved performance status, liver function,

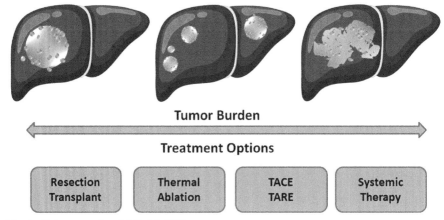

Fig. 1. Heterogeneity of BCLC B HCC.

and with tumor burden ≤5 cm, either greater than 3 tumor nodules or with intrahepatic venous invasion or >5 cm, but ≤3 tumor nodules and no venous invasion).[15]

In a large series of patients undergoing liver resections, 737 of which were performed for BCLC B HCC, the 1- and 5-year overall survival (OS) rates were 88% and 57%, respectively.[16] A series of 434 liver resections for patients with Child-Pugh A (CP A) liver function and multinodular disease achieved 5-year OS of 56%.[17] Of note, much of these data comes from Asian countries and may not be generalizable to Western populations.

Liver Transplantation

Intermediate-stage HCC is, by definition, beyond traditional Milan criteria for liver transplantation (LT). However, expanded criteria and downstaging protocols may allow LT to be a successful treatment option for BCLC B HCC.

Multiple expanded criteria for LT have been proposed including the University of California, San Francisco (UCSF) criteria and the Metroticket 2.0 systems.[18,19] Adoption of these expanded LT criteria yields comparable outcomes in terms of 5-year post-LT survival and, importantly, allows for an increase in the number of HCC patients eligible for LT, particularly the subgroup of BCLC stage B patients with well-defined nodules.

Downstaging protocols consist of administering various locoregional treatments with the goal of decreasing tumor burden to fall within LT criteria. These strategies, to be described in subsequent sections, have yielded promising results with up to 70% of carefully selected patients being successfully downstaged to LT criteria and subsequent post-transplant 1- and 4-year survival rates of 96% and 92% respectively.[20] Although patient selection is a key component to successful downstaging, these therapies have significantly expanded the pool of patients eligible for LT.

LOCOREGIONAL THERAPY FOR INTERMEDIATE-STAGE HEPATOCELLULAR CARCINOMA
Transarterial Chemoembolization

Transarterial chemoembolization (TACE) was historically the recommended treatment for intermediate-stage HCC and still stands as the recommended treatment for patients with well-defined nodules beyond extended LT criteria. TACE involves careful selection and infusion of cytotoxic agents and embolic particles (typically 100–300 μm) into the hepatic arteries feeding HCC tumors. When technically successful, TACE allows high-dose treatment delivery to tumors, resulting in both cytotoxicity and ischemia.[21]

Technical Considerations

There are 2 common variants of the TACE technique: conventional (c-TACE) and drug-eluding beads (DEB-TACE). c-TACE involves injecting an emulsion of cytotoxic agent (commonly doxorubicin or cisplatin) and iodinated oily contrast (ethiodized oil) followed by injection of embolic particles. Theoretically, the small delay between administration of the emulsion and the particles allows some of the cytotoxic drug to leak into systemic circulation.[22] In response, DEB-TACE was developed, which involves loading microspheres with a cytotoxic agent (commonly doxorubicin) prior to infusion. DEB-TACE delivers drug and embolic simultaneously, theoretically allowing higher doses and more sustained release of cytotoxic agent in the embolized tissue.[22,23]

Despite important technical differences between c-TACE and DEB-TACE, clinical outcomes may be comparable overall. A randomized-controlled trial (RCT) of 201 patients found, in a subgroup of patients with CP B liver disease, DEB-TACE resulted in higher overall response rate and fewer severe adverse events compared with c-TACE.[24] However, multiple subsequent studies have failed to demonstrate any benefit of DEB-TACE over c-TACE.[25,26] Meta-analysis comparing c-TACE and DEB-TACE demonstrated a nonsignificant trend toward increased OS in patients who received DEB-TACE; however, comparison of patients with BCLC B HCC was not specifically performed.[27] Ultimately, DEB-TACE appears to be at least equivalent to c-TACE, and the preferred technical approach remains variable and institution-dependent.

Efficacy

Initial RCTs established benefit of TACE over supportive care for unresectable HCC.[28,29] Over 100 TACE studies on over 10,000 patients have been conducted, and the objective response rate after TACE is reported at 52.5% (95% confidence interval [CI]: 43.6–61.5).[30] One-year and 5-year OS rates after TACE are 70% and 32%, respectively, with median survival time of 19.4 months (95% CI: 16.2–22.6). Nevertheless, current literature regarding outcomes after TACE is somewhat difficult to interpret given the heterogeneity of patients with intermediate-stage HCC. Although guidelines recommend TACE for treatment of distinct HCC tumors in BCLC B disease, it is generally not beneficial in the subgroup of patients with extensive, infiltrative HCC.[31]

Several models (eg STATE, "six-and-twelve") have been proposed to help predict which patients may benefit from TACE.[32,33] One example is the ALBI-TAE model, which categorizes patients by their albumin-bilirubin (ALBI) grade, alpha-fetoprotein (AFP), and tumor burden.[34] In this model, the best prognosis group had OS over 5 years, and the worst prognosis group had OS of 6 months. Additionally, TACE is often applied multiple times over the lifetime of a patient with BCLC B HCC. On average, the duration of response after initial TACE is roughly 8.5 months before repeat treatment is required.[35] Several predictive models (eg ART, ABCR) have also been developed to determine whether repeat treatment with TACE is appropriate.[36,37]

Adverse Events

TACE is ideally performed in a fashion that selectively delivers therapeutic dose to the target tumor, but some degree of injury to surrounding liver tissue is unavoidable. Ischemia in the embolized tissue can induce cells to upregulate signaling proteins such as vascular endothelial growth factor (VEGF), changing the tumor microenvironment and activating unfavorable angiogenic pathways.[38] Additionally, tissue ischemia after embolization frequently causes a systemic release of cytokines resulting in postembolization syndrome. Accordingly, the most common adverse events following TACE are: fever (57% of patients), liver function test (LFT) abnormalities (52%), abdominal pain (42%), fatigue (40%), and nausea/vomiting (34%).[30] Higher-grade adverse events are less common but include hepatic artery injury (7.2%), new-onset ascites (6.1%), hepatic decompensation or failure (1.0%), hepatic abscess (0.9%), and acute renal injury (0.6%).[30]

Transarterial Radioembolization

Transarterial radioembolization (TARE) is another catheter-derived therapy now recommended for treatment of early stage HCC not amenable to surgery or ablation.[8] Despite its absence from BCLC recommendations for treatment of intermediate-stage HCC, there is an increase in institutions that have started to adopt TARE in lieu of TACE.[39] TARE is a form of brachytherapy that delivers radiation locally to liver tumors while minimizing damage to extrahepatic structures.

Technical Considerations

TARE involves infusing microspheres (either glass or resin) loaded with a radioactive isotope, typically Yttrium-90 (Y90) into arteries feeding the tumor. Radioactive decay of the Y90 results in β particles irradiating the surrounding tissues within a range of a few millimeters. The microspheres themselves are much smaller (30–60 μm) than those used in TACE and do not cause as much ischemia, an important consideration as oxygen-free radicals are critical to the tumoricidal effect of radiation.[40]

TARE was initially used to treat entire hepatic lobes and can be used to treat large, multifocal, or infiltrative tumors with tolerable levels of radiation-induced liver toxicity.[41] The advent of radiation segmentectomy, or very selective administration (similar to TACE) of Y90, was a major advancement for TARE that allowed for selective treatment of HCC tumors while preserving surrounding normal liver tissue.[42] These angiographic techniques in TARE have been applied in BCLC B patients such that even advanced disease subgroups can be treated safely.[43]

TARE dosimetry is critical to the efficacy of the treatment as demonstrated on correlative pathology studies.[44] The thresholds for tumoricidal and safety doses have evolved over time and have led to increased dose delivery in practice.[45–47] Perhaps the most impactful advancement in terms of TARE dosimetry, however, is the advent of advanced, personalized dosimetry models, which offer patients improved objective response rates.[48] Overall, TARE continues to evolve in terms of angiographic technique and radiation dosimetry.

Efficacy

High-quality evidence based on large studies for TARE in patients with intermediate-stage HCC is lacking. An early RCT with 45 patients demonstrated TARE provided longer time to progression (>26 versus 6.8 months) compared with c-TACE but similar OS (18.9 versus 17.7 months).[49] A single-center RCT with 72 patients demonstrated significantly longer time to progression (17.1 versus 9.5 months) and OS (30.2 versus 15.6 months) with TARE compared to DEB-TACE.[50] A global, retrospective study of 209 patients, largely with BCLC B and C HCC (32.5% and 54.5%, respectively), found median OS of 20.3 months (95% CI 16.7–26.4 months).[47] A cohort study of 325 patients with BCLC B disease receiving TARE reported median OS of 16.9 months (95% CI 12.8–22.8 months), similar to that of TACE.[51] A prospective cohort of 86 patients with intermediate-stage HCC undergoing TARE or TACE found similar median OS (16.4 versus 18 months) despite significantly higher tumor burden in the TARE group.[52] Meta-analysis of comparative trials between TARE and TACE in treatment of HCC (irrespective of stage) also demonstrated similar OS.[53]

Although clinical data support TARE being at least as effective TACE, cost-effectiveness and patient-reported outcomes may help determine choice of therapy. Economic modeling from the perspective of US and UK health systems suggests that TARE may be cost-effective compared with TACE in patients with unresectable HCC.[54,55] Although TARE costs more per treatment, the durability of response compared with TACE results in fewer repeat treatments and, therefore, lower lifetime costs. In a prospective trial of 56 patients, those treated with TARE reported better scores on social and functional questionnaires compared with those treated with TACE at 4 weeks after treatment.[56]

Adverse Events

TARE has lower rates of post-treatment abdominal pain, vomiting, and fatigue compared with TACE, but overall adverse event rates are similar.[49,53] TARE carries the added risk of radiation-induced liver injury, which is characterized by jaundice, ascites, and LFT abnormalities 4 to 8 weeks after treatment.[57] In practice, however, use of more selective segmental treatments and personalized dosimetry techniques minimizes these risks.[47,58] Accordingly, studies report the risk of grade 3 and 4 adverse events (eg, hyperbilirubinemia) at 5% to 15%.[49,51]

LOGOREGIONAL TREATMENT FOR DOWNSTAGING OR BRIDGING TO SURGICAL THERAPY

Locoregional treatments such as TACE and TARE, if applied correctly, can help patients with intermediate-stage HCC gain curative intent with surgical approaches. Studies have found TARE can treat HCC and induce contralateral hepatic lobe hypertrophy, which can aid in planning future liver resection.[59] A single-institution review of 31 patients who received TARE prior to resection of HCC demonstrated significant liver remnant hypertrophy and disease control in all patients leading to 1- and 3-year OS rates of 96% and 86%, respectively.[60] As a result, TARE can be applied safely as a bridge therapy to surgical resection.

TACE and TARE have also been successfully applied in select subgroups of patients with intermediate-stage HCC to downstage their disease, making them eligible for LT. A single institution review of 86 patients demonstrated higher percentage of patients successfully downstaged to transplant criteria (58% TARE versus 31% TACE).[61] Subsequent meta-analyses have found that downstaging success rates are similar between TACE and TARE with a pooled success rate of 0.48 (95% CI 0.39–058).[62]

Thermal Ablation

Use of thermal ablation with microwave (MWA) in intermediate-stage HCC is somewhat limited, largely because of technical difficulties ablating large or numerous tumors. However, studies have demonstrated feasibility of MWA in BCLC B HCC, with a multicenter study of 215 patients reporting 1-,3-, and 5-year OS rates of 89%, 60%, and 21%, respectively.[63] MWA can also be combined with intra-arterial treatments such as TACE and can achieve similar radiologic response and survival to TARE.[64]

Systemic Therapy for Intermediate-Stage Hepatocellular Carcinoma

Systemic treatment of HCC has changed dramatically over the last 6 years. Sorafenib was the only systemic treatment option for HCC for over a decade until multiple, large phase 3 RCTs demonstrated benefits in OS with new systemic agents, leading to an explosion of approved drugs (**Fig. 2**).[65] For intermediate-stage HCC, however, systemic therapy is often only applied in patients with infiltrative or bilobar disease.

Molecular Targeted Therapies

Sorafenib is an oral tyrosine kinase inhibitor (TKI) that was shown in 2 separate studies to offer a 3-month OS benefit over placebo.[66,67] However, time to progression was not significantly different, and there was a higher rate of adverse events in the sorafenib group, including diarrhea, weight loss, skin reactions, and alopecia. Nevertheless, sorafenib became the first approved systemic therapy for advanced HCC in 2007.

Several subsequent phase 3 trials attempted to improve patient prognosis compared with sorafenib. Lenvatinib, a multitarget inhibitor, was the first new agent to demonstrate noninferiority in OS compared with sorafenib and also offered longer progression-free survival.[68] Subsequently, regorafenib, cabozantinib, and ramucirumab were found to improve OS in patients who had progressed on

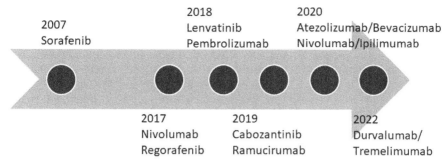

Fig. 2. US Food Drug Administration drug approval in hepatocellular carcinoma.

sorafenib, resulting in their approvals as second- or third-line treatments for advanced HCC.[69–71]

Immune Checkpoint Inhibitors

Nivolumab is a monoclonal antibody that blocks programmed cell death protein-1 (PD-1) signaling and was found to offer a higher objective response rate than sorafenib but with similar OS.[72,73] Similarly, pembrolizumab was found to improved OS and overall response rate in patients progressing on sorafenib.[74] However, despite initial excitement, subsequent studies did not show significant improvement in OS, and only a few patients seem to respond to single-agent immunotherapy.

Combination Therapies

The combination of atezolizumab (antiprogrammed cell death-ligand 1[PDL1] antibody) and bevacizumab (anti-VEGF antibody) was compared with sorafenib in the treatment of unresectable HCC and demonstrated improved median survival (19.2 months versus 13.4 months, respectively).[75] Approximately 15% of these patients had BCLC B HCC, and this subgroup achieved an OS of 25.8 months. Of note, treatment of patients with high bleeding risk was contraindicated because of the potential adverse effects from bevacizumab.

The combination of durvalumab (anti-PDL1) and tremelimumab (anti-cytotoxic T-lymphocyte-associated protein 4 [CTLA4] antibody) was compared with sorafenib in the treatment of unresectable HCC and also demonstrated improved median OS (16.4 months versus 13.8 months respectively).[76] Accordingly, both combination therapies were approved for the first-line treatment of advanced HCC.

COMPARING LOCOREGIONAL VERSUS SYSTEMIC TREATMENTS FOR INTERMEDIATE-STAGE HEPATOCELLULAR CARCINOMA

Because of the heterogeneity and complexity of this patient population, comparison studies of locoregional versus systemic treatment for BCLC B HCC are limited and difficult to translate into clinical practice.

Two international RCTs, SARAH and SIRveNIB, evaluated TARE versus sorafenib in patients with unresectable HCC. SARAH included 467 patients from a Western population; 31.6% and 32.9% of patients had BCLC B HCC disease (TARE versus sorafenib, respectively).[77] SIRveNIB included 360 patients from an Asia-Pacific population; 45.1% and 38.8% of patients had BCLC B HCC disease (TARE versus sorafenib, respectively).[78] Both studies demonstrated no significant difference in OS, but lower frequency of adverse events with TARE. Of note, both studies had relatively high rates of drop-out from TARE (22% and 28.6%, SARAH and SIRveNIB, respectively).

A retrospective, propensity-matched study of 30 patients on lenvatinib versus 60 patients who received c-TACE for intermediate-stage HCC found better OS in the lenvatinib group (37.9 versus 21.3 months).[79] Although retrospective, this study was foundational for RCTs evaluating locoregional versus systemic treatment in the intermediate-stage HCC population. Indeed, several trials are currently enrolling, including a multicenter phase 3 RCT comparing atezolizumab/bevacizumab with TACE.[80]

Combining Modalities

Locoregional treatments (TACE in particular) can cause tissue hypoxia and affect tumor microenvironment, resulting in angiogenesis and potentially tumor proliferation and metastasis. This provides scientific rationale for combining ischemia-inducing treatments like TACE with agents that block neovascularization when treating HCC.[81] There is also early evidence that locoregional treatments such as TACE or ablation can enhance protein expression or induce a local immune response that can have a synergistic effect with immunotherapy.[82,83]

The TACTICS multicenter RCT compared combination TACE and sorafenib versus TACE alone for patients with unresectable HCC.[84] Patients treated with TACE and sorafenib had longer progression-free survival (25.2 versus 13.5 months) and longer time to progression that was untreatable by repeat TACE (26.7 versus 20.6 months). However, the TACTICS trial was the first positive trial of TACE in combination with a molecular targeted agent. Multiple preceding trials demonstrated negative results in terms of efficacy and have suggested increased toxicity with these strategies. The phase 2 single-arm SOCRATES trial combined TACE and sorafenib in patients with intermediate-stage HCC but found a 15% rate of grade 3 or 4 toxicity and 12% patient mortality in the study period.[85] A phase 3 RCT evaluating DEB-TACE combined with sorafenib versus placebo in 313 patients was terminated at interim analysis because of lack of significant difference in progression-free survival.[86] Similarly, the SPACE trial randomized patients with intermediate-stage HCC to DEB-TACE with sorafenib versus placebo, failed to reach its primary efficacy endpoint, and found more patients in the sorafenib arm had grade 5 events.[87]

Early studies of combination atezolizumab/bevacizumab in combination with TACE in the treatment of intermediate-stage HCC have reported encouraging results in terms of overall response rates.[88] Currently, numerous studies combining systemic agents with TACE and TARE are underway and enrolling patients.

SUMMARY

Intermediate-stage HCC comprises a heterogeneous group of patients with varying levels of tumor burden. TACE was traditionally the mainstay of treatment for intermediate-stage HCC for almost 2 decades. New and emerging treatment options have revolutionized HCC therapy, allowing for broader application to patients with intermediate- and advanced-stage disease. Accordingly, new guidelines acknowledge these options, and intermediate-stage HCC can now be treated with surgical, locoregional or systemic therapies, or a combination thereof. Patients will continue to benefit from the development of complex treatment strategies in a multidisciplinary setting to optimize individual outcomes.

CLINICS CARE POINTS

- Management of intermediate-stage HCC requires an individualized patient profile to determine an optimal treatment strategy.
- Locoregional treatments such as TACE and TARE can be applied in intermediate-stage HCC to downstage to curative options or as destination therapy.
- Systemic therapy is often only applied in intermediate-stage HCC in the presence of infiltrative or bilobar disease.
- New and emerging treatment options have revolutionized HCC therapy, allowing for broader application to patients with intermediate-stage disease.

CONFLICTS OF INTEREST

Financial support: None.

DISCLOSURES

M. Patel is on the medical advisory board of Boston Scientific Incorporated. A. Pillai is on the medical advisory board of Exelixis, Genentech, AstraZeneca, Eisai Incorporated and on the safety advisory board for Replimune.

ACKNOWLEDGEMENTS

Specific author contributions: MP drafted initial article. AP provided critical revision of the article. All authors approved the final article submitted.

REFERENCES

1. Villanueva A. Hepatocellular carcinoma. N Engl J Med 2019;380(15):1450–62.
2. Llovet JM, Kelley RK, Villanueva A, et al. Hepatocellular carcinoma. Nat Rev Dis Prim 2021;7(1):6.
3. McGlynn KA, Petrick JL, El-Serag HB. Epidemiology of hepatocellular carcinoma. Hepatology 2021;73(1):4–13.
4. Njei B, Rotman Y, Ditah I, et al. Emerging trends in hepatocellular carcinoma incidence and mortality. Hepatology 2015;61(1):191–9.
5. Tabrizian P, Holzner ML, Mehta N, et al. Ten-year outcomes of liver transplant and downstaging for hepatocellular carcinoma. JAMA Surg 2022;157(9):779–88.
6. Llovet JM, Bru C, Bruix J. Prognosis of hepatocellular carcinoma: the BCLC staging classification. Semin Liver Dis 1999;19(3):329–38.
7. Giannini EG, Moscatelli A, Pellegatta G, et al. Application of the intermediate-stage subclassification to patients with untreated hepatocellular carcinoma. Am J Gastroenterology 2016;111(1):70–7.
8. Rieg M, Forner A, Rimola J, et al. BCLC strategy for prognosis prediction and treatment recommendation: The 2022 update. Hepatology 2022;76(3):681–93.
9. Cabibbo G, Enea M, Attasio M, et al. A meta-analysis of survival rates of untreated patients in randomized clinical trials of hepatocellular carcinoma. Hepatology 2010;51(4):1274–83.
10. Giannini EG, Farinati F, Ciccarese F, et al. Prognosis of untreated hepatocellular carcinoma. Hepatology 2015;61(1):184–90.

11. Bolondi L, Burroughs A, Dufour J-F, et al. Heterogeneity of patients with intermediate (BCLC B) hepatocellular carcinoma: proposal for a subclassification to facilitate treatment decisions. Semin Liver Dis 2012;32(4):348–59.

12. Kudo M, Arizumi T, Ueshima K, et al. Subclassification of BCLC B stage hepatocellular carcinoma and treatment strategies: proposal of modified Bolondi's subclassification (Kinki criteria). Dig Dis 2015;33(6):751–8.

13. Yamakado K, Miyayama S, Hirota S, et al. Prognosis of patients with intermediate-stage hepatocellular carcinomas based on the Child-Pugh score: subclassifying the intermediate stage (Barcelona Clinic Liver Cancer stage B). Jpn J Radiol 2014;32(11):644–9.

14. Wallace MC, Huang Y, Preen DB, et al. HKLC triages more hepatocellular carcinoma patients to curative therapies compared to BCLC and is associated with better survival. Dig Dis Sci 2017;62(8):2182–92.

15. Yau T, Tang VY, Yao TJ, et al. Development of Hong Kong Liver Cancer staging system with treatment stratification for patients with hepatocellular carcinoma. Gastroenterology 2014;146(7):1691–700.

16. Torzilli G, Belghiti J, Kokudo N, et al. A snapshot of the effective indications and results of surgery for hepatocellular carcinoma in tertiary referral centers: Is it adherent to the EASL/AASLD recommendations? An observational study of the East-West study group. Ann Surg 2013;257(5):929–37.

17. Ishizawa T, Hasegawa K, Aoki T, et al. Neither multiple tumors nor portal hypertension are surgical contraindications for hepatocellular carcinoma. Gastroenterology 2008;134(7):1908–16.

18. Yao FY, Ferrell L, Bass NM, et al. Liver transplantation for hepatocellular carcinoma: expansion of the tumor size limits does not adversely impact survival. Hepatology 2001;33(6):1394–403.

19. Mazzaferro V, Sposito C, Zhou J, et al. Metroticket 2.0 model for analysis of competing risks of death after liver transplantation for hepatocellular carcinoma. Gastroenterology 2018;154(1):128–39.

20. Yao FY, Kerlan RK, Hirose R, et al. Excellent outcome following down-staging of hepatocellular carcinoma prior to liver transplantation: an intention-to-treat analysis. Hepatology 2008;48(3):819–27.

21. Liu Z, Zhang X, Xu W, et al. Targeting the vasculature in hepatocellular carcinoma treatment: starving versus normalizing blood supply. Clin Transl Gastroenterol 2017;8(6):e98.

22. Varela M, Real MI, Burrel M, et al. Chemoembolization of hepatocellular carcinoma with drug eluting beads: efficacy and doxorubicin pharmacokinetics. J Hepatol 2007;46(3):474–81.

23. Lencioni R, De Baere T, Burrel M, et al. Transcatheter treatment of hepatocellular carcinoma with doxorubicin-loaded DC bead (DEBDOX): technical recommendations. Cardiovasc Intervent Radiol 2010;35(5):980–5.

24. Lammer J, Malagari K, Vogl T, et al. Prospective randomized study of doxorubicin-eluting-bead embolization in the treatment of hepatocellular carcinoma: results of the PRECISION V study. Cardiovasc Intervent Radiol 2010; 33(1):41–52.

25. Facciorusso A, Mariani L, Sposito C, et al. Drug-eluting beads versus conventional chemoembolization for the treatment of unresectable hepatocellular carcinoma. J Gastroenterol Hepatol 2016;31(3):645–53.

26. Golfieri R, Giampalma E, Renzulli M, et al. Randomised controlled trial of doxorubicin-eluting beads vs conventional chemoembolisation for hepatocellular carcinoma. Br J Cancer 2014;111(2):255–64.

27. Facciorusso A, Di Maso M, Muscatiello N. Drug-eluting beads versus conventional chemoembolization for the treatment of unresectable hepatocellular carcinoma: a meta-analysis. Dig Liver Dis 2016;48(6):571–7.
28. Llovet JM, Real MI, Montana X, et al. Arterial embolisation or chemoembolisation versus symptomatic treatment in patients with unresectable hepatocellular carcinoma: a randomised controlled trial. Lancet 2002;359(9319):1734–9.
29. Lo CM, Ngan H, Tso WK, et al. Randomized controlled trial of transarterial lipiodol chemoembolization for unresectable hepatocellular carcinoma. Hepatology 2002;35(5):1164–71.
30. Lencioni R, de Baere T, Soulen MC, et al. Lipiodol transarterial chemoembolization for hepatocellular carcinoma: a systematic review of efficacy and safety data. Hepatology 2016;64(1):106–16.
31. Reig M, Darnell A, Forner A, et al. Systemic therapy for hepatocellular carcinoma: the issue of treatment stage migration and registration of progression using the BCLC-refined RECIST. Semin Liver Dis 2014;34(4):444–55.
32. Hucke F, Pinter M, Graziadei I, et al. How to STATE suitability and START transarterial chemoembolization in patients with intermediate stage hepatocellular carcinoma. J Hepatol 2014;61(6):1287–96.
33. Wang Q, Xia D, Bai W, et al. Development of a prognostic score for recommended TACE candidates with hepatocellular carcinoma: a multicenter observational study. J Hepatol 2019;70(5):893–903.
34. Lee IC, Hung YW, Liu CA, et al. A new ALBI-based model to predict survival after transarterial chemoembolization for BCLC stage B hepatocellular carcinoma. Liver Int 2019;39(9):1704–12.
35. Terzi E, Golfieri R, Piscaglia F, et al. Response rate and clinical outcome of HCC after first and repeated cTACE performed "on demand.". J Hepatol 2012;57(6):1258–67.
36. Sieghart W, Hucke F, Pinter M, et al. The ART of decision making: retreatment with transarterial chemoembolization in patients with hepatocellular carcinoma. Hepatology 2013;57(6):2261–73.
37. Adhoute X, Penaranda G, Naude S, et al. Retreatment with TACE: the ABCR SCORE, an aid to the decision-making process. J Hepatol 2015;62(4):855–62.
38. Liu K, Min XL, Peng J, et al. The changes of HIF-1α and VEGF expression after TACE in patients with hepatocellular carcinoma. J Clin Med Res 2016;8:297–302.
39. Salem R, Gabr A, Riaz A, et al. Institutional decision to adopt Y90 as primary treatment for hepatocellular carcinoma informed by a 1000-patient 15 your expe rience. Hepatology 2018;68(4):1429–40.
40. Patel MV, McNiel D, Brunson C, et al. Prior ablation and progression of disease correlate with higher tumor-to-normal liver 99mTc-MAA uptake ratio in hepatocellular carcinoma. Abdominal Radiol 2022;48(2):752–7.
41. Lakhoo J, Perez TH, Borgmann AJ, et al. Lobar radioembolization for intermediate and advanced hepatocellular carcinoma: retrospective and prospective data. Semin Intervent Radiol 2021;38(4):412–8.
42. Lewandowski RJ, Gabr A, Abouchaleh N, et al. Radiation segmentectomy: potential curative therapy for early hepatocellular carcinoma. Radiology 2018;287(3):1050–8.
43. Ranganathan S, Gabr A, Entezari P, et al. Radioembolization for intermediate-stage hepatocellular carcinoma maintains liver function and permits systemic therapy at progression. J Vasc Intervent Radiol 2023;34(6):968–75.

44. Gabr A, Riaz A, Johnson GE, et al. Correlation of Y90-absorbed radiation dose to pathological necrosis in hepatocellular carcinoma: confirmatory multicenter analysis in 45 explants. Eur J Nucl Med Mol Imag 2021;48(2):580–3.

45. Vouche M, Habib A, Ward TJ, et al. Unresectable solitary hepatocellular carcinoma not amenable to radiofrequency ablation: multicenter radiology-pathology correlation and survival or radiation segmentectomy. Hepatology 2014;60(1):192–201.

46. Toskich B, Vidal LL, Olson MT, et al. Pathologic response of hepatocellular carcinoma treated with Yttrium-90 glass microsphere radiation segmentectomy prior to liver transplantation: a validation study. J Vasc Intervent Radiol 2021;32(4):518–26.

47. Lam M, Garin E, Maccauro M, et al. A global evaluation of advanced dosimetry in transarterial radioembolization of hepatocellular carcinoma with Yttrium-90: the TARGET study. Eur J Nucl Med Mol Imag 2022;49(10):3340–52.

48. Garin E, Tselikas L, Guiu B, et al. Personalised versus standard dosimetry approach of selective internal radiation therapy in patients with locally advanced hepatocellular carcinoma (DOSISPHERE-01): a randomised, multicenter, open-label phase 2 trial. Lancet Gastroenterol Hepatol 2021;6(1):17–29.

49. Salem R, Gordon AC, Mouli S, et al. Y90 radioembolization significantly prolongs time to progression compared with chemoembolization in patients with hepatocellular carcinoma. Gastroenterology 2016;151(6):1155–63.

50. Dhondt E, Lambert B, Hermie L, et al. 90Y radioembolization versus drug-eluting bead chemoembolization for unresectable hepatocellular carcinoma: Results from the TRACE phase II randomized controlled trial. Radiology 2022;303(3):699–710.

51. Sangro B, Carpanese L, Cianni R, et al. Survival after yttrium-90 resin microsphere radioembolization of hepatocellular carcinoma across Barcelona Clinic Liver Cancer stages: a European evaluation. Hepatology 2011;54(3):868–78.

52. El Fouly A, Ertle J, El Dorry A, et al. In intermediate stage hepatocellular carcinoma: radioembolization with yttrium 90 or chemoembolization? Liver Int 2015;35(2):627–35.

53. Lobo L, Yakoub D, Picado O, et al. Unresectable hepatocellular carcinoma: radioembolization versus chemoembolization: a systematic review and meta-analysis. Cardiovasc Intervent Radiol 2016;39(11):1580–8.

54. Rostambeigi N, Dekarske AS, Austin EE, et al. Cost effectiveness of radioembolization compared with conventional transarterial chemoembolization for treatment of hepatocellular carcinoma. J Vasc Intervent Radiol 2014;25(7):1075–84.

55. Manas D, Bell JK, Mealing S, et al. The cost-effectiveness of Therasphere in patients with hepatocellular carcinoma who are eligible for transarterial embolization. Eur J Surg Oncol 2021;47(2):401–8.

56. Salem R, Gilbertsen M, Butt Z. Increased quality of life among hepatocellular carcinoma patients treated with radioembolization compared with chemoembolization. Clin Gastroenterol Hepatol 2013;11(10):1358–65.

57. Sangro B, Gil-Alzugaray B, Rodriguez J, et al. Liver disease induced by radioembolization of liver tumors: description and possible risk factors. Cancer 2008;112(7):1538–46.

58. Riaz A, Gates VL, Atassi B, et al. Radiation segmentectomy: a novel approach to increase safety and efficacy of radioembolization. Int J Radiat Oncol Biol Phys 2011;79(1):163–71.

59. Garlipp B, de Baere T, Damm R, et al. Left –liver hypertrophy after therapeutic right-liver radioembolization is substantial but less than after portal vein embolization. Hepatology 2014;59(5):1864–73.
60. Gabr A, Abouchaleh N, Ali R, et al. Outcomes of surgical resection after radioembolization for hepatocellular carcinoma. J Vasc Intervent Radiol 2018;29(11):1502–10.
61. Lewandowski RJ, Kulik LM, Riaz A, et al. A comparative analysis of transarterial downstaging for hepatocellular carcinoma: chemoembolization versus radioembolization. Am J Transplant 2009;9(8):1920–8.
62. Parikh ND, Waljee AK, Singal AG. Downstaging hepatocellular carcinoma: a systematic review and pooled analysis. Liver Transplant 2015;21(9):1142–52.
63. Giorgio A, Gatti P, Montesarchio L, et al. Microwave ablation in intermediate hepatocellular carcinoma in cirrhosis: an Italian multicenter prospective study. J Clin Transl Hepatol 2018;6(3):251–7.
64. Yu Q, Thapa N, Karani K, et al. Transarterial radioembolization versus transarterial chemoembolization plus percutaneous ablation for unresectable, solitary hepatocellular carcinoma of >3cm: a propensity score-matched study. J Vasc Intervent Radiol 2022;33(12):1570–7.
65. Brar G, Kesselman A, Malhotra A, et al. Redefining intermediate-stage HCC treatment in the era of immune therapies. JCO Oncol Pract 2021;18(1):35–41.
66. Llovet JM, Ricci S, Mazzaferro V, et al. Sorafenib in advanced hepatocellular carcinoma. N Engl J Med 2008;359(4):378–90.
67. Cheng AL, Kang YK, Chen Z, et al. Efficacy and safety of sorafenib in patients in the Asia-Pacific region with advanced hepatocellular carcinoma: a phase III randomised, double-blind, placebo-controlled trial. Lancet Oncol 2009;10(1):25–34.
68. Kudo M, Finn RS, Qin S, et al. Lenvatinib versus sorafenib in first-line treatment of patients with unresectable hepatocellular carcinoma: a randomised phase 3 noninferiority trial. Lancet 2018;391(10126):1163–73.
69. Bruix J, Qin S, Merle P, et al. Regorafenib for patients with hepatocellular carcinoma who progressed on sorafenib treatment (RESORCE): a randomised, double-blind, placebo-controlled, phase 3 trial. Lancet 2017;389(10064):56–66.
70. Abou-Alfa GK, Meyer T, Cheng AL, et al. Cabozantinib in patients with advanced and progressing hepatocellular carcinoma. N Engl J Med 2018;379(1):54–63.
71. Zhu AX, Kang YK, Yen CJ, et al. Ramucirumab after sorafenib in patients with advanced hepatocellular carcinoma and increased α-fetoprotein concentrations (REACH-2): a randomised, double-blind, placebo-controlled, phase 3 trial. Lancet Oncol 2019,20(2).202–90.
72. El-Khoueiry AB, Sangro B, Yau T, et al. Nivolumab in patients with advanced hepatocellular carcinoma (CheckMate 040): an open-label, non-comparative, phase 1/2 dose escalation and expansion trial. Lancet 2017;389(10088):2492–502.
73. Yau TPJ, Finn RS, Cheng A-L, et al. CheckMate 459: A randomized, multi-center phase III study of nivolumab vs sorafenib as first-line treatment in patients with advanced hepatocellular carcinoma. Ann Oncol 2019;30:v874–5.
74. Philippe Merle JE, Bouattour M, Cheng A-L, et al. Pembrolizumab vs placebo in patients with advanced hepatocellular carcinoma previously treated with sorafenib: Updated data from the randomized, phase III KEYNOTE-240 study. J Clin Oncol 2021;39(s33):268.
75. Finn RS, Qin S, Ikeda M, et al. Atezolizumab plus bevacizumab in unresectable hepatocellular carcinoma. N Engl J Med 2020;382(20):1894–905.

76. Abou-Alfa GH, Chan SL, Kudo M, et al. Phase 3 randomized, open-label multicenter study of tremelimumab and durvalumab as first-line therapy in patients with unresectable hepatocellular carcinoma: HIMALAYA. J Clin Oncol 2022; 40(4):379.

77. Vilgrain V, Pereira H, Assenat E, et al. Efficacy and safety of selective internal radiotherapy with yttrium-90 resin microspheres compared with sorafenib in locally advanced and inoperable hepatocellular carcinoma (SARAH): an open-label randomised controlled phase 3 trial. Lancet Oncol 2017;18(12):1624–36.

78. Chow PKH, Gandhi M, Tan SB, et al. SIRveNIB: selective internal radiation therapy versus sorafenib in Asia-Pacific patients with hepatocellular carcinoma. J Clin Oncol 2018;36(19):1913–21.

79. Kudo M, Ueshima K, Chan S, et al. Lenvatinibi as an initial treatment in patients with intermediate-stage hepatocellular carcinoma beyond up-to-seven criteria and Child-Pugh A liver function: a proof-of-concept study. Cancers 2019;11(8): 1084.

80. Foerster F, Kloeckner R, Reig M, et al. ABC-HCC: A phase IIIb, randomized, multicenter, open-label trial of atezolizumab plus bevacizumab versus transarterial chemoembolization (TACE) in intermediate-stage hepatocellular carcinoma. J Clin Oncol 2022;40(4):TPS498.

81. Liu K, Zhang X, Xu W, et al. Targeting the vasculature in hepatocellular carcinoma treatment: Starving versus normalizing blood supply. Clin Transl Gastroenterol 2017;8(6):e98.

82. Montasser A, Beaufrere A, Cauchy F, et al. Transarterial chemoembolization enhances programmed death-1 and programmed death-ligand 1 expression in hepatocellular carcinoma. Histopathology 2021;79(1):36–46.

83. Duffy AG, Ulahannan SV, Makorova-Rusher O, et al. Tremelimumab in combination with ablation in patients with advanced hepatocellular carcinoma. J Hepatol 2017;66(3):545–51.

84. Kudo M, Ueshima K, Ikeda M, et al. Randomised, multicenter prospective trial of transarterial chemoembolization (TACE) plus sorafenib as compared with TACE alone in patients with hepatocellular carcinoma: TACTICS trial. Gut 2020;69(8): 1492–501.

85. Erhardt A, Kolligs F, Dollinger M, et al. TACE plus sorafenib for the treatment of hepatocellular carcinoma: results of the multicenter, phase II SOCRATES trial. Cancer Chemother Pharmacol 2014;74(5):947–54.

86. Meyer T, Fox R, Ma YT, et al. Sorafenib in combination with transarterial chemoembolisation in patients with unresectable hepatocellular carcinoma (TACE 2): a randomised placebo-controlled, double-blind, phase 3 trial. Lancet Gastroenterol Hepatol 2017;2(8):565–75.

87. Lencioni R, Llovet JM, Han G, et al. Sorafenib or placebo plus TACE with doxorubicin-eluting beads for intermediate stage HCC: the SPACE trial. J Hepatol 2016;64(5):1090–8.

88. Wang K, Zhu H, Yu H, et al. Early experience of TACE combined with atezolizumab plus bevacizumab for patients with intermediate-stage hepatocellular carcinoma beyond up-to-seven criteria: a multicenter, single-arm study. JAMA Oncol 2023;6353047.

Role of Stereotactic Body Radiation Therapy in Hepatocellular Carcinoma

Aseel Y. Abualnil, MD[a], Ritesh Kumar, MD[a],
Mridula A. George, MD[b], Alexander Lalos, MD[c],
Mihir M. Shah, MD[d], Matthew P. Deek, MD[a,1],
Salma K. Jabbour, MD[a,1,*]

KEYWORDS

- Hepatocellular carcinoma (HCC) • Stereotactic body radiation therapy (SBRT)
- Radiation therapy • Transarterial chemoembolization • Bridge-therapy

KEY POINTS

- The use of SBRT in HCC has been shown to have excellent local control rates and minimal toxicity compared to conventional radiation therapy.
- SBRT is a promising treatment option for patients with HCC who are not surgical candidates.
- SBRT can be safely combined with other treatment modalities, including Transarterial chemoembolization and immunotherapy.
- While SBRT has demonstrated its efficacy and safety in treating HCC, future studies are needed to address dose and fractionation schemes, patient selection criteria, and incorporation of systemic therapies.

INTRODUCTION

Stereotactic body radiation therapy (SBRT) is a promising treatment option for patients with hepatocellular carcinoma (HCC), the most common type of primary liver cancer.[1] This advanced radiation therapy (RT) technique delivers ablative doses of radiation to the tumor while minimizing radiation exposure to surrounding healthy tissues, which may lead to improved outcomes and fewer side effects.[2,3] Compared

[a] Department of Radiation Oncology, Rutgers Cancer Institute of New Jersey, Rutgers Robert Wood Johnson Medical School, Rutgers University, New Brunswick, NJ 08901, USA; [b] Department of Medical Oncology, Rutgers Cancer Institute of New Jersey, Rutgers Robert Wood Johnson Medical School, Rutgers University, New Brunswick, NJ 08901, USA; [c] Division of Gasteroenterology and Hepatology, Rutgers Robert Wood Johnson Medical School, Rutgers University, New Brunswick, NJ 08901, USA; [d] Division of Surgical Oncology, Department of Surgery, Emory University School of Medicine, Atlanta, GA 30342, USA
[1] Co-Senior Authors.
* Corresponding author.
E-mail address: jabbousk@cinj.rutgers.edu

Surg Oncol Clin N Am 33 (2024) 173–195
https://doi.org/10.1016/j.soc.2023.06.012

to traditional conventionally fractionated RT techniques, which typically require many sessions of treatment over several weeks, SBRT delivers a higher dose of radiation in fewer sessions, typically 5 or fewer sessions, and its convenience can improve quality of life.[2] Other advantages of SBRT for HCC include conformal targeting of the tumor, which is important for tumors that are difficult to access or are near critical structures such as the gastrointestinal tract, lungs, or spinal cord. Also, it is particularly effective for patients with small or early-stage HCC in terms of local control owing to dose-escalated approaches. In addition, it may be used in combination with other therapies, such as surgery or systemic therapy, to enhance their effectiveness.[4,5] Despite its potential benefits, SBRT may not be appropriate for all patients with HCC, particularly those with advanced liver disease or decompensated cirrhosis. Therefore, careful patient selection and individualized treatment planning are essential for maximizing the benefits of SBRT while minimizing the risks.[6,7]

STEREOTACTIC BODY RADIATION THERAPY
Definition and Main Components of Stereotactic Body Radiation Therapy

In a multidisciplinary setting, the decision to treat HCC with a locoregional therapy (LRT) is assessed, a particular LRT selected is determined by the treatment intent—such as bridge-to-transplant, down-staging for transplant, definitive/curative treatment, and/or palliation—as well as underlying patient clinical factors.[8] SBRT is an external beam radiotherapy (EBRT) technique that accurately delivers a high dose of radiation to an extracranial target in one or a few treatment fractions.[3,9–11] Several crucial elements of the SBRT definition are described in greater detail later in discussion.[3,9–12]

Indications of stereotactic body radiation therapy and outcomes
Despite the fact that SBRT as a radiation technique has historically been used to treat patients with HCC and poor prognosis deemed inappropriate for other therapies and other treatment lines, it has shown promising results in various trials and research.[13] The use of SBRT as a promising alternative therapy for HCC is supported by expanding retrospective and prospective evidence (**Table 1**). In a retrospective study, Yuan and colleagues [26] compared the outcomes of 48 patients with HCC treated between 2006 and 2011 with microscopic complete resection (n = 26, 88% Child Pugh-A, 12% Child Pugh-B, median tumor size 4.6 cm, median dose 45 Gy, range 39-54 Gy in 3-8 fractions) versus SBRT (n = 22, 45% CP-A, 45% CP-B, 10% CP-C, median tumor size 4.3 cm, median dose 45 Gy, range 39-54.[26] and reported favorable side effect profile with SBRT and resulting in one-, two-, and three-year local control rates of 92.9%, 90.0%, and 67.7%, respectively. Overall survival rates of the surgical treatment were 88.5%, 73.1%, and 69.2% at 1, 2, and 3 years, while those of SBRT were 72.7%, 66.7%, and 57.1%, respectively. Although the results with SBRT are numerically lower, patients with Child A cirrhosis and good functional status are more likely to undergo surgical treatment, confounding these results with bias towards surgical resection.

A Phase 3 study performed by Dawson, and colleagues[5] (NRG/RTOG 1112, 2023), sought to improve overall survival (OS), progression-free survival (PFS), and quality of life (QOL) in patients with HCC who were ineligible for surgery, ablation, or TACE. The trial compared the efficacy of SBRT followed by sorafenib (SBRT + sorafenib) to sorafenib alone (S). Patients with new or recurrent HCC, Zubrod performance status (PS) 0-2, Child-Pugh (CP) A, BCLC stage B or C, at least 5 HCCs, a total number of hepatic HCCs of less than 20 cm, and distant metastases of less than 3 cm were included in the study. With 292 patients, 238 OS events, an HR of 0.72, 80% power, and a 1-sided = 0.05, the desired sample size was 292 patients. Due to a modification in the HCC standard of care, planned accrual of 292 patients was prematurely

Table 1
Prospective and retrospective studies for SBRT technique in HCC with different outcomes

Reference Year	Study Design	N	Dose	Dose Type	Fractions	Tumor Size	LC	OS	Follow-up (months)
Cardenas et al,[14] 2010	Prospective	17	36–48 Gy	Variable	3–5 fr.	NA	100% (1 yr.)	75% (1 yr.)	24
Choi et al,[15] 2006	Retrospective	20	50 Gy	Fixed	5–10 fr.	38 mm	100% (1 yr.)	70% (1 yr.)	23
Choi et al,[16] 2008	Retrospective	27	30–39 Gy	Variable	3 fr.	NA	100% (1 yr.)	81% (1 yr.)	11
Louis et al,[17] 2010	Retrospective	25	45 Gy	Fixed	3 fr.	NA	95% (1 yr.)	79% (1 yr.)	13
Kwon et al,[18] 2010	Retrospective	42	30–39 Gy	Variable	3 fr.	NA	72% (1 yr.)	93% (1 yr.)	29
Seo et al,[19] 2010	Retrospective	38	33–57 Gy	Variable	3–4 fr.	NA	66% (2 yr.)	61% (2 yr.)	15
Honda et al,[20] 2013	Retrospective	30	48 Gy 60 Gy	Fixed	4 fr. 8 fr.	16 mm	100% (1 yr.)	100% (1 yr.)	12
Bae et al,[21] 2013	Retrospective	35	30–60 Gy	Variable	3–5 fr.	NA	69% (1 yr.)	52% (1 yr.)	14
Sanuki et al,[22] 2014	Retrospective	185	40 or 35 Gy	Fixed	5 fr.	NA	91% (3 yr.)	70% (3 yr.)	24
Mendez et al,[23] 2006	Retrospective	45	25–37.5 Gy	Variable	3–5 fr.	NA	94% (1 yr.)	75% (1 yr.)	13
Wahl et al,[24] 2015	Retrospective	224	30–50 Gy	Variable	5 fr.	32 mm	NA	74% (1 yr.)	13
Sapir et al,[25] 2016	Retrospective	48	NA	NA	NA	22 mm	97% (1 yr.)	63% (1 yr.)	10
Yuan et al,[26] 2013	Retrospective	48	39–54 Gy	Variable	3–8 fr.	46 mm	92.9% (1 yr.)	73.1% (1 yr.)	23

Abbreviations: LC, local control; N, number of patients; N.B: fr., fractions; NA, not available; and OS, overall survival.

terminated, and the statistics were modified to reflect data as of July 1, 2022, forecasting 155 OS occurrences with 65% power and the same α. According to the study, SBRT + Sorafenib improved median OS to 15.8 months compared to 12.3 months with sorafenib alone (HR=0.77, p = .0554) in 177 eligible patients who were randomly assigned to receive S (n = 92) or SBRT + S (n = 85). After adjusting for performance status, stage, CP A5 vs. 6, and degree of macrovascular invasion, OS was statistically significantly improved for SBRT + Sorafenib (HR=0.72, p = .042). Median PFS was improved to 9.2 months with SBRT + Sorafenib as compared to 5.5 months with sorafenib alone (HR=0.55, p = .0001).[5]

In 2006, Mendez-Romero and colleagues.[23] published the first prospective outcomes of SBRT for HCC. They treated 8 patients with HCC who were not suitable for other local therapies, with a median tumor size of 3.2 cm and 63% were CP-A. Patients with tumors less than 4 cm received 37.5 Gy in 3 fractions and those with tumors greater than or equal to 4 cm received 25 Gy in 5 fractions. The one-year rates of LC and OS were both 75%. and local failure was observed in 4 patients who were in the 25 Gy treatment arm[23]; however, this radiation dose provides a lower biologically effective dose.

Additionally, a retrospective study was performed by Sapir and colleagues[25] (2016) in 48 patients with 50 HCC lesions (see **Table 1**). SBRT was used for patients with liver cancer, specifically those who had undergone prior Transarterial Chemoembolization (TACE). The study found that whole post-TACE cavity treatment with SBRT was the most common approach, and there was no significant difference in survival rates between patients with TACE-naive and those who underwent TACE. Local failure was observed in 9 cases, and a higher number of active lesions was associated with decreased local control rates. Portal vein thrombosis, increasing number of active lesions, and tumor size were associated with decreased OS rates. Three patients in each group experienced grade 3+ toxicity. The authors concluded, SBRT to be safe and effective treatment for patients with HCC, whether used as a primary treatment or following TACE.[25]

Inclusion and exclusion criteria for stereotactic body radiation therapy

While the utilization of SBRT for liver cancer (HCC) has increased, its role in treating HCC remains less well-defined and there is a need for additional phase III studies to best define its position within the landscape of HCC therapies. Patient selection is crucial, and a multidisciplinary approach is necessary, with all viable treatment options weighed and discussed[13] The eligibility requirements for SBRT treatment are listed in **Table 2**. SBRT is appropriate for lesions that are not amenable for surgical therapy such as those located in the central liver at the bifurcation of the main portal area, close to the biliary

Table 2
Eligibility criteria for using SBRT as a treatment for HCC

Eligibility Criteria for Using SBRT in HCC Treatment	
Criteria	SBRT Treatment
Tumor Size	40 or 50 mm
No. of lesions	Not more than 3
Location	Away from luminal organs and central biliary tree
LC (2 yr.)	> 90%
Level of evidence	Low

Adapted from Sanuki N, Takeda A, Kunieda E. Role of stereotactic body radiation therapy for hepatocellular carcinoma. World journal of gastroenterology. Mar 28 2014;20(12):3100-11. doi:10.3748/wjg.v20.i12.3100.

system, or invading major vessels supplying both lobes of the liver.[27] SBRT may be helpful for patients who cannot be treated with other local treatments. Moreover, SBRT has been studied as a transitional therapy, allowing patients to stay on the transplant list while awaiting the availability of donated livers. The viability and safety of utilizing SBRT as a stopgap measure before transplantation have been demonstrated in several trials. When contemplating SBRT as a therapeutic option, thorough patient selection and multidisciplinary team discussion are required.[28–30]

Alternatively, SBRT can be used as a definitive, salvage, or bridge therapy for HCC. Patient selection for SBRT depends on factors such as the extent of disease, tumor location, and prior treatments.[31,32] Traditionally, SBRT has been used for patients who are not suitable for surgical resection or other forms of LRT. However, recent evidence suggests good LC and OS with SBRT, leading to increased use of this treatment modality for the definitive treatment of HCC with comparable results to ablative technologies even for small tumors. Patients with moderately good liver function are generally suitable for SBRT,[14] although caution should be exercised for those with advanced cirrhosis or poor liver function due to the risk of radiation-associated liver toxicity.[33,34]

Tumors that are not amenable to percutaneous ablation or tumors located adjacent to large vessels or the biliary system can be treated with SBRT. In these cases, hypofractionated regimens or laparoscopically placed tissue expanders can be used. In cases where liver tolerance cannot be met with photon radiation, protons may offer superior liver sparing and reduced risk of radiation-associated liver toxicity.[35–39]

The safe delivery of liver radiation is dependent on several factors, including the evaluation of the patient's baseline liver function and extent of disease, clear delineation of the tumor using a triple-phase contrast CT and/or an MR liver with contrast, motion management to limit the amount of normal liver parenchyma in the radiation field, and creation of a radiation plan that respects known liver tolerances to mitigate the risk of acute and late toxicity.[35] Daily image guidance is also required for precise and accurate alignment of the target.[35] It is critical to understand the implications of the mean liver dose as well as the consideration of the low dose splash to the uninvolved liver parenchyma. Strategies such as fiducial markers for gated treatment and alignment, abdominal compression, or controlled breath-hold techniques should be utilized to limit liver, respiratory motion, and tumor motion.[35,39–42]

Optimal doses and fractions of stereotactic body radiation therapy

There is little research on the ideal therapeutic doses for HCC, hence there are a variety of prescription doses and treatment planning techniques reported for HCC (see **Table 1**; **Table 3**). Small tumors ranging from < 2-3 cm located in anatomically favorable positions can often be treated with ablative regiments (ie, 50 Gy/5 fractions, 54 Gy/3 fractions). As the size of the tumor increases or the location becomes less favorable with respect to organs at risk, dose de-escalation can be used to as low as 27.5 Gy/5 fractions to meet normal tissue constraints. Other reported hypofractionated regimens include 36 Gy/3 fractions or 40 Gy/5 fractions.[3,4,14,17,19,20,51,59,60]

With increasingly large tumor size or concern for normal liver toxicity other hypofractionated regimens can be used (see **Tables 1** and **3**). Using normal tissue complication probability models, prospective assigned prescription doses can be calculated while retaining the same projected risk of liver complication. This method was used to create an iso-toxic SBRT regimen at Princess Margaret Hospital at the University of Toronto, which administered doses of 54 Gy (9 Gy x 6) for low effective volume of normal liver irradiated (Veff 25%) and doses of 30-45 Gy (5 to 7.5 Gy x 6) for high Veff (25%-60%). The 1-year LC rate was 87% in their phase I study of 102 patients with HCC.[61,62] Additional 15 fraction regimens have been prospectively studied. Hong and colleagues

Table 3
Side effects and toxicity degree of SBRT in HCC treatment

Author	N	Study Design	CP-score		Follow-up (Months)	Side Effects	Toxicity (Grade-3)
			A	B			
Mendez et al,[23] 2006	45	Retrospective	NA	NA	13	Tolerable	0%
Wu et al.[18]	38	Prospective	NA	NA	45.8	Severe	79%
Que et al,[43] 2014	115	Retrospective	104	11	15.5	Tolerable	None
Sanuki et al,[22] 2014	185	Retrospective	158	27	24	Worsening of CP	13%
Lee et al,[34] 2020	85	Retrospective	NA	NA	32.9	RILD	2.6%
Bujold et al,[4] 2013	102	Retrospective	102	0	31.4	Death of 2 pt.	30%
Wei et al,[44] 2023	24	Retrospective	NA	NA	NA	Inflammation	NA
Takahashi et al,[45] 2012	68	Retrospective	56	12	10.5	Biliary stenosis	NA
Jung et al,[46] 2013	92	Retrospective	68	24	25.7	RILD	6.5%
Son et al,[47] 2010	47	Retrospective	23	3	NA	33% grade2	11%
Jun et al,[48] 2018	117	Retrospective	89	28	22.5	RILD (CP>7)	NA
Lee et al,[49] 2022	302	Retrospective	276	27	45	Enzyme deterioration	3%
Kimura et al,[50] 2021	36	Prospective	33	3	20.8	NA	3%
Tse et al,[51] 2008	41	Prospective	31	10	31.4	High liver enzymes	10 pt.
Jang et al,[52] 2020	65	Retrospective	64	1	12.9	GIT toxicity	6%
Kim et al,[53] 2021	72	Prospective	33	6	27	None	0%
Labrunie et al,[54] 2020	43	Prospective	37	6	48	High liver enzymes	31%
Hara et al,[55] 2019	143	Retrospective	214	16	30.2	NA	8.2%
Fang et al,[56] 2018	90	Prospective	NA	NA	37	Decline in CP score	7%
Park et al,[57] 2020	290	Prospective	250	40	38.2	Deterioration in CP	2.3%
Jeong et al,[58] 2018	119	Prospective	108	11	25.8	RILD	2%

Abbreviations: CP, child-Paugh score; GIT, gastrointestinal tract; N.B: RILD, radiation-induced liver damage; NA, not available.

enrolled patients with HCC tumors with median size of 6 cm (range, 2.2 cm – 10.9 cm) and treated with a hypofractionated proton approach using doses of 67.5 Gy/15 fractions for peripheral tumors and 58.05 Gy/15 fractions for central tumors. Further dose de-escalation was allowed in order to meet normal tissue constraints (mean liver–GTV ≤ 24 Gy). At two years, the local control was 94.8% using this approach.[63]

It is crucial to comprehend the variations in treatment aim (curative or semi-radical) and objectives when using fixed-dose and variable-dose prescription techniques for the treatment of HCC (early or advanced). The prescribed radiation dose is defined by two possible theories: the first is to give the organs at risk the highest acceptable exposure while still adhering to dose restrictions to optimize anticancer effects, particularly for bigger tumors. The second option is to apply the ALARA (as low as reasonably possible) concept and deliver the lowest effective dose with enough efficacy, which may be feasible for tiny HCCs.[64,65] **Figure 1** shows SBRT plan of a representative patient treated with SBRT (45 Gy in 5 fractions), showing tumor volumes, radiation beam arrangement, PTV coverage and low isodose lines.

Side effects and toxicity post SBRT
Historically, radiation-induced liver disease (RILD) was a concerning side effect that limited the potential use of radiation in HCC. Ascites, high levels of alkaline phosphatase (ALP), and anicteric hepatomegaly are symptoms of RILD that commonly appear 2–12 months following treatment. Fortunately, despite concerns for this toxicity, modern treatment techniques show the risk of serious liver injury following radiation is low.

Although gastrointestinal toxicity is a potential risk, SBRT is usually considered to be safe. The risk of developing a gastric or duodenal ulcer or perforation can be reduced

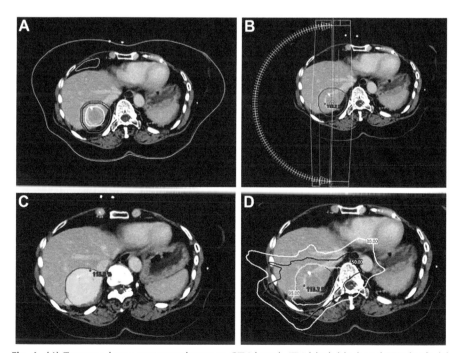

Fig. 1. (A) Tumor volume contours shown as GTV (*cyan*), ITV (*dark blue*) and PTV (*red*): (B) VMAT beam arrangement; (C) Dose color wash showing PTV coverage with 95% isodose line; (D) Low dose fall shown with 50% isodose line (*blue*) and 30% isodose line (*yellow*).

by adhering to dose constraints and optimizing motion management.[28] Tumors within or abutting to the biliary system can be treated with SBRT or a moderate hypofractionated approach as a precautionary measure.[3,21] Studies have revealed that 13–30% of individuals who had SBRT experience immediate but temporary grade 3 toxicity.[22] In these investigations, a small percentage of deaths (1.3–7%) that may have been caused by the therapy occurred 1.1–7.7 months after SBRT. Two patients (1.3%) developed grade 5 liver failure in a retrospective study of 185 patients HCC who received SBRT of 35 or 40 Gy in 5 fractions and is most expected with poor baseline liver function (CP-B8 or worse), whereas 13% of patients exhibited acute but temporary grade 3 toxicities.[51]

Retrospective data analysis were performed by Roquette and colleagues[66] in 318 patients with 375 HCC diagnoses who were treated between June 2007 and December 2018. The study discussed acute and late toxicities as well as efficacy criteria such as OS, relapse-free survival, and LC. The average number of follow-up months was 70.2. Radiation dose of 45 Gy in 3 fractions was given to most patients. The planning target volume (PTV) had a 90.7 (2.6-1067.6) cubic centimeter median (range) volume. The LC was 94% (91-97%) at 24 months and 94% (91-97%) at 60 months, respectively. Relapse-free survival was 62% (55-67%), 29% (23-36%), and 13% (8-19%) at 12, 24, and 60 months, respectively. The OS rate was 72% (95%CI 67-77%), 44% (38-50%), and 11% (7-15%) at 12, 24, and 60 months, respectively. Acute and late toxicities were experienced by about 51% and 38% of individuals respectively. CP score B-C, a high BCLC score, portal thrombosis, a high gross tumor volume (GTV) volume, and a larger PTV volume as indicated on the total liver volume ratio were all substantially associated with OS. SBRT has a low toxicity profile and is an effective therapeutic option for HCC. Treatment results are significantly influenced by the underlying cirrhosis and its natural progression. **Table 4** shows the side effects and toxicity of SBRT treatment in multiple retrospective studies.

In conclusion, owing to low treatment toxicity and few interruptions, SBRT is considered a very safe and effective therapy option for HCC. High GTV volume and high PTV volume reported on the total hepatic volume ratio were found to be predictive factors of grade > 1 toxicity. Given the normal course of HCC and underlying cirrhosis, it may be challenging to link the incidence of late toxicities, such as fatigue and ascites, to SBRT alone. The difficulties in treating HCC as a multifocal illness are highlighted by the discovery that out-of-field hepatic relapse is the primary reason for treatment failure. Further studies may be required to investigate how to enhance local control and guard against out-of-field hepatic recurrence.[59,72,73]

Role of Stereotactic Body Radiation Therapy as First-Line Treatment of Hepatocellular Carcinoma

There is growing literature to support the use of SBRT in the initial treatment of HCC. **Table 4** documents several studies examining this question. An early study was performed by Andolino and colleagues [59] at Indiana University where 60 patients with liver-confined HCC were treated with upfront SBRT with 36 patients having CTP Class A and 24 CTP Class B. Median dose and fraction number was 44 Gy/3 fractions and 40 Gy/5 fractions for CTP Class A and B, respectively.[59] With median follow up of 27 months, two-year LC, PFS, and OS of 90%, 48%, and 67%, respectively, and a median time to progression of 47.8 months. Importantly, 23 patients underwent liver transplant successfully at a median time of 7 months.[59]

Kang and colleagues[60](2012) investigated the effectiveness of SBRT as a treatment option for inoperable HCC in 302 patients that had not responded to TACE. Patients with tumors less than 10 cm in size were included in the study, and SBRT doses

Table 4
Selected studies for the use of SBRT as first-line treatment of HCC

Reference Year	Study Design	N	CP Score	Dose	Fractions	Tumor Size	LC	OS	Toxicity Grade-3%	Previous Treatment
Andolino et al,[59] 2011	Phase I/II	60	CP-A (36) CP-B (24)	42–60 Gy	3 fr.	31 mm	94.6% (2 yr.)	68.7% (2 yr.)	10%	100%
Kang et al,[60] 2012	Phase II	47	CP-A (41) CP-B (6)	24–48 Gy	3 fr.	29 mm	90% (2 yr.)	67% (2 yr.)	25%	NA
Bujold et al,[4] 2013	Phase I/II	102	CP-A (102) CP-B (0)	24–54 Gy	6 fr.	72 mm	87% (2 yr.)	34% (2 yr.)	30%	52%
Yoon et al,[67] 2013	Phase I/II	93	CP-A (69) CP-B (24)	30–60 Gy	3–4 fr.	20 mm	92% (3 yr.)	54% (3 yr.)	6.5%	NA
Qiu et al,[43] 2014	NA	63	CP-A (53%) CP-B (35%)	50–60 Gy	5–10 fr.	44 mm	94%	NA	10%	72%
Sanuki et al,[22] 2014	NA	185	CP-A (158) CP-B (27)	35–40 Gy	5 fr.	24–27 mm	91% (2 yr.)	70%	13%	70%
Lasely et al,[68] 2015	Phase II	59	CP-A (38) CP-B (21)	48 Gy 40 Gy	3 fr. 5 fr.	NA	91% 82%	61% 26%	11% 38%	NA
Marta et al,[69] 2015	NA	43	CP-A (23) CP-B (20)	36–60 Gy	6 fr.	48 mm	85.5% (1 yr.)	77.9% (1 yr.)	16%	65%
Takeda et al,[70] 2016	Phase II	90	CP-A (82) CP-B (8)	40 or 35 Gy	5 fr.	23 mm	96.3% (3 yr.)	66.7% (3 yr.)	15%	64%
Jeong et al,[58] 2018	NA	119	CP-A (108) CP-B (11)	30–60 Gy	3–4 fr.	17 mm	97% (3 yr.)	84% (3 yr.)	2%	97.5%
Jang et al,[52] 2020	Phase II	55	CP-A (64) CP-B (1)	42–60 Gy	3 fr.	24 mm	95% (3 yr.)	76% (3 yr.)	2%	100%
Durand et al,[54] 2020	Phase II	43	CP-A (37) CP-B (6)	43 Gy	3 fr.	28 mm	94% (2 yr.)	69% (2 yr.)	31%	0%

(continued on next page)

Table 4
(continued)

Reference Year	Study Design	N	CP Score	Dose	Fractions	Tumor Size	LC	OS	Toxicity Grade-3%	Previous Treatment
Mathew et al,[71] 2020	NA	297	CP-A (225) CP-A (59)	27–60 Gy	3–6 fr.	27 mm	13% (3 yr.)	39% (3 yr.)	16%	NA
Kimura et al,[50] 2021	Phase II	36	CP-A (33) CP-B (3)	40 Gy	5 fr.	23 mm	90% (3 yr.)	76% (3 yr.)	11%	0%

Abbreviations: fr., dose fraction; N.B: CP, child-Pugh class; NA, not available; yr., year.

ranged from 42 to 60 Gy in 3 fractions. The results of the study showed that 38.3% of patients achieved complete remission within 6 months of completing SBRT, and 38.3% experienced a partial response. The 2-LC was 94.6%, OS rate was 68.7%, and PFS rate was 33.8% (see **Table 4**). Gastrointestinal toxicity was experienced by 6.4% of patients, and gastric ulcer perforation was experienced by 4.3% of patients.[60]

Bujold and colleagues[4](2013) reported on two prospective trials of SBRT in HCC unsuitable for standard locoregional therapies. The primary endpoints were toxicity and LC at 1 year. A total of 102 patients were evaluated, and the results showed that SBRT was associated with an 87% LC rate at 1 year, and a median OS of 17 months. Toxicity ≥ grade 3 was seen in 30% of patients, and death of 7 patients was possibly related to treatment[4](see **Table 4**).

Qiu and colleagues[43](2014), reported on a retrospective cohort from Taiwan. Where 22 patients with large, unresectable HCC (>10 cm) unsuitable for other lines of treatment were included(2009-2011). The tumor response rate was 86.3% (complete and partial response), with a 1-year LC rate of 55.5% and an OS rate of 50%, indicating the effectiveness of the treatment even in very large tumors. Patients with a CP score of A and those receiving doses of at least 40 Gy had 1-year LC of 66.7% and 71.4%, respectively (see **Table 4**). Mild and tolerable acute toxicities were observed (only one grade 3 toxicity).[43]

Marta and colleagues [69] reported on patients with 1-3 HCC lesions, diameter ≤6 cm and CP class A or B disease treated with SBRT using 2 prescription regimens (48-75 Gy in 3 consecutive fractions, or 36-60 Gy in 6 fractions). The primary endpoints were in-field LC and toxicity, and the secondary endpoints were OS and PFS. The study included 43 patients with 63 HCC lesions, and the median follow-up was 8 months. The actuarial LC at 6, 12, and 24 months was 94.2%, 85.8%, and 64.4%, respectively, and the median OS was 18.0 months (see **Table 4**). The study found SBRT to be a safe and effective therapeutic option for inoperable HCC lesions with acceptable local control rates and low treatment-related toxicity.[69]

Lasely and colleagues[68] reported on 38 patients with CPC-A and 21 patients with CPC-B with HCC treated with SBRT. Results showed that local control at 6 months was 92% for CPC-A and 93% for CPC-B, and median OS was 44.8 months for patients with CPC-A and 17.0 months for patients with CPC-B. However, 11% of patients with CPC-A and 38% of patients with CPC-B experienced grade III/IV liver toxicity (see **Table 4**), and there was a correlation between higher liver toxicity and increased risk of death in patients with CPC-A.[68]

Takeda and colleagues,[70] reported on a retrospective cohort of 63 untreated solitary patients with HCC who received SBRT preceded by TACE between 2005 and 2012. The prescribed dose of SBRT was 35-40 Gy in 5 fractions. The LC rates at 1, 2, and 3 years were 100%, 95%, and 92%, respectively, and OS rates were 100%, 87%, and 73%, respectively (see **Table 4**).[70]

Durand and colleagues [54] investigated in a prospective phase 2 trial of patients with single HCC lesions unsuitable for standard locoregional therapies. The primary endpoint was LC of irradiated HCC at 18 months. The patients received SBRT with a dose of 45 Gy in 3 fractions. All 43 patients had cirrhosis, and 37 (88%) were CP-A. Results showed that the 18-month LC rate was 98%, and the 18-month OS rate was 72%. Median OS was 3.5 years. Thirteen patients (31%) experienced grade ≥3 acute adverse events, including 8 patients with abnormal liver function tests (19%). Three patients (10%) experienced a decline in CP at 3 months post-SBRT (see **Table 4**).[54]

A multicenter phase II trial performed by Jang and colleagues[52] enrolled patients with unresectable HCC who received SBRT with 45 to 60 Gy in 3 fractions. The primary endpoint was treatment-related severe toxicity at 1 year after SBRT, and secondary endpoints were LC, PFS, and OS rates at 2 years. Out of 65 eligible patients, only 1 patient experienced acute grade ≥3 toxicity, and the actuarial rate of treatment-related severe toxicity at 1 year was 3%. The 2-year and 3-year LC rates were 97% and 95%, respectively (see **Table 4**). The PFS and OS rates were 48% and 84% at 2 years and 36% and 76% at 3 years, respectively.[52]

Another multicenter study performed by Kimura and colleagues[50] investigated the effectiveness and safety of SBRT in patients with primary solitary HCC who were inel-igible for surgery and radiofrequency ablation. The primary endpoint was 3-year OS, and the secondary endpoints were PFS, LC, and adverse events (see **Table 4**). Thirty-six patients were enrolled, and the results showed that SBRT had acceptable toxicity with comparable LC and OS rates for previously untreated solitary HCC. The study suggests that SBRT may be a viable alternative treatment option for early HCC in patients who are unsuitable for resection and RFA. Several other studies[22,57,67,72,74,75] of SBRT in HCC are summarized in **Table 4**.

Finally, NRG/RTOG 1112 reported a prospective trial of Sorafenib ± SBRT. This trial enrolled 193 patients many of whom had advanced disease (74% with macrovascu-lanvasion, median tumor diameter of 8.2 cm). Median OS was significantly improved from 12.3 months with Sorafenib alone to 15.8 months with SBRT and Sorafenib (HR = 0.72, p = 0.042). Treatment was well tolerated with no difference in rates of grade 3 or higher toxicity between the two groups.

Stereotactic Body Radiation Therapy as Bridge Treatment in Advanced Cases of Hepatocellular Carcinoma

For individuals with early-stage HCC who meet the Milan criteria, liver transplantation (LT) is the recommended course of treatment. Unfortunately, patients may have to wait many months before receiving a transplant due to the restricted supply of organs. Bridging therapies including Transarterial chemoembolization (TACE), radiofrequency ablation/microwave ablation (RFA/MWA), or Transarterial radioembolization (TARE) are utilized to stop tumor growth during this waiting period.[30,76,77] For patients with HCC awaiting LT, SBRT has also demonstrated promise as a bridge therapy.[30]

The effectiveness of SBRT as a bridging therapy for LT has been assessed in a num-ber of retrospective investigations.[27,30,76–82] Several studies (**Table 5**) have demon-strated that, with different dose-fraction schedules, SBRT has an OS range of 75 to 100%, a disease-free survival of roughly 75%, when using SBRT as a bridge to trans-plant. In one study, Sapisochin and colleagues[77] contrasted RFA (36 patients), SBRT (36 patients), and TACE (244 patients) as a bridge to transplant using the rigorous intention-to-treat analysis. With rates ranging from 69% to 75%, the 5-year OS after LT was comparable among the SBRT, TACE, and RFA groups. The drop-out rates, which ranged from 16.7% to 20.2%, were also comparable among the 3 groups. Due to selection bias, such as poor liver function and not meeting the Milan criteria in the SBRT group, the rate of impaired liver function was considerably greater in the SBRT group (38.9%) than in the TACE (19.4%) and RFA groups (13%).

For patients with HCC awaiting LT, SBRT has been demonstrated to be a safe and effective bridging therapy overall. When traditional bridging therapies, including TACE and RFA, are ineffective or fail to control tumors, it may be employed as a substitute. Patients with questionable liver function who might not tolerate TACE or RFA may benefit from SBRT as well. SBRT has had encouraging results, although LT continues to be the predominant factor in this population's strong outcomes.[2]

Table 5
SBRT as a bridge treatment for HCC liver transplantation

Reference Year	Study Design	N	Dose	Fr.	Tumor Size	Free Survival	OS	Months to LT	CR Rate
Sandroussi et al,[81] 2010	Retrospective	10	33 Gy	6 fr.	79 cc	NA	NA	5	NA
O' Cannar et al,[30] 2012	Retrospective	10	51 Gy	3 fr.	34 mm	NA	100% (5 yr.)	3.5	27%
Katz et al,[27] 2012	Retrospective	18	50 Gy	10 fr.	40 mm	NA	NA	6	18.2%
Barry et al,[78] 2016	Retrospective	38	36 Gy	6 fr.	60.5 mm	79% (5 yr.)	76% (5 yr.)	NA	NA
Mannina et al,[80] 2017	Retrospective	38	40 Gy	5 fr.	24 mm	74% (5 yr.)	77% (3 yr.)	8.1	23.5%
Sapisochin et al,[77] 2017	Retrospective	36	36 Gy	6 fr.	45 mm	74% (3 yr.)	75% (5 yr.)	13.7	13.3%
Moore et al,[76] 2017	Retrospective	23	54 Gy	3 fr.	25 mm	NA	NA	4.8	27.3%
Gresswell et al,[79] 2018	Retrospective	15	40 Gy	5 fr.	23 mm	NA	NA	5	46%
Wang et al,[83] 2020	Retrospective	14	45 Gy	5 fr.	44.5 mm	18 months	37.8 months	8.4	23.1%
Wong et al,[84] 2021	Retrospective	40	40 Gy	5 fr.	28 mm	NA	88.1% (1 yr.)	NA	45–53%

Abbreviations: CR, pathological complete response; N.B: LT, liver transplantation.

Stereotactic Body Radiation Therapy as a Combined Therapy of Hepatocellular Carcinoma

The available evidence for the efficacy of SBRT compared to other liver-directed therapies such as surgical resection, RFA, and TACE in early stage HCC is limited to RCTs and a recent non-inferiority Phase 3 RCT. No large RCTs have been conducted to directly compare the outcomes of SBRT with those of other liver-directed therapies commonly used in early stage HCC.[85] (**Table 6**).

In a phase 2 trial performed by Buckstein and colleagues,[86] individuals with a solitary HCC measuring 4 to 7 cm who were not candidates for surgery were evaluated for the effects of TACE and SBRT. The best objective response rate (ORR) by modified Response Evaluation Criteria in Solid Tumors was the primary endpoint, and 32 eligible patients were enrolled at one institution (mRECIST). With a median duration to complete response (CR) of 10.1 months, the ORR in the target lesion was 91%. The PFS was 35 months, and the median OS was not yet attained. Those who experienced a full response generally had better PFS. Low toxicity was observed. The combination of TACE and SBRT may be a successful therapy strategy for large, unresectable HCC, according to these encouraging data. It is necessary to conduct larger phase 2 and 3 clinical trials for further research.[86]

A study performed by Bauer and colleagues,[87] aimed to investigate the effectiveness of TACE and SBRT as bridging therapies to liver transplantation for patients with HCC. The study analyzed the histopathological response of liver explants of 27 patients who received either TACE or SBRT alone, or a combination of TACE and SBRT. The results showed that the combination of TACE and SBRT resulted in a significantly higher rate of complete histopathological response (89%) compared to TACE (0%) or SBRT (25%) alone. The study suggests that a combination of TACE and SBRT may be a more effective bridging therapy option for patients with HCC awaiting liver transplantation.[87]

Another study was performed by Wahl and colleagues,[24] in 2015 at the University of Michigan where 224 patients treated with unresectable, nonmetastatic HCC underwent RFA (n = 161) or image-guided SBRT (n = 63). This study was performed to evaluate the efficacy of both SBRT or RFA for the treatment of HCC (see **Table 1**). The SBRT group had more prior liver-directed treatments and more pretreatment alphafetoprotein levels, as well as lower pretreatment CP scores.[24] One- and two-year freedom from local progression (FFLP) was 97.4% and 83.8% for patients treated with SBRT, compared to 83.6% and 80.2% in patients treated with RFA. In patients receiving RFA, tumor size was a predictor of FFLP (hazard ratio [HR] = 1.54 per cm, p = 0.006), but not in those receiving SBRT (HR = 1.21 per cm, p = 0.62). For tumors larger than 2 cm, there was decreased FFLP with RFA compared to SBRT (HR = 3.35).

Table 6						
SBRT combined with other techniques for HCC treatment						
Author Year	**N**	**Study Design**	**Combined Technique**	**ORR**	**CR**	**Follow-up (months)**
Buckstein et al,[86] 2022	32	Prospective	TACE	91%	63%	37
Bauer et al,[87] 2021	27	Retrospective	TACE	NA	88%	NA
Su et al,[93] 2016	115	Retrospective	TAE, TACE	75.5%	NA	20.5
Chinage et al,[88] 2019	185	Retrospective	TACE	100%	40%	14.9
Juloori et al,[89] 2023	119	Prospective	Immunotherapy	57%	NA	NA

Abbreviations: CR, complete response; N.B: ORR, overall response rate.

RFA and SBRT were both well tolerated with acute grade 3+ toxicity occurring in 11% vs. 5% of patients, respectively. At one- and two years following treatment, the OS rates were 74% and 46% for SBRT treatment. This study concluded SBRT was a good first-line treatment for unresected HCC, but further prospective studies were recommended.[24]

According to Chiang and colleagues,[88] for individuals with large tumors, the traditional treatment for unresectable HCC have limits in terms of efficacy and safety. In this retrospective case series, 5 patients with advanced HCC and sizable tumors (median size 9.8 cm; range:9-16.1 cm) who were ineligible for curative intervention were treated with SBRT and anti-PD-1 therapy. Before receiving SBRT, TACE was administered to 4 of these patients in a single dosage. Two CR and 3 PR were observed in all patients, and no patient experienced tumor progression throughout the course of a median follow-up of 14.9 months. Both the LC and OS at one year were 100%. There were grade 3 toxicities in one patient, but no traditional radiation-induced liver damage. More prospective trials are required to validate these findings, but these results imply that the combination of SBRT and checkpoint inhibitors may be a promising therapeutic option for large tumors.[88]

Su and colleagues,[90] reported on HCC with a diameter greater than 5 cm treated with SBRT alone or in combination with TAE or TACE. The study aimed to compare the results and identify prognostic factors. Fifty patients had SBRT alone, whereas 77 patients received SBRT with TAE/TACE. The typical tumor size was 8.5 cm, and the median follow-up time was 20.5 months. According to the study, TAE/TACE + SBRT significantly improved both distant metastasis-free survival (DMFS) and OS compared to SBRT alone. In the whole patient population, a biologically effective dose (BED10) of less than 100 Gy and an equivalent dose in two fractions (EQD2) of less than 74 Gy were important prognostic variables for OS, PFS, LRFS, and DMFS. According to the results, TAE/TACE combined with SBRT may be an efficient supplementary therapy strategy for HCC with a diameter more than 5 cm.[90]

Another study by Juloori and colleagues,[89] aimed to determine whether SBRT and immunotherapy were safe and effective for treating individuals with advanced or incurable HCC. The primary outcome of the experiment, a multicenter phase 1 randomized trial, was dose-limiting toxicity occurring within 6 months of SBRT. Fourteen individuals were enrolled across 3 centers before the study was prematurely terminated due to slow accrual. The findings revealed that when compared to immunotherapy alone, the combination of SBRT with nivolumab and ipilimumab demonstrated adequate safety. The findings support additional research into this multimodal therapy.[89]

The effectiveness of combining SBRT with TACE is another topic of interest. For tiny HCC with a median tumor size of less than 20 mm, Kimura and colleagues[91,92] retrospectively compared 28 patients treated with SBRT alone and 122 patients treated with SBRT + TACE. According to the research, there was no significant difference in the 2-year OS and local progression-free survival (LPFS) rates between the SBRT alone group and the SBRT + TACE group (78.6% vs. 80.3%; p = 0.6583 and 71.4% vs. 80.8%; p = 0.9661, respectively).[91]

Imaging After Stereotactic Body Radiation Therapy Treatment of Hepatocellular Carcinoma

A variety of imaging characteristics are used to assess the effectiveness of LRT for HCC using multiphasic CT or dynamic post-contrast MRI, depending on the treatment response categorization method being employed. These imaging characteristics include APHE (arterial phase hyperenhancement), WO (washout) appearance, pretreatment-like enhancement, and size change. While current classification systems do not strictly incorporate auxiliary MRI parameters such as diffusion restriction and T2-weighted hyperintensity for treatment response assessment, HCC response to SBRT frequently makes use of a combination of these findings. The duration between RT and the imaging examination must be considered when evaluating SBRT response since imaging features in the post-SBRT context change over time. Moreover, it can be difficult to discern between a treated tumor, a viable tumor, and the surrounding parenchyma due to radiation-induced alterations in the liver's surrounding parenchyma after SBRT.[93]

Following LRT, the effectiveness of the therapy is assessed using either contrast-enhanced CT or MRI. While follow-up schedule for patients who have received SBRT varies, imaging should normally take place every three months after treatment. Imaging tests should not be performed until three months have passed since microvascular radiation-induced veno-occlusive alterations may cause widespread arterial phase hyperenhancement throughout the treatment zone, which may make it difficult to evaluate the treated lesion.[57]

SBRT often results in a modest shrinkage of HCC, making it challenging to spot a measurable size shift between quick imaging studies.[94] HCCs treated with SBRT show size reductions of 35% after 3 months, 48% after 9 months, and 54% after 12 months.[95] Another study demonstrated that none of the 67 HCCs treated with SBRT showed an increase in size over the first 12 months after therapy, instead, all remained the same size or declined.[96] As the size of these lesions has not changed, they should not be regarded as viable. On the other hand, it is strongly suggestive of persistent or recurrent viable illness if a treated tumor shows an increase in size after SBRT.[97] **Figure 2** shows representative MRI images of a patient of HCC treated with SBRT, comparing pre-treatment and post-treatment follow-up images.

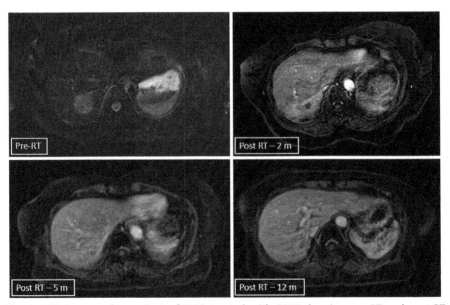

Fig. 2. MRI images of a patient of HCC treated with SBRT showing pre-RT and post-RT follow-up images at 2-month, 5 month and 12 months showing radiological response.

SUMMARY

SBRT has emerged as an effective treatment option for HCC in both early and late stages of the disease. It has traditionally been used as a last-line therapy in patients who are ineligible for surgical resection or have already undergone other LRTs. However, recent studies have shown that SBRT can be an effective first-line treatment for HCC.

In addition, SBRT can be used in combination with other treatment techniques such as TACE or RFA to improve treatment outcomes and achieve higher rates of complete response. Furthermore, SBRT has been shown to be comparable or even superior to other LRTs in terms of overall survival rates and response rates, allowing for bridging and downstaging of tumors for liver transplant.

Overall, SBRT has emerged as an important treatment option for HCC, particularly for patients who are not surgical candidates or who have failed other LRTs. It has shown promising results both as a standalone treatment and in combination with other techniques, and future research is likely to further define its role in the management of HCC.

DISCLOSURE

Dr S.K. Jabbour received National Institutes of Health, USA grant funding number 1R50CA275877-01.

CLINICS CARE POINTS

- SBRT is an effective treatment option for both early and late stage HCC.
- SBRT can be used in combination with LRT (TACE, RFA) and systemic therapies including immumotherapy to improve treatment outcomes and achieve higher rates of complete response.
- SBRT is comparable to other LRTs in terms of OS and RR, allowing for bridging and downstaging of tumors for liver transplant.
- Future studies will elucidate dose and fractionation schemes, patient selection criteria and incorporation of systemic therapies.

REFERENCES

1. Clark I, Maximin S, Meier J, et al. Hepatocellular carcinoma: review of epidomi ology, screening, imaging diagnosis, response assessment, and treatment. Curr Probl Diagn Radiol 2015;44(6):479–86.
2. Kimura T, Fujiwara T, Kameoka T, et al. The current role of stereotactic body radiation therapy (SBRT) in hepatocellular carcinoma (HCC). Cancers 2022;14(18). https://doi.org/10.3390/cancers14184383.
3. Huang WY, Jen YM, Lee MS, et al. Stereotactic body radiation therapy in recurrent hepatocellular carcinoma. Int J Radiat Oncol Biol Phys 2012;84(2):355–61.
4. Bujold A, Massey CA, Kim JJ, et al. Sequential phase I and II trials of stereotactic body radiotherapy for locally advanced hepatocellular carcinoma. J Clin Oncol 2013;31(13):1631–9.
5. Dawson LA, Winter KA, Knox JJ, et al. NRG/RTOG 1112: Randomized phase III study of sorafenib vs. stereotactic body radiation therapy (SBRT) followed by sorafenib in hepatocellular carcinoma (HCC). J Clin Oncol 2023;41(4_suppl):489.

6. Ueno M, Takabatake H, Itasaka S, et al. Stereotactic body radiation therapy versus radiofrequency ablation for single small hepatocellular carcinoma: a propensity-score matching analysis of their impact on liver function and clinical outcomes. J Gastrointest Oncol 2021;12(5):2334–44.

7. Reig M, Forner A, Rimola J, et al. BCLC strategy for prognosis prediction and treatment recommendation: the 2022 update. J Hepatol 2022;76(3):681–93.

8. Shampain KL, Hackett CE, Towfighi S, et al. SBRT for HCC: overview of technique and treatment response assessment. Abdominal radiology (New York) 2021; 46(8):3615–24.

9. Kirkbride P, Cooper T. Stereotactic body radiotherapy. Guidelines for commissioners, providers and clinicians: a national report. Clin Oncol 2011;23(3):163–4.

10. Potters L, Kavanagh B, Galvin JM, et al. American society for therapeutic radiology and oncology (ASTRO) and American college of radiology (ACR) practice guideline for the performance of stereotactic body radiation therapy. Int J Radiat Oncol Biol Phys 2010;76(2):326–32.

11. Sahgal A, Roberge D, Schellenberg D, et al. The Canadian Association of Radiation Oncology scope of practice guidelines for lung, liver and spine stereotactic body radiotherapy. Clin Oncol 2012;24(9):629–39.

12. Guckenberger M, Andratschke N, Alheit H, et al. Definition of stereotactic body radiotherapy: principles and practice for the treatment of stage I non-small cell lung cancer. Strahlenther Onkol 2014;190(1):26–33.

13. Sayan M, Yegya-Raman N, Greco SH, et al. Rethinking the role of radiation therapy in the treatment of unresectable hepatocellular carcinoma: a data driven treatment algorithm for optimizing outcomes. Front Oncol 2019;9:345.

14. Cárdenes HR, Price TR, Perkins SM, et al. Phase I feasibility trial of stereotactic body radiation therapy for primary hepatocellular carcinoma. Clin Transl Oncol 2010;12(3):218–25.

15. Choi BO, Jang HS, Kang KM, et al. Fractionated stereotactic radiotherapy in patients with primary hepatocellular carcinoma. Jpn J Clin Oncol 2006;36(3):154–8.

16. Choi BO, Choi IB, Jang HS, et al. Stereotactic body radiation therapy with or without transarterial chemoembolization for patients with primary hepatocellular carcinoma: preliminary analysis. BMC Cancer 2008;8:351.

17. Louis C, Dewas S, Mirabel X, et al. Stereotactic radiotherapy of hepatocellular carcinoma: preliminary results. Technol Cancer Res Treat 2010;9(5):479–87.

18. Kwon JH, Bae SH, Kim JY, et al. Long-term effect of stereotactic body radiation therapy for primary hepatocellular carcinoma ineligible for local ablation therapy or surgical resection. Stereotactic radiotherapy for liver cancer. BMC Cancer 2010;10:475.

19. Seo YS, Kim MS, Yoo SY, et al. Preliminary result of stereotactic body radiotherapy as a local salvage treatment for inoperable hepatocellular carcinoma. J Surg Oncol 2010;102(3):209–14.

20. Honda Y, Kimura T, Aikata H, et al. Stereotactic body radiation therapy combined with transcatheter arterial chemoembolization for small hepatocellular carcinoma. J Gastroenterol Hepatol 2013;28(3):530–6.

21. Bae SH, Kim MS, Cho CK, et al. Feasibility and efficacy of stereotactic ablative radiotherapy for barcelona clinic liver cancer-C stage hepatocellular carcinoma. J Korean Med Sci 2013;28(2):213–9.

22. Sanuki N, Takeda A, Oku Y, et al. Stereotactic body radiotherapy for small hepatocellular carcinoma: a retrospective outcome analysis in 185 patients. Acta oncologica (Stockholm, Sweden) 2014;53(3):399–404.

23. Méndez Romero A, Wunderink W, Hussain SM, et al. Stereotactic body radiation therapy for primary and metastatic liver tumors: a single institution phase i-ii study. Acta oncologica (Stockholm, Sweden) 2006;45(7):831–7.

24. Wahl DR, Stenmark MH, Tao Y, et al. Outcomes after stereotactic body radiotherapy or radiofrequency ablation for hepatocellular carcinoma. J Clin Oncol 2016;34(5):452–9.

25. Sapir E, Jackson W, Bazzi L, et al. Efficacy of liver stereotactic body radiation therapy as primary treatment or following transarterial chemoembolization (TACE) in patients with HCC. Int J Radiat Oncol Biol Phys 2016;96(2):E176–7.

26. Yuan Z, Tian L, Wang P, et al. Comparative research on the efficacy of CyberKnife® and surgical excision for Stage I hepatocellular carcinoma. OncoTargets Ther 2013;6:1527–32.

27. Katz AW, Chawla S, Qu Z, et al. Stereotactic hypofractionated radiation therapy as a bridge to transplantation for hepatocellular carcinoma: clinical outcome and pathologic correlation. Int J Radiat Oncol Biol Phys 2012;83(3):895–900.

28. Eriguchi T, Takeda A, Sanuki N, et al. Acceptable toxicity after stereotactic body radiation therapy for liver tumors adjacent to the central biliary system. Int J Radiat Oncol Biol Phys 2013;85(4):1006–11.

29. Facciuto ME, Singh MK, Rochon C, et al. Stereotactic body radiation therapy in hepatocellular carcinoma and cirrhosis: evaluation of radiological and pathological response. J Surg Oncol 2012;105(7):692–8.

30. O'Connor JK, Trotter J, Davis GL, et al. Long-term outcomes of stereotactic body radiation therapy in the treatment of hepatocellular cancer as a bridge to transplantation. Liver Transplant 2012;18(8):949–54.

31. Gerum S, Jensen AD, Roeder F. Stereotactic body radiation therapy in patients with hepatocellular carcinoma: a mini-review. World J Gastrointest Oncol 2019; 11(5):367–76.

32. Zeng ZC, Seong J, Yoon SM, et al. Consensus on stereotactic body radiation therapy for small-sized hepatocellular carcinoma at the 7th Asia-Pacific primary liver cancer expert meeting. Liver Cancer 2017;6(4):264–74.

33. Jackson WC, Tang M, Maurino C, et al. Individualized adaptive radiation therapy allows for safe treatment of hepatocellular carcinoma in patients with child-turcotte-Pugh B liver disease. Int J Radiat Oncol Biol Phys 2021;109(1):212–9.

34. Lee P, Ma Y, Zacharias I, et al. Stereotactic body radiation therapy for hepatocellular carcinoma in patients with child-Pugh B or C cirrhosis. Advances in Radiation Oncology 2020;5(5):889–96.

35. Crane CH, Koay LJ. Solutions that enable ablative radiotherapy for large liver tumors: Fractionated dose painting, simultaneous integrated protection, motion management, and computed tomography image guidance. Cancer 2016; 122(13):1974–86.

36. Fukuda K, Okumura T, Abei M, et al. Long-term outcomes of proton beam therapy in patients with previously untreated hepatocellular carcinoma. Cancer Sci 2017; 108(3):497–503.

37. Sanford NN, Pursley J, Noe B, et al. Protons versus photons for unresectable hepatocellular carcinoma: liver decompensation and overall survival. Int J Radiat Oncol Biol Phys 2019;105(1):64–72.

38. Yoon K, Kwak J, Cho B, et al. Gated volumetric-modulated arc therapy vs. Tumor-tracking CyberKnife radiotherapy as stereotactic body radiotherapy for hepatocellular carcinoma: a dosimetric comparison study focused on the impact of respiratory motion managements. PLoS One 2016;11(11):e0166927.

39. Yoon SS, Aloia TA, Haynes AB, et al. Surgical placement of biologic mesh spacers to displace bowel away from unresectable liver tumors followed by delivery of dose-intense radiation therapy. Practical Radiation Oncology 2014;4(3): 167–73.
40. Miften M, Vinogradskiy Y, Moiseenko V, et al. Radiation dose-volume effects for liver SBRT. Int J Radiat Oncol Biol Phys 2021;110(1):196–205.
41. Riou O, Llacer Moscardo C, Fenoglietto P, et al. SBRT planning for liver metastases: a focus on immobilization, motion management and planning imaging techniques. Rep Practical Oncol Radiother 2017;22(2):103–10.
42. Toesca DAS, Osmundson EC, von Eyben R, et al. Assessment of hepatic function decline after stereotactic body radiation therapy for primary liver cancer. Practical Radiation Oncology 2017;7(3):173–82.
43. Que JY, Lin LC, Lin KL, et al. The efficacy of stereotactic body radiation therapy on huge hepatocellular carcinoma unsuitable for other local modalities. Radiat Oncol 2014;9:120.
44. Wei L, Simeth J, Aryal MP, et al. The effect of stereotactic body radiation therapy for hepatocellular cancer on regional hepatic liver function. Int J Radiat Oncol Biol Phys 2023;115(3):794–802.
45. Takahashi S, Kimura T, Nishibuchi I, et al. Portal vein and bile duct toxicity following stereotactic body radiation therapy (SBRT) for hepatocellular carcinoma (HCC). Int J Radiat Oncol Biol Phys 2012;84(3):S331.
46. Jung J, Yoon SM, Kim SY, et al. Radiation-induced liver disease after stereotactic body radiotherapy for small hepatocellular carcinoma: clinical and dose-volumetric parameters. Radiat Oncol 2013;8(1):249.
47. Son SH, Choi BO, Ryu MR, et al. Stereotactic body radiotherapy for patients with unresectable primary hepatocellular carcinoma: dose-volumetric parameters predicting the hepatic complication. Int J Radiat Oncol Biol Phys 2010;78(4): 1073–80.
48. Jun BG, Kim YD, Cheon GJ, et al. Clinical significance of radiation-induced liver disease after stereotactic body radiation therapy for hepatocellular carcinoma. Korean J Intern Med 2018;33(6):1093–102.
49. Lee S, Jung J, Park J-h, et al. Stereotactic body radiation therapy as a salvage treatment for single viable hepatocellular carcinoma at the site of incomplete transarterial chemoembolization: a retrospective analysis of 302 patients. BMC Cancer 2022;22(1):175.
50. Kimura T, Takeda A, Sanuki N, et al. Multicenter prospective study of stereotactic body radiotherapy for previously untreated solitary primary hepatocellular carcinoma: the STRSPH study. Hepatol Res 2021;51(4):461–71.
51. Tse RV, Hawkins M, Lockwood G, et al. Phase I study of individualized stereotactic body radiotherapy for hepatocellular carcinoma and intrahepatic cholangiocarcinoma. J Clin Oncol 2008;26(4):657–64.
52. Jang WI, Bae SH, Kim MS, et al. A phase 2 multicenter study of stereotactic body radiotherapy for hepatocellular carcinoma: safety and efficacy. Cancer 2020; 126(2):363–72.
53. Kim N, Cheng J, Huang W-Y, et al. Dose-response relationship in stereotactic body radiation therapy for hepatocellular carcinoma: a pooled analysis of an Asian liver radiation therapy group study. Int J Radiat Oncol Biol Phys 2021; 109(2):464–73.
54. Durand-Labrunie J, Baumann AS, Ayav A, et al. Curative irradiation treatment of hepatocellular carcinoma: a multicenter phase 2 trial. Int J Radiat Oncol Biol Phys 2020;107(1):116–25.

55. Hara K, Takeda A, Tsurugai Y, et al. Radiotherapy for hepatocellular carcinoma results in comparable survival to radiofrequency ablation: a propensity score analysis. Hepatology 2019;69(6):2533–45.

56. Feng M, Suresh K, Schipper MJ, et al. Individualized adaptive stereotactic body radiotherapy for liver tumors in patients at high risk for liver damage: a phase 2 clinical trial. JAMA Oncol 2018;4(1):40–7.

57. Park S, Jung J, Cho B, et al. Clinical outcomes of stereotactic body radiation therapy for small hepatocellular carcinoma. J Gastroenterol Hepatol 2020;35(11): 1953–9.

58. Jeong Y, Jung J, Cho B, et al. Stereotactic body radiation therapy using a respiratory-gated volumetric-modulated arc therapy technique for small hepatocellular carcinoma. BMC Cancer 2018;18(1):416.

59. Andolino DL, Johnson CS, Maluccio M, et al. Stereotactic body radiotherapy for primary hepatocellular carcinoma. Int J Radiat Oncol Biol Phys 2011;81(4): e447–53.

60. Kang JK, Kim MS, Cho CK, et al. Stereotactic body radiation therapy for inoperable hepatocellular carcinoma as a local salvage treatment after incomplete transarterial chemoembolization. Cancer 2012;118(21):5424–31.

61. Ben-Josef E, Normolle D, Ensminger WD, et al. Phase II trial of high-dose conformal radiation therapy with concurrent hepatic artery floxuridine for unresectable intrahepatic malignancies. J Clin Oncol 2005;23(34):8739–47.

62. Dawson LA, Eccles C, Craig T. Individualized image guided iso-NTCP based liver cancer SBRT. Acta oncologica (Stockholm, Sweden) 2006;45(7):856–64.

63. Hong TS, Wo JY, Yeap BY, et al. Multi-institutional phase II study of high-dose hypofractionated proton beam therapy in patients with localized, unresectable hepatocellular carcinoma and intrahepatic cholangiocarcinoma. J Clin Oncol 2016;34(5):460.

64. Okuwaki Y, Nakazawa T, Shibuya A, et al. Intrahepatic distant recurrence after radiofrequency ablation for a single small hepatocellular carcinoma: risk factors and patterns. J Gastroenterol 2008;43(1):71–8.

65. Sanuki N, Takeda A, Kunieda E. Role of stereotactic body radiation therapy for hepatocellular carcinoma. World J Gastroenterol 2014;20(12):3100–11.

66. Roquette I, Bogart E, Lacornerie T, et al. Stereotactic body radiation therapy for the management of hepatocellular carcinoma: efficacy and safety. Cancers 2022; 14(16). https://doi.org/10.3390/cancers14163892.

67. Yoon SM, Lim YS, Park MJ, et al. Stereotactic body radiation therapy as an alternative treatment for small hepatocellular carcinoma. PLoS One 2013;8(11): e79854.

68. Lasley FD, Mannina EM, Johnson CS, et al. Treatment variables related to liver toxicity in patients with hepatocellular carcinoma, Child-Pugh class A and B enrolled in a phase 1-2 trial of stereotactic body radiation therapy. Pract Radiat Oncol 2015;5(5):e443–9.

69. Scorsetti M, Comito T, Cozzi L, et al. The challenge of inoperable hepatocellular carcinoma (HCC): results of a single-institutional experience on stereotactic body radiation therapy (SBRT). J Cancer Res Clin Oncol 2015;141(7):1301–9.

70. Takeda A, Sanuki N, Tsurugai Y, et al. Phase 2 study of stereotactic body radiotherapy and optional transarterial chemoembolization for solitary hepatocellular carcinoma not amenable to resection and radiofrequency ablation. Cancer 2016;122(13):2041–9.

71. Mathew AS, Atenafu EG, Owen D, et al. Long term outcomes of stereotactic body radiation therapy for hepatocellular carcinoma without macrovascular invasion. Eur J Cancer 2020;134:41–51.

72. Liu HY, Lee Y, McLean K, et al. Efficacy and toxicity of stereotactic body radiotherapy for early to advanced stage hepatocellular carcinoma - initial experience from an australian liver cancer service. Clin Oncol 2020;32(10):e194–202.

73. Lo CH, Yang JF, Liu MY, et al. Survival and prognostic factors for patients with advanced hepatocellular carcinoma after stereotactic ablative radiotherapy. PLoS One 2017;12(5):e0177793.

74. Loi M, Comito T, Franzese C, et al. Stereotactic body radiotherapy in hepatocellular carcinoma: patient selection and predictors of outcome and toxicity. J Cancer Res Clin Oncol 2021;147(3):927–36.

75. Yeung R, Beaton L, Rackley T, et al. Stereotactic body radiotherapy for small unresectable hepatocellular carcinomas. Clin Oncol 2019;31(6):365–73.

76. Moore A, Cohen-Naftaly M, Tobar A, et al. Stereotactic body radiation therapy (SBRT) for definitive treatment and as a bridge to liver transplantation in early stage inoperable Hepatocellular carcinoma. Radiat Oncol 2017;12(1):163.

77. Sapisochin G, Barry A, Doherty M, et al. Stereotactic body radiotherapy vs. TACE or RFA as a bridge to transplant in patients with hepatocellular carcinoma. An intention-to-treat analysis. J Hepatol 2017;67(1):92–9.

78. Barry AS, Sapisochin G, Russo M, et al. The use of stereotactic body radiotherapy as a bridge to liver transplantation for hepatocellular carcinoma. J Clin Oncol 2016;34(4_suppl):418.

79. Gresswell S, Tobillo R, Hasan S, et al. Stereotactic body radiotherapy used as a bridge to liver transplant in patients with hepatocellular carcinoma and Child-Pugh score ≥8 cirrhosis. J Radiosurg SBRT 2018;5(4):261–7.

80. Mannina EM, Cardenes HR, Lasley FD, et al. Role of stereotactic body radiation therapy before orthotopic liver transplantation: retrospective evaluation of pathologic response and outcomes. Int J Radiat Oncol Biol Phys 2017;97(5):931–8.

81. Sandroussi C, Dawson LA, Lee M, et al. Radiotherapy as a bridge to liver transplantation for hepatocellular carcinoma. Transpl Int 2010;23(3):299–306.

82. Wang Y-F, Dai Y-H, Lin C-S, et al. Clinical outcome and pathologic correlation of stereotactic body radiation therapy as a bridge to transplantation for advanced hepatocellular carcinoma: a case series. Radiat Oncol 2021;16(1):15.

83. Wang L, Ke Q, Huang Q, et al. Stereotactic body radiotherapy versus radiofrequency ablation for hepatocellular carcinoma: a systematic review and meta-analysis. Int J Hyperthermia 2020;37(1):1313–21.

84. Wong TC-L, Lee VH-F, Law AL-Y, et al. Prospective study of stereotactic body radiation therapy for hepatocellular carcinoma on waitlist for liver transplant. Hepatology 2021;74(5):2580–94.

85. Mathew AS, Dawson LA. Current understanding of ablative radiation therapy in hepatocellular carcinoma. J Hepatocell Carcinoma 2021;8:575–86.

86. Buckstein M, Kim E, Özbek U, et al. Combination transarterial chemoembolization and stereotactic body radiation therapy for unresectable single large hepatocellular carcinoma: results from a prospective phase 2 trial. Int J Radiat Oncol Biol Phys 2022;114(2):221–30.

87. Bauer U, Gerum S, Roeder F, et al. High rate of complete histopathological response in hepatocellular carcinoma patients after combined transarterial chemoembolization and stereotactic body radiation therapy. World J Gastroenterol 2021;27(24):3630–42.

88. Chiang CL, Chan ACY, Chiu KWH, et al. Combined stereotactic body radiotherapy and checkpoint inhibition in unresectable hepatocellular carcinoma: a potential synergistic treatment strategy. Front Oncol 2019;9:1157.

89. Juloori A, Katipally RR, Lemons JM, et al. Phase 1 randomized trial of stereotactic body radiation therapy followed by nivolumab plus ipilimumab or nivolumab alone in advanced/unresectable hepatocellular carcinoma. Int J Radiat Oncol Biol Phys 2023;115(1):202–13.

90. Su T-S, Liang P, Liang J, et al. Long-term survival analysis of stereotactic ablative radiotherapy versus liver resection for small hepatocellular carcinoma. Int J Radiat Oncol Biol Phys 2017;98(3):639–46.

91. Kimura T, Aikata H, Doi Y, et al. Comparison of stereotactic body radiation therapy combined with or without transcatheter arterial chemoembolization for patients with small hepatocellular carcinoma ineligible for resection or ablation therapies. Technol Cancer Res Treat 2018;17. https://doi.org/10.1177/1533033818783450. 1533033818783450.

92. Huo YR, Eslick GD. Transcatheter arterial chemoembolization plus radiotherapy compared with chemoembolization alone for hepatocellular carcinoma: a systematic review and meta-analysis. JAMA Oncol 2015;1(6):756–65.

93. Mastrocostas K, Jang HJ, Fischer S, et al. Imaging post-stereotactic body radiation therapy responses for hepatocellular carcinoma: typical imaging patterns and pitfalls. Abdominal radiology (New York) 2019;44(5):1795–807.

94. Brook OR, Thornton E, Mendiratta-Lala M, et al. CT imaging findings after stereotactic radiotherapy for liver tumors. Gastroenterology research and practice 2015;2015:126245.

95. Haddad MM, Merrell KW, Hallemeier CL, et al. Stereotactic body radiation therapy of liver tumors: post-treatment appearances and evaluation of treatment response: a pictorial review. Abdominal radiology (New York) 2016;41(10): 2061–77.

96. Mendiratta-Lala M, Masch W, Shankar PR, et al. Magnetic resonance imaging evaluation of hepatocellular carcinoma treated with stereotactic body radiation therapy: long term imaging follow-Up. Int J Radiat Oncol Biol Phys 2019; 103(1):169–79.

97. Mendiratta-Lala M, Masch W, Owen D, et al. Natural history of hepatocellular carcinoma after stereotactic body radiation therapy. Abdominal radiology (New York) 2020;45(11):3698–708.

Moving?

Make sure your subscription moves with you!

To notify us of your new address, find your **Clinics Account Number** (located on your mailing label above your name), and contact customer service at:

Email: journalscustomerservice-usa@elsevier.com

800-654-2452 (subscribers in the U.S. & Canada)
314-447-8871 (subscribers outside of the U.S. & Canada)

Fax number: 314-447-8029

Elsevier Health Sciences Division
Subscription Customer Service
3251 Riverport Lane
Maryland Heights, MO 63043

*To ensure uninterrupted delivery of your subscription, please notify us at least 4 weeks in advance of move.

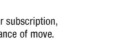

Printed and bound by CPI Group (UK) Ltd, Croydon, CR0 4YY

03/10/2024

01040467-0001